The Blood-Retinal Barriers

NATO ADVANCED STUDY INSTITUTES SERIES

A series of edited volumes comprising multifaceted studies of contemporary scientific issues by some of the best scientific minds in the world, assembled in cooperation with NATO Scientific Affairs Division.

Series A: Life Sciences

Recent Volumes in this Series

The series is published by an international board of publishers in conjunction with NATO Scientific Affairs Division

A Life Sciences	Plenum Publishing Corporation
B Physics	London and New York
C Mathematical and Physical Sciences	D. Reidel Publishing Company Dordrecht, Boston and London
D Behavioral and Social Sciences	Sijthoff & Noordhoff International Publishers
E Applied Sciences	Alphen aan den Rijn, The Netherlands, and Germantown U.S.A.

The Blood-Retinal Barriers

Edited by
Jose G. Cunha-Vaz
*Abraham Lincoln School of Medicine, University of Illinois College of Medicine
and University of Illinois Eye and Ear Infirmary, Chicago, Illinois
and University of Coimbra, Portugal*

PLENUM PRESS • NEW YORK AND LONDON
Published in cooperation with NATO Scientific Affairs Division

Library of Congress Cataloging in Publication Data

Nato Advanced Study Institute on the Blood-Retinal Barriers, Espinho, Portugal, 1979.
   The blood-retinal barriers.

   (NATO advanced study institutes series: Series A, Life sciences; v. 32)
   Includes index.
   1. Retina—Blood-vessels—Permeability. 2. Blood-brain barrier. 3. Biological transport.
4. Retina—Blood-vessels—Diseases. I. Cunha-Vaz, Jose G. II. North Atlantic Treaty Organization. III. Title. IV. Series.
QP479.N37 1979   617.7'3   80-10517
ISBN 0-306-40430-0

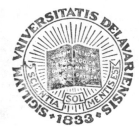

QP
479
. N37
1979

Lectures presented at a NATO Advanced Study Institute on the
Blood—Retinal Barriers, held in Espinho, Portugal, September 10-19, 1979

© 1980 Plenum Press, New York
A Division of Plenum Publishing Corporation
227 West 17th Street, New York, N.Y. 10011

PREFACE

The concept of a blood-retinal barrier is still relatively new in the ophthalmic literature. Whereas work on the blood-brain barrier was initiated in the first decade of this century, the blood-retinal barrier has only recently been defined. Information accumulated during the last 10 years has shown that the function of the blood-ocular barriers may be better understood if two main barrier systems are considered to exist in the eye. The blood-aqueous barrier regulates the exchanges between the blood and the intraocular fluids, and the blood-retinal barrier separates the neural tissue from the blood.

Recent studies have shown that the blood-retinal barrier plays a fundamental role in controlling the microenvironment of the retina. Similarly, the significance of the blood-retinal barrier in retinal disease has become increasingly clear. Fluorescein angiography has demonstrated an intricate series of relationships between alterations of the blood-retinal barrier and diverse retinal diseases, particularly vascular retinopathies and pigment epitheliopathies. Finally, in the past few years, vitreous fluorophotometry has provided a new and accurate index of the alteration of the blood-retinal barrier.

The blood-retinal barrier is a rapidly developing field of research. It is at a stage now in which the number of research workers is growing very fast but the information available is still dispersed. There is, therefore, a need for a reference book on the blood-retinal barriers that gives an integrated review of the new information available on the anatomy, ultrastructure, biochemistry, physiology, and pathophysiology of the blood-retinal barrier. This would be particularly useful not only for those currently working in this field, but for others who are attempting their first steps in this area of research. There is also a need to review the present knowledge on the blood-retinal barriers under the light of the available information on the blood-brain barrier. These barrier systems have many similarities, but whereas the blood-brain barrier shows a much greater wealth of research work, the blood-retinal barrier offers a different approach to examine similar problems.

v

Communication between research workers in these areas is evidently of mutual interest.

These were the main objectives of the Advanced Study Institute on "the Blood-Retinal Barriers" that was held in Espinho, Portugal, from September 10 to September 19, 1979. This book is comprised of the lectures given at the meeting.

The first chapter reviews the basic mechanism of membrane permeability. It examines biochemical aspects, with special emphasis on active transport, followed by a review on the mathematical analysis of the passive mechanisms.

The second chapter explores the sites and functions of the blood-brain and blood-retinal barriers, particularly the morphological aspects of the barriers.

The physiology and pharmacology of both barriers are then considered at some length, with particular emphasis on the relationship of the blood-retinal barriers with intraocular fluid dynamics. The role the blood-retinal barrier takes in maintaining retinal homeostasis opens an entirely new and extensive area of research.

The methods available to examine barrier permeability are critically evaluated. Fluorescein angiography has proved invaluable in showing how frequent the alteration of the barrier is in retinal disease. Vitreous fluorophotometry, on the other hand, is a more recent quantitative method that has opened interesting possibilities in early diagnosis of barrier alteration. It appears to be a research tool of much potential.

Finally, the pathology of the blood-retinal barrier is examined with particular emphasis on the role of alterations of the barrier in the pathophysiological mechanisms of retinal disease. An attempt is made to separate the retinal pathology associated with alterations of the inner blood-retinal barrier from that characterized by breakdown of the outer blood-retinal barrier.

We hope this book will serve as a much needed reference source for students of the blood-retinal barriers and show the present limitations of our understanding of the basic mechanism of the blood-retinal barrier in both health and disease.

I would like to thank especially Professors Norman Ashton and Paul Henkind who, with their experience and knowledge, helped significantly in the scientific organization of the meeting.

The meeting was made possible by substantial financial support from NATO. The Instituto Nacional de Investigacao Cientifica of Portugal also contributed with its support to the success of the meeting. I wish to thank their representatives for their oustanding generosity and help.

Jose G. Cunha-Vas

LECTURERS

DESMOND ARCHER
Professor and Chairman, Department of Ophthalmology, the
Queen's University of Belfast, Royal Victoria Hospital,
Belfast, N. Ireland, U.K.

ANDERS BILL
Professor, Department of Physiology and Medical Biophysics
Uppsala University, Uppsala, Sweden.

LASZLO BITO
Associate Professor, Laboratory of Ocular Physiology,
Research Division, Department of Ophthalmology, Columbia
University, College of Physicians and Surgeons, New York,
U.S.A.

MILTON BRIGHTMAN
Director, Laboratory of Neuropathology and Neuroanatomical
Sciences, National Institute of Neurological and Communi-
cative Diseases and Stroke, National Institutes of Health,
Bethesda, Maryland, U.S.A.

ARCELIO CARVALHO
Professor and Director, Center for Cell Biology, Department
of Zoology, University of Coimbra, Portugal.

GABRIEL COSCAS
Professor and Director, Clinique Ophtalmologique, Universite
de Paris, Hopital Communale de Creteil, Paris, France.

JOSE CUNHA-VAZ
Professor, Department of Ophthalmology, the Abraham Lincoln
School of Medicine, University of Illinois College of
Medicine; Director, Retina Service, University of Illinois
Eye and Ear Infirmary, Chicago, Illinois, U.S.A.
Professor and Chairman, Department of Ophthalmology,
University of Coimbra, Portugal.

x

AUGUST DEUTMAN
Professor and Head, Department of Ophthalmology, University
Of Nijmegen, Nijmegen, Netherlands.

DANIEL FINKELSTEIN
Associate Professor, Retinal Vascular Center, Wilmer
Ophthalmological Institute, Johns Hopkins Hospital,
Baltimore, Maryland, U.S.A.

MORTON GOLDBERG
Professor and Head, Department of Ophthalmology, the
Abraham Lincoln School of Medicine, University of Illinois
College of Medicine; Ophthalmologist-in-Chief, University
of Illinois Eye and Ear Infirmary, Chicago, Illinois, U.S.A.

PAUL HENKIND
Professor and Chairman, Department of Ophthalmology, Albert
Einstein College of Medicine; Montefiore Hospital and
Medical Center; Bronx, New York, U.S.A.

ABEL LAJTHA
Director, Center for Neurochemistry, Rockland Research
Institute, Ward's Island, New York, U.S.A.

ALAN LATIES
Professor, Department of Ophthalmology, Scheie Eye Institute,
University of Pennsylvania, Philadelphia, Pennsylvania, U.S.A.

JOAO P. DE LIMA
Associate Professor, Department of Physics, University of
Coimbra, Portugal; Senior Researcher, Faculty of Medicine,
University of Coimbra, Portugal.

DAVID MAURICE
Adjunct Professor of Surgery, Department of Surgery, Division
of Ophthalmology, Stanford University School of Medicine,
Stanford, California, U.S.A.

STANLEY RAPOPORT
Director, Laboratory of Neurosciences, National Institute
on Aging, Gerontology Research Center, Baltimore City
Hospitals, Baltimore, Maryland, U.S.A.

MARK TSO
Professor, Department of Ophthalmology, the Abraham Lincoln
School of Medicine, University of Illinois College of
Medicine; Director, Georgiana Theobald Ophthalmic Pathology
Laboratory; Director, Macula Clinic, University of Illinois
Eye and Ear Infirmary, Chicago, Illinois, U.S.A.

CONTENTS

xi

STRUCTURE AND FUNCTION OF CELL MEMBRANES

Transport Across Single Biological Membranes

Arsélio P. Carvalho

Center for Cell Biology, Department of Zoology

University of Coimbra, Portugal

SUMMARY

Cellular membranes are composed of a phospholipid bilayer interrupted by intrinsic proteins embedded in the lipid layers. The membranes are asymmetric with respect to the disposition of the lipids and the proteins. The Ca^{2+}-ATPase of sarcoplasmic reticulum is an example of an intrinsic protein with enzymatic activity. This enzyme requires lipid for ATP hydrolysis which is coupled to the transport of Ca^{2+} in exchange for H^+, K^+ and Mg^{2+}. The primary events of the transport process are the phosphorylation of the enzyme, the formation of a proton gradient and, possibly, the development of a membrane potential. The Ca^{2+}-ATPase is similar to the Na^+-K^+-ATPase in that both enzymes form a phosphorylated intermediate (E~P) in the process of generating ion gradients and these gradients can synthesize ATP. Electrochemical gradients generated across cell membranes drive the flow of other substances against their chemical gradients through specific "carriers" or porters which link the various transport systems.

INTRODUCTION

The cell membrane is a lipid bilayer with proteins embedded deeply into the lipid (3,7,10,20). The lipid bilayer is highly impermeable to ions and cell metabolites in general, but specific proteins, which span the entire thickness of the membrane, form pores or "carriers" (porters) which facilitate the transfer of substances across the membrane structure (20,78,82,90). Nevertheless, biological membranes remain highly selective permeability barriers (3,10,48).

1

The molecular basis of several transmembrane transport
processes is rapidly being elucidated (48,49,80,81,90,94), and some
clear generalizations are now possible. Thus, it appears that energy
derived from ATP or from electron transport, or even directly from
light, is preserved, in many cases, in the form of ion and electric
gradients across cell membranes which can then be utilized to drive
the transport of many substances and to synthesize ATP (48,49,80,95).
Therefore, "energization" of the membrane results in the
development of an electrochemical potential due to the pumping of
ions (49).

In mitochondria, the electron transport chain generates a
proton and an electric gradient across the inner mitochondrial
membrane during respiration, and this constitutes a store of energy
which can be utilized to synthesize ATP or to transport other
substances (49,88,91). Chloroplasts and photosynthetic bacteria
capture energy from light part of which they also convert into an
electrochemical gradient capable of synthesizing ATP and transporting
metabolites (80,81,87-90).

Another general process utilized by the cell to generate
electrochemical gradients involves the utilization of ATP as the
energy source. The reaction is catalized by an ATPase (Na^+-K^+-ATPase
or Ca^{2+}-ATPase) which is a protein inserted in the lipid bilayer of
the cell membrane (10,73,74,78,82,84,94). The energy of ATP is first
captured in an intermediate step by phosphorylation of the ATPase
and, subsequently, dephosphorylation occurs in a process which is
tightly coupled to the transfer of ions across the membrane (73,78,
82,84,88,94). The system may, generally, be viewed as indicated in
Fig. 1.

One important characteristic of this system is its reversibility,
so that ATP promotes the formation of ion gradients which in turn
promote the synthesis of ATP (15,31,47,55,84,88,94). The following

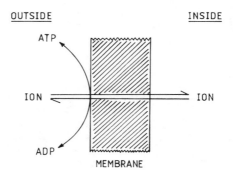

Fig. 1. Coupling between ATP hydrolysis and ion transport.

general reaction can be written:

$$ION_1 + E + ATP \xrightleftharpoons[\text{ADP}]{\text{ADP}} ION - E{\sim}P \rightleftharpoons E + P + ION_2$$

where ION_1 and ION_2 refer to the ions in the two sides of the
membrane, E is the ATPase and E~P is the phosphorylated
intermediate.

     I shall present here some of the principal current concepts of
cell membrane organization, and then I shall describe some details
of the Ca^{2+}-ATPase of sarcoplasmic reticulum of skeletal muscle as
an example of a membrane bound enzyme which is part of one of the
simplest biological membranes capable of reversibly forming an ion
gradient and synthesizing ATP. I shall also compare the properties
of the Ca^{2+}-ATPase with those of the better known membrane bound
enzyme, the Na^+-K^+-ATPase. Finally, I shall briefly describe the
principle of the relationship which exists between the
electrochemical gradients across biological membranes and their
capacity to transport solutes.

MEMBRANE ORGANIZATION

Danielli-Davson Membrane Model

     The classical picture of a biomembrane, before 1972, was that
of an uninterrupted lipid bilayer with proteins on its surfaces
(Fig. 2).

     It is only of limited interest to review here the experimental
evidence which supported this arrangement of lipids and proteins in
biological membranes. The older literature reviews this aspect
extensively (63,64), and it will be of more interest to concentrate
on the recent developments which have changed the immage of
biological membranes, especially with respect to the organization
of the proteins in the lipid bilayer. It is now accepted that,
although some proteins sit on the surface of the lipid, many
penerate the bilayer partially or completely (Fig. 3).
     The concept of the lipid bilayer, which was put forward in 1925
by Gorter and Grendel (1) on the basis of sketchy evidence, has
survived close analysis by modern technology. Gorter and Grendel
found that if they spread   all the lipid molecules of a red cell
membrane side by side on a water surface they occupied an area
about twice the area of the red cell membrane from which they had
been extracted. On this basis, these investigators postulated that
the lipids must be organized in the membrane as a bilayer with the

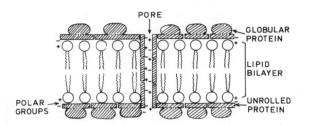

Fig. 2. Classical Danielli-Davson conception of a biomembrane. The lipid bilayer was sandwiched between two layers of "unrolled" protein. The unrolled protein would interact with the lipid through both polar and nonpolar forces. In addition, globular proteins would bind to the surface. Pores are lined with proteins and could contain charges on their walls.

apolar side chains of the lipids sequestered together away from contact with water, whereas the polar head groups of the lipids would be in direct contact with the aqueous phase on either side of the membrane (1). Subsequently, Danielli and Harvey (61) concluded that the surface tension of lipid globules in the aqueous part of mackerel eggs was very low, and suggested that the lipid must adsorb some emulsifying agent on its surface. Early chemical analysis showed that isolated membranes contain proteins and Danielli and Davson (60-62) postulated that such proteins would exist on the surface of the lipid bilayer of the cell membrane, as indicated in Fig. 2. Danielli explained the rapid diffusion of some types of molecules, which are lipid insoluble, by postulating the existence of "pores" in the lipid bilayer, lined with protein molecules (Fig. 2). This concept, which originated in the 1930's, was to remain basically unchanged until the early 1970's (3).

Fluid Mosaic Membrane Model

All recent membrane models include the idea that the lipid is in the form of a bilayer, but the proteins, although some may sit on the surface, penetrate the lipid bilayer partially or totally (3). Some of these proteins are tightly associated with the lipids and an integral part of the membrane continuum. These proteins are designated integral or intrinsic proteins, whereas those proteins more loosely bound to the rest of the membrane structure are designated peripheral or extrinsic proteins. This is really an operational definition proposed by Singer and Nicolson (3) which can be summarized as follows:

Extrinsic (or peripheral) Proteins (constitute about 30% of the total membrane protein).

1. Are dissociated from the membrane by mild treatment such

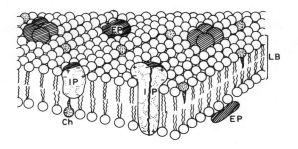

LB LIPID BILAYER   IP INTRINSIC PROTEIN
Ch CHOLESTEROL   EP EXTRINSIC PROTEIN

Fig. 3. The fluid mosaic model membrane. The phospholipids are
arranged in a discontinuous bilayer with their polar heads in
contact with water. The integral proteins are globular polypeptide
chains partially embedded in the lipid bilayer and partially
protruding. The protruding parts have charges and are in contact
with water, while the nonpolar residues are buried in the
hydrophobic part of the lipid bilayer. Cholesterol molecules are
dispersed in the lipid bilayer.

as increase in ionic strength and chelating agents.
2. Are easily obtained free of lipid.
3. Once dissociated, they are soluble in neutral aqueous
buffers.
Intrinsic (or Integral) Proteins (constitute about 70% of the
total protein).
1. Can be dissociated from membranes only by very drastic
treatments with detergents or organic solvents.
2. In many instances they remain associated with lipids when
isolated.
3. If isolated completely free of lipids, they are insoluble
in aqueous buffers.

Examples of peripheral proteins are the cytochrome **c** of the
internal membrane of mitochondria and spectrin of the erythrocyte
membrane both of which can be removed by chelating agents under mild
conditions (10,11,65). The Na^+-K^+-ATPase and the Ca^{2+}-ATPase of
various sources constitute the best examples of integral proteins
(6,32,11). The distinction between peripheral and integral proteins
is useful in that it is assumed that only the integral proteins are
critical to the structural integrity of biological membranes. Thus,
the interactions of peripheral proteins with the membranes, although
of interest, are not of central importance to understand the basic
membrane structure.

Unfortunately, not all extrinsic membrane proteins can be
removed by mild conditions. Proteins localized exclusively on the

outside of the lipid bilayer can make hydrophobic contacts with
proteins that are themselves intrinsic to the membrane continuum,
and these would require breaking the hydrophobic bounds to be
released. The mitochondrial ATPase (5) and the calsequestrin of
sarcoplasmic reticulum (6,32) are among the extrinsic membrane
proteins which require chaotropic salts or detergents to be released.
Probably the basic difference between extrinsic and intrinsic
membrane proteins resides in the properties of their surfaces, the
intrinsic proteins being much more hydrophobic than the extrinsic
proteins.

A membrane according to the model postulated by Danielli and
Davson (62) would necessarily be unstable because the unfolded
layer of protein would have many nonpolar residues exposed to water
and would cover the hydrophilic ends of the lipid molecules whose
interaction with water is essential for the stability of the
monolayer. Furthermore, recent studies indicate that about 40% of
the length of integral membrane proteins is not unfolded, but rather
assumes a α-helix configuration, which suggests that the integral
proteins probably are globular (4). If these globular proteins
existed on the surface of the membrane, attached to the lipid, the
membrane would have to be much thicker than the 70-100 Å usually
measured.

The fluid mosaic model (Fig. 3) proposed by Singer and
Nicolson (3) takes into account these difficulties. In this model
it is assumed that the globular proteins are amphipathic, i.e.,
possess hydrophobic and hydrophilic ends. The hydrophobic end is
embedded in the interior of the lipid bilayer which is hydrophobic,
while the hydrophilic end projects into the aqueous medium
surrounding the membrane. In some cases, the intrinsic proteins span
the entire thickness of the membrane in which case they have two
hydrophilic ends protruding out of the lipid bilayer and an
hydrophobic middle portion embedded in the lipid (3,7).

The State of the Lipid Bilayer

It has been shown that under physiological conditions the
lipids of a functional cell membrane are in a fluid rather than
in a gel state (11,12,20). The intrinsic proteins inserted in the
fluid lipid bilayer are free to undergo lateral diffusion within
the membrane, at rates determined by the viscosity of the membrane
(8-11). In principle, other movements are also possible, as
indicated in   Fig. 4.
When the temperature of a pure crystalline lipid is raised, an
endothermic transition occurs at a temperature which is specific
for each lipid. At this temperature, the hydrocarbon chains of the
fatty acids "melt" and become liquid-like in mobility, while the
polar ends are still in a rigid, quasi-crystalline structure (9-12).

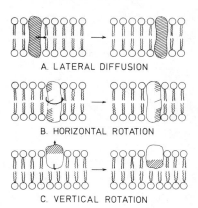

A. LATERAL DIFFUSION

B. HORIZONTAL ROTATION

C. VERTICAL ROTATION

Fig. 4. Proteins are free to move in the fluid lipid bilayer by: A. Lateral diffusion; B. Rotation in the plane of the membrane, and C. Rotation perpendicular to the plane of the membrane (11,12).

The increase in disorder (or entropy) at the melting point occurs at the expense of an enthalpy change at a constant pressure, since the free-energy change is zero.

This melting phenomenon can be detected by differential scanning calorimetry. By this technique, the sample and reference materials are kept at equal temperatures and the differential power needed to maintain the temperatures is recorded. This difference in power reflects the heat absorbed during the endothermic transition (Fig. 5).

The transition temperature depends on both the polar and apolar parts of the lipids (phospholipids). The more unsaturated the lipid, the lower the transition temperature, since cis bonds decrease chain cohesion. Increase in chain length increases the interaction between chains and the transition occurs at higher temperature (12). The polar heads of the phospholipids also influence the transition temperature. Thus, dimyristoyl phosphatidyl ethanolamine melts at 45°C, whereas dimyristoyl phosphatidyl choline melts at 25°C (13). Apparently, the interaction between the polar heads affects the melting temperature of the hydrocarbon chains. Therefore, it is not surprising that the ionic environment of the lipids has a strong influence on the transition temperatures. For example Ca^{2+} and H^+ induce a better packing of the fatty chains and increase the transition temperature of anionic phospholipids (14).

The lipids of the membrane are free to difuse laterally in the plane of the membrane. Devaux and McConnell (41) showed that PE in sarcoplasmic reticulum vesicles have a diffusion constant of about 7×10^{-8} cm^2/sec at 40°C which is close to the value obtained in lecithin bilayers. This suggests that the interaction of the lipid

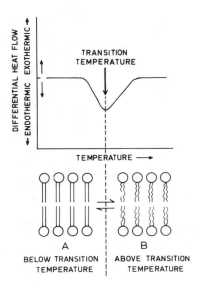

Fig. 5. Thermotropic transition of lipids from (A) crystalline to (B) liquid-crystalline phase. At the top is represented the recording of the differential heat flow over a range of temperatures. The peak occurs at the transition temperature. Above this temperature the lipids are in a fluid state.

molecules with the Ca^{2+}-ATPase molecules of sarcoplasmic reticulum does not greatly affect their rates of lateral diffusion. However, the lipids in the sarcoplasmic reticulum membrane probably are not free to "flip-flop". This was demonstrated for artificial phospholipid vesicles (42,43) and probably is also true for natural membranes. For a phospholipid molecule to jump from one monolayer to the other, the motion of flip-flop has to take place, which requires that the polar head passes through the hydrophobic core of the membrane (Fig. 6). This is indeed very improbable so that a given molecule, on the average, makes the passage only about once a month. However, the rapid lateral diffusion of the molecules in the fluid lipid makes the membrane an extremely dynamic system.

Interaction Between Lipids and Proteins

In natural membranes up to 1/3 of the area of the membrane may be occupied by intrinsic proteins inserted in the lipid bilayer (11). One layer of phospholipid one molecule thick is directly in contact with the intrinsic proteins, while the remaining lipids are in free bilayer form, not in direct contact with proteins (11,68,69). Therefore, the lipid molecules immediately in contact with the intrinsic proteins have their phase transition behavior altered.

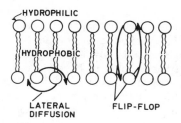

Fig. 6. Bilayer of phospholipids. The phospholipids diffuse laterally but do not "flip-flop" from one layer to the other.

Thus, approximately 25% of the lipids of the membranes of A. laidlawii do not undergo the normal calorimetric transition (70). The intrinsic proteins also have an immobilizing effect on the neighboring lipid layer with which they come in contact as was shown with spin labels of lipids in membranes and in extracted lipids (11,12,71). Fig. 7 represents the boundary lipid layer, one molecule thick, around an intrinsic membrane protein, such as an enzyme. The influence of this lipid "annulus" on the enzyme is now in debate (101-103).

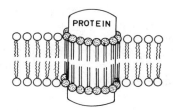

Fig. 7. Representation of an intrinsic membrane protein surrounded by a lipid boundary one molecule thick. This layer of lipid does not undergo a normal phase transition because of its interaction with the protein.

ENZYMATIC ACTIVITY OF INTRINSIC PROTEINS: THE EXAMPLE OF SARCOPLASMIC RETICULUM (SR)

Whether we are considering membrane enzymes or membrane "carriers", the environment in which they operate is rich in lipid. Therefore, let ue consider the effect of lipids on the enzymatic activity of intrinsic proteins. The enzyme we have studied most is the Ca^{2+}-ATPase of sarcoplasmic reticulum (15-18,37,38,47,51,52, 56-59). The SR membrane is a very simple membrane isolated from

muscle cells where it forms a network of tubules surrounding the
myofibrils. The membranes of SR can be isolated in vesicular form
by differential centrifugation and the vesicles obtained transport
Ca^{2+} coupled to the hydrolysis of ATP (15,51,55,74,78,94). This
membrane is composed of a lipid bilayer in which is embedded
predominantly a single protein, the Ca^{2+}-ATPase, with a molecular
weight of about 105,000, which constitutes as much as 85% of the
total membrane protein (Fig. 8). Other minor proteins also present
are a high affinity Ca^{2+} binding protein (HAP) with a molecular
weight of about 54,000 and calsequestrin with a molecular weight of
about 46,000 (CAL). In addition, there is a small band of proteolipids
(PL) of molecular weight of about 12,000 (6,32).

The lipid present in SR is mostly of the phospholipid type
(Table I), in which phosphatidylcholine (70%) and phosphatidylethanolamine (17%) predominate. The ratio of total lipid to protein
is about 1:2, i.e., about 1/3 by weight of SR is lipid (15). Thus,
the lipid bilayer is densily populated with Ca^{2+}-ATPase molecules
which are embedded in the lipid bilayer (Figs. 11 and 12).

TABLE I

LIPID COMPOSITION OF RABBIT AND LOBSTER SR

The lipids were extracted in $CHCl_3$: CH_3OH mixtures and separated by TLC in silica gel G with a solvent mixture containing:
$CHCl_3$: CH_3OH: 25% NH_4OH: H_2O (70:30:4:1, v/v). Inorganic phosphate
was determined in the scraped spots previously digested with 70%
$HClO_4$. The values are the mean of two experiments. The molar ratios
were estimated assuming that SR protein is 50% and 65% ATPase
(M.W. 100,000 daltons) for rabbit and lobster SR, respectively (15).

Component	Rabbit SR		Lobster SR	
Total Lipid				
mg/mg protein	0.68		0.99	
mg/mg Ca^{2+}-pump	1.36		1.52	
Phospholipid Classes	% total Pi	mol/mole of Ca^{2+} - pump	% total Pi	mol/mole of Ca^{2+} - pump
Phosphatidylcholine	68.9	54.6	69.4	70.5
Phosphatidylethanolamine	17.9	14.2	16.5	16.7
Phosphatidylserine	6.5	5.2	6.5	6.6
Sphingomyelin	3.5	2.8	3.7	3.1
Lysolecithin	2.4	1.9	2.3	2.3
Origin on Chromatogram	1.5	1.2	2.2	2.2

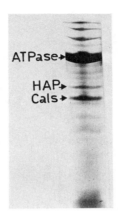

Fig. 8. Gel electrophoresis profile of SR isolated from rabbit skeletal muscle. The membranes were dissolved in Pi buffer, at pH 7.0, containing 1% SDS and 1% β-mercaptoethanol. About 70 μg of protein were applied in gels containing 10% acrylamide, 0.135% bisacrylamide and 0.1% SDS, and electrophoresis was carried out at 8 mA per gel for about 6 hrs. Gels were stained with Coomassie blue. HAP, high affinity protein; CAL, calsequestrin.

In Table I we compare the lipid composition of SR isolated from rabbit, an animal which maintains constant the temperature of its body with that of SR isolated from lobster, an animal whose body temperature fluctuates with that of the environment. There is a higher lipid content in lobster SR than in rabbit SR, but the phospholipid classes are similar (15). However, the activity of the Ca^{2+}-ATPase of the two preparations differs in its response to temperature variations. Fig. 9 shows that the Ca^{2+} ATPase of lobster SR is inactivated at 10°C lower than is the case for the ATPase of rabbit SR (17). We also found that Arrhenius plots of the Ca^{2+}-ATPase activity show a break at 16.7°C for rabbit SR, but at 11.5°C for lobster SR (15,16) as shown in Fig. 10.

Recently, further work carried out in our laboratory by Madeira and Antunes-Madeira (18) showed that the lobster SR phospholipids contain large amounts of unsaturated fatty acids which are present in low amounts in rabbit SR membranes. The total unsaturated fatty acids of phosphatidylcholines (PC) represent about 53% and 73% of the total fatty chains of rabbit and lobster, respectively. The values for the unsaturated fatty acids of phosphatidylethanolamines (PE) are 56% and 64%, respectively.

The activities of many lipid-dependent enzymes are largely influenced by the physical state of the associated lipids (10,11,19)

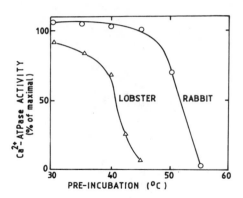

Fig. 9. Thermal inactivation of the Ca^{2+}-ATPase isolated from rabbit or lobster skeletal muscles (see reference 17 for experimental conditions).

and, generally, the enzymes require the lipids in a fluid state for optimal activity. Therefore, changes in the physical state of the membrane lipids can be detected as alterations of the parameters of enzyme activities and other membrane associated phenomena (19, see references 10 and 20 for review). Arrhenius plots of lipid dependent enzyme activities are known to show breaks which can be correlated with the phase transition temperature of the lipids (10). This is in contrast to most soluble enzymes which give a rectilinear relationship predicted by the equation of Arrhenius:

$$E_A = 2.303 \ RT^2 \ \frac{d \ log \ k}{dT} \qquad\qquad [1]$$

where E_A is the energy of activation and k is the rate constant. E_A is related to the enthalpy difference ΔH^* between the transition state and the reactant by:

$$E_A = \Delta H^* + RT \qquad\qquad [2]$$

In membrane bound enzymes, there occur sudden increases of the value of E_A. Below the break, the value of E_A usually increases 2-4 fold (10). Breaks in Arrhenius plots also occur for other cellular functions such as permeability properties, transport systems, hormone binding to membranes, hormone-stimulated adenylate cyclase, and physiological activities that are the result of complex biochemical reactions (10,11,19,21-23).

The interpretation given to the discontinuities in Arrhenius plots assumes that two independent processes having different E_A are required to produce the discontinuity, with the process having

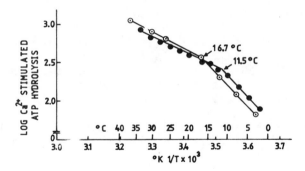

Fig. 10. Arrhenius plots for the Ca^{2+}-ATPase activity of SR isolated from rabbit and lobster skeletal muscle. See references 15 and 16 for experimental conditions. Calculated energies of activation above the break are 10.115 and 8.714 cal/mol for rabbit and lobster SR, respectively. Below the break the values are 19.423 and 19.658 cal/mol. Rabbit SR, o—o; Lobster SR, ●—●.

the higher E_A operating exclusively at temperatures below the discontinuity. It is assumed that the system undergoes a phase change at the break temperature, and that this change in the environment induces a conformational change in the protein, so that the conformation with higher E_A exists below the critical temperature (24). The phase change is ascribed to the lipid of the membrane and the breaks in the Arrhenius plots usually coincide with critical temperatures associated with phase transition of the lipids. However, this correlation cannot always be made, and the interpretation of the results is complex (9-12,19,25), especially since cations and other environmental factors affect fluidity of the membranes (26).

I should like to return to our results with rabbit and lobster SR. The difference in breaking points in the Arrhenius plots very likely reflect differences in fluidity of the lipids of the two membrane systems at various temperatures. As noted, the lipids of the lobster SR are more unsaturated than the lipids of the SR of the rabbit (18). Therefore, it is expected that these lipids will remain in the fluid state until lower temperatures than those at which the phase transition occurs for the rabbit SR membranes, i.e., the membranes of the lobster provide sufficient fluidity for normal Ca^{2+}-ATPase activity at relatively low temperatures which are likely to be encountered by the lobster's tissues. Adaptation of various organisms to grow at low temperatures usually involves increase in unsaturation of the membrane lipids and, therefore, increase in fluidity at low temperatures (19).

Lipid is Necessary for Ca^{2+}-ATPase Activity

Several methods have been utilized to isolate the purified
Ca^{2+}-ATPase of SR (29,30). Invariably, the enzyme retains bound to
its structure about 90 phospholipid molecules per molecule of
enzyme (29). This is about the same ratio of lipid to protein found
in the intact membrane (15,29) as can be seen in Table I. When the
lipid to protein ratio is decreased, the Ca^{2+}-ATPase activity
decreases, but can be recovered if the lipid is added back. However,
some lipid must always be present if the activity is not to be lost
irreversibly (Fig. 11).

The purified enzyme, in conjunction with its lipid environment
reassembles itself in membranes, in the form of vesicles, which are
nearly indistinguishable from the original vesicles which form upon
fragmenting the membranes of the sarcoplasmic reticulum (27-32).

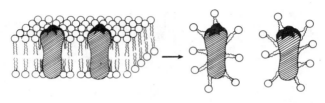

SR MEMBRANE Ca^{2+}ATPase MOLECULES

Fig. 11. Schematic representation of the SR membrane and of the
Ca^{2+}-ATPase molecules in situ and isolated. Each Ca^{2+}-ATPase retains
about 90 molecules of lipid bound which is essential for activity.

ASYMMETRY OF THE SR MEMBRANE

Asymmetry of the Proteins in the SR Membranes

Recent studies show that the SR membrane is asymmetric with
respect to the proteins (33,34,39) and the lipids (38,39). The evidence is still controversial, but it now appears that the Ca^{2+}-ATPase
molecule, although mostly embedded in the lipid bilayer, is exposed
to the outside since it can be digested with trypsin (33,34,45). If
the membranes are previously treated with phospholipase A, the
trypsin digestion occurs to a greater extent (17), which suggests
that the phospholipase makes the Ca^{2+}-ATPase molecule more accessible to trypsin, probably because it removes some of the lipid
molecules which surround the enzyme.

Furthermore, when ATP-γ^{32}P is incubated with SR membranes, the
Ca^{2+}-ATPase is phosphorylated and the part of the molecule which is
phosphorylated is removed by trypsin (72) which suggests that the
phosphoryl accepting group is located externally. In fact, the location of the whole Ca^{2+}-ATPase molecule in the membrane seems very
asymmetric, as was shown recently by electron microscopy studies
using glutaraldehyde supplemented by 1% tannic acid as fixatives
(33). Thin sections of pelleted preparations show triple-layered
membranes which from inside the vesicle to the outside, are 22, 21
and 70 Å thick, i.e., the outer layer is much thicker than the
inner layer. This is not characteristic of other membranes which
show the layers of about equal thickness.

Freeze fracture studies of SR vesicles also show that the
membrane particles embedded in the lipid bilayer are predominantly
attached to the outer lipid layer of the membrane (33,35). In Fig.12,
I represent the general picture for the arrangement of the
Ca^{2+}-ATPase molecule in the SR membrane vesicles.

Several workers have observed by negative staining of SR
vesicles that there are particles of about 35-40 Å on the surface
of the SR membrane (31,34-36), whereas the particles seen on the
interior of the membrane by the freeze-fracture technique are about
80-90 Å in diameter and their number is about 1/4 of that of the
surface particles (31,34). It is believed that the two types of
particles represent different views of the Ca^{2+}-ATPase molecule.
This discrepancy between their densities and sizes is attributed to
the fact that the molecule is composed of four subunits (33,34,37)
which on the outside appear individually when seen by negative
staining   but appear as a cluster on the hydrophobic region of the
membrane when seen by the freeze-fracture technique (31,33,35).

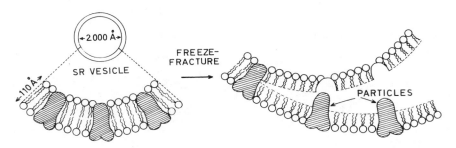

Fig. 12. Schematic representation of the asymmetric arrangement
of the Ca^{2+}-ATPase molecules in SR membranes. The thickness of the
membrane takes into account recent findings by electron microscopy
using glutaraldehyde supplemented by 1% tannic acid as fixatives
(33).

In any case, it appears that the Ca^{2+}-ATPase molecule is strongly anchored in the outer lipid layer. It has been calculated that there are about 5,700 Ca^{2+}-ATPase molecules/μm^2 of membrane (34).

The calsequestrin and the high affinity Ca^{2+} binding proteins are generally considered to be localized on the internal surface of the membrane, where they bind Ca^{2+} after it is transported by the Ca^{2+}-ATPase (32).

Asymmetry of the Lipids in the SR Membrane

The amino phospholipids, phosphatidylethanolamine (PE) and phosphatidylserine (PS), of the SR membrane are distributed unequally on the internal and external lipid layers of the membrane (38-40). The approach used in our laboratory to study this asymmetry was to label the amino groups of the external phospholipids with 2,4,6-trinitrobenzenesulfonate (TNBS), a chemical probe for amino groups which does not penetrate the membrane. Similarly, the amino groups of the phospholipids located on the internal side of the membrane were labelled with 1-fluoro-2,4-dinitrobenzene (FDNB), which readily penetrates the membrane (38). The studies with both probes were also performed with solubilized membranes. After reacting with TNBS or FDNB, the phospholipids were extracted and separated by thin layer chromatography and the amino phospholipids were identified by their yellow colour (38).

The reactions between these probes and the primary amino groups are indicated below:

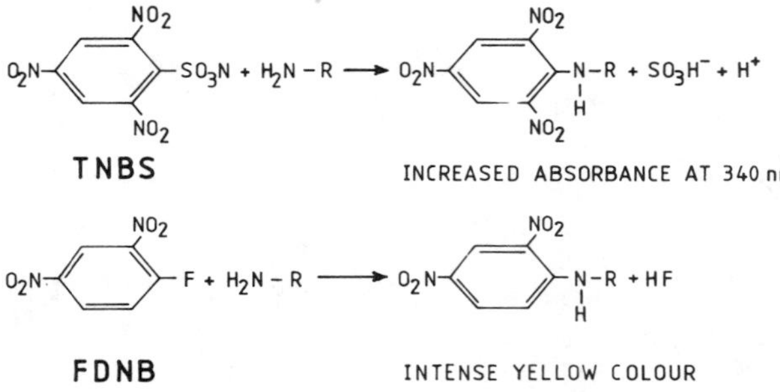

The results show that about 70% of the total PE is located on the external surface of the membrane, about 20% is on the internal surface, and about 10% is not accessible to the probe. In contrast, most of the PS is located on the inner surface of the membrane (38).

Fig. 13 represents schematically the asymmetric arrangement of

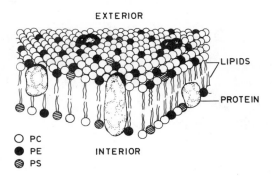

Fig. 13. Schematic representation of the SR membrane to show asymmetric distribution of the phosphatidylethanolamine (PE) and phosphatidylserine (PS). About 70% of the total PE is located on the external surface. Most of the PS is located on the internal surface (38).

the amino phospholipids in the SR membrane. The large protein shown in cross section represents the Ca^{2+}-ATPase which is shown here to completely span the thickness of the membrane and protruding to the exterior. We conclude, therefore, that the SR membrane is highly asymmetric with respect to the location of its proteins and amino phospholipids. The phosphatidylcholine (PC) probably is distributed uniformly throughout the bilayer.

COUPLING OF Ca^{2+}-ATPase ACTIVITY AND OF Ca^{2+} TRANSPORT IN SARCOPLASMIC RETICULUM

The Nature of the Ca^{2+}-Pump in SR

The basic function of sarcoplasmic reticulum membranes of muscle cells is to transport Ca^{2+} from the sarcoplasm into to the longitudinal tubules forming the SR (31,73). The SR membrane has been extensively studied in recent years, and much is known about the mechanism of the Ca^{2+} transport across this membrane. The SR is an ideal membrane system to study because of its simplicity and homogeneity in composition, especially when compared to the mitochondrial membrane which for many years was the membrane preferred by biochemists.

During Ca^{2+} transport by SR vesicles formed from fragmented SR, the ATPase activity is stimulated as indicated in Fig. 14. Mg^{2+} is a necessary cofactor (15,31,55,73,74).

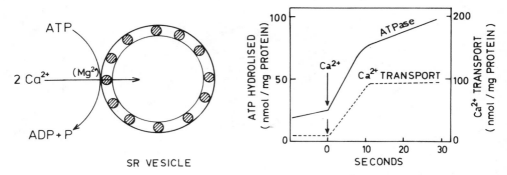

Fig. 14. Sarcoplasmic reticulum vesicles transport Ca^{2+} in the presence of ATP and Mg^{2+}. The external Ca^{2+} stimulates the Ca^{2+}-ATPase of the SR and 1 ATP molecule is hydrolysed per 2 Ca^{2+} transported. A. Schematic representation of Ca^{2+} transport by SR vesicles. B. Recording of the ATPase activity. See reference (15) for experimental conditions. ATPase remains stimulated only during Ca^{2+} transport.

The lipid bilayer is relatively impermeable to Ca^{2+}, but a bilayer in which the Ca^{2+}-ATPase is introduced becomes selectively permeable to Ca^{2+} as determined by an increase in conductance of the bilayer (44,45). Furthermore, after partial digestion of the Ca^{2+}-ATPase with trypsin, a fragment with a molecular weight of 20,000 is obtained which when inserted in PC-cholesterol membranes induces the following selectivity sequence $Ba^{2+} > Ca^{2+} > Sr^{2+} > Mn^{2+}$, Mg^{2+} (44,45). Another fragment of 45,000 molecular weight also increases the membrane conductance, but without any apparent selectivity for Ca^{2+} (46). A third fragment of the Ca^{2+}-ATPase, with a molecular weight of 30,000, is phosphorylated by ATP and constitutes the enzyme center (72).

In Fig. 15 we show the gradual fragmentation of the Ca^{2+}-ATPase by trypsin and its effect of the Ca^{2+}-ATPase activity and on Ca^{2+} transport. Under these conditions the calsequestrin, an internal protein, is not digested by trypsin and the high affinity protein (HAP) is coincident with F_1 in the gels (17).

This information is taken as suggestive evidence that the "carrier" or "pore", for Ca^{2+} in the SR membrane is localized in the Ca^{2+}-ATPase itself and that only a small part of this molecule has hydrolitic activity. The 30,000 molecular weight fragment, which is phosphorylated by ATP, apparently couples its action with that of the ionophoric components, i.e., the 45,000 (non-specific) and the 20,000 (specific for Ca^{2+}). It has been suggested that this latter peptide acts as the "gate" to the transmembrane pore formed by the large non-specific ionophoric peptide (45,46) (Fig. 16).

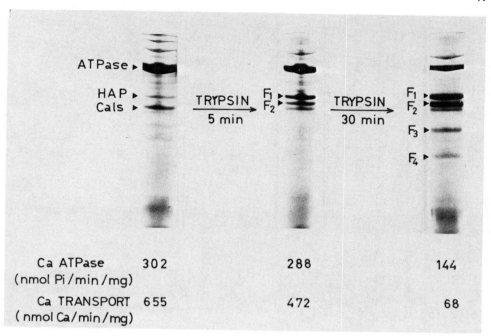

Ca ATPase	302	288	144
(nmol Pi/min/mg)			
Ca TRANSPORT	655	472	68
(nmol Ca/min/mg)			

Fig. 15. Fragmentation of SR by trypsin. First, two poly-peptides (F_1 and F_2), are formed of M.W. 55,000 and 45,000 without loss of activity. When the 55,000 polypeptide is fragmented into two peptides (F_3 and F_4) of 30,000 (phosphorylating peptide) and 20,000 (ionphoric peptide) the Ca^{2+}-ATPase is uncoupled from Ca^{2+} transport. See references (17,72) for experimental conditions. Calsequestrin is not affected by trypsin under these conditions, which suggests that it is not exposed to the surface.

A fixed pore mechanism, in which a conformational change within the protein-lined pore translocates the binding site across the membrane is preferred to a mobile carrier mechanism in which the binding site gets from one side of the membrane to the other by rotation of the entire transport protein across the membrane. The latter process would require the passage through the hydrophobic membrane interior of the hydrophilic parts of the proteins which, thermodynamically, is a highly unfavorable process.

Dutton et al (104) have carried out experiments which eliminate the possibility of the existence in the SR membrane of a mobile carrier for Ca^{2+} transport. These workers attached antibodies to the Ca^{2+}-ATPase and found that this produced no significant effect on the kinetics of the transport process. The attachment of a large molecule to the "carrier" should inhibit its activity.

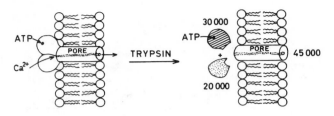

Fig. 16. Diagramatic representation of the hydrolytic and ionophoric components of the SR membrane. The 20,000 M.W. fragment represents the "gate" which leads into the non-specific trans-membrane pore, a polypeptide of M.W. of 45,000. The 30,000 and the 20,000 M.W. polypeptides are coupled in their functions, i.e., the hydrolysis of ATP is catalized by the 30,000 polypeptide and the energy liberated is utilized by the 20,000 fragment to transport Ca^{2+} in conjunction with the 45,000 fragment (45,46).

During Ca^{2+} transport by SR, ATP is hydrolysed and in the process a phosphorylated intermediate is formed according to the following equation which is a simplified version of the process:

$$ATP + E + 2\ Ca^{2+}_o \underset{Mg^{2+}}{\rightleftharpoons} \boxed{\begin{array}{c} ADP \\ + \\ \underset{Ca}{\overset{Ca}{\diagup}} E \sim P \end{array}} \rightleftharpoons E + P + 2\ Ca^{2+}_i$$

Phosphorylated
intermediate

Many details are know about the phosphorylation and dephospho-rylation mechanism, but the issue remains still controversial (31, 55,73-76). It suffices for our purposes to consider the above reaction in its simplest form, since the fundamental mechanism of energy transduction in, the SR membrane is not known.

The complete process of ATP hydrolyses requires Mg^{2+} and phospholipids (73,74). The phosphorylated intermediate, E~P, binds 2 Ca^{2+} ions which are translocated from one side of the membrane to the other. Thus, the two Ca^{2+} on each side of the equation are in different compartments. The reaction is reversible and, therefore, increasing the Ca^{2+}_i concentration on the right (inside the SR vesicle) causes the reaction to reverse, which means that a gradient of Ca^{2+} can synthesize ATP, as has in fact been observed in many laboratories (31,47,55,73,75).

Fig. 17 shows the results of experiments in which we used a Ca^{2+} gradient across the SR membrane to synthesize ATP (47). The SR vesicles were initially loaded with Ca^{2+} by prolonged suspension in 20 mM $CaCl_2$. Sudden 20-fold dilution of the SR suspension in media of 4 mM EGTA, 1 mM ADP and Pi, caused a release of Ca^{2+}, which was ADP dependent, i.e., the release did not take place in the absence of ADP, which suggests that the efflux of Ca^{2+} from SR is tightly coupled to the ATP synthesis. About 1 molecule of ATP was synthesized per each 2 Ca^{2+} that diffused out (47). Similar experiments showing this coupling between Ca^{2+} efflux and ATP synthesis can be carried out with SR vesicles loaded with Ca^{2+} by several different means (55).

Therefore, the overall mechanism of Ca^{2+} transport with ATP utilization, and of ATP synthesis at the expense of a pre-formed Ca^{2+} gradient, can be visualized as depicted schematically in Fig 18.

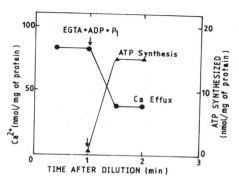

Fig. 17. Coupling between ATP synthesis and Ca^{2+} release from passively loaded SR vesicles. See reference 47 for experimental conditions.

The Balance of Charge During Ca^{2+} Transport by SR

The Ca^{2+} transport by SR is an example of active transport in which a charged species is carried across the membrane. The SR membrane must either have a tightly-coupled exchange-diffusion system for exchanging cations for the Ca^{2+} transported, or anions must accompany the Ca^{2+} transported. Evidently, the two systems could also operate simultaneously.

This balance of charge can be made either through a "pore" in the membrane, or through a "carrier", which may be any substance in the membrane which facilitates the passage of the ions through the lipid barrier. Although the term carrier as utilized presently does not specify a mechanism, and may include transfer across the membrane

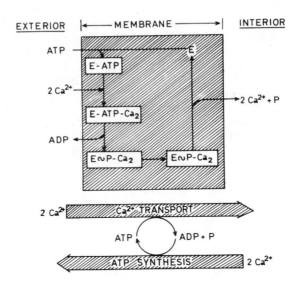

Fig. 18. Diagram to show coupling between Ca^{2+} transport and ATP hydrolysis and between ATP synthesis and the efflux of Ca^{2+}. The diagram is simplified since it omits the role of Mg^{2+}. It has been proposed that following the release of Ca^{2+} at the interior, the phosphorylated enzyme changes its configuration, binds Mg^{2+} and carries it to the outside where the Pi is also liberated (73,77-79). Thus, both ADP and Pi would be liberated on the outside, whereas Ca^{2+} would be transported to the outside.

through mere alteration in conformation of the carrier molecule, the original concept implied that the carrier was <u>mobile</u> within the membrane lipid structure (48). This mobility now is considered in most cases to be restricted to parts of the carrier molecules bearing the binding sites. Thus, carriers are understood to be proteins inserted in the lipid bilayer which provide recognition sites for the substances being transferred (48). It should be noted that the size of many "carriers" and "pumps" is sufficiently large to span the entire thickness of the membrane, being exposed on both surfaces by hydrophilic groups. Such carriers do not move across the membrane, and their rotation is also restricted by their hydrophilic ends which cannot easily penetrate the hydrophobic core of the membrane.

The term <u>porter</u> was introduced to distinguish from true enzymes the "catalysts" for the mediated transfer of solutes across membranes by processes which do not truly involve enzymatic reactions (e.g., the classic case of exchange-diffusion), thus, avoiding the termination "ase" reserved for the names of enzymes, and generally denoting covalent bond labelization (49,50). The sym--coupled and anti-coupled translocations are designated as symport and antiport, respectively (Fig. 19). Furthermore, non-coupled solute translocation can also occur and is designated as uniport. In the latter case, if the solute transferred is charged, an electric potential difference ($\Delta\Psi$) develops across the membrane, and the tranfer is designated as electrogenic (Fig. 20).

The membrane potential generated by an electrogenic pump can be utilized to electrophoretically drive those cations and anions to which the membrane is permeable and, as a result, there will occur accumulation of cations and anions against their chemical gradient on either side of the membrane, with a consequent collapse of the membrane potential. Therefore, an electrogenic pump will generate a permanent membrane only if the membrane is relatively impermeable to ions.

We observed (51) twelve years ago that isolated sarcoplasmic reticulum releases Mg^{2+}, K^+ and H^+ during accumulation of Ca^{2+} in the presence of ATP (Figs. 21 and 22). The technique which we utilized to measure the cation exchange that took place during Ca^{2+} transport did not permit measurement of the cation distribution immediately after Ca^{2+} transport, so that we could not follow the time course of the reaction. Also, we did not determine whether a transmembrane potential developed across the SR membrane.

We also observed that Mg^{2+} and K^+ are bound by the membranes of SR vesicles in the absence of ATP, and that this binding was pH dependent in a manner which suggested that H^+ competes with Mg^{2+}

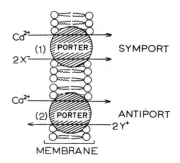

Fig. 19. Balance of charge during Ca^{2+} transport. Porter (1) is designated a symport, whereas porter (2) is an antiport. The transfer of Ca^{2+} is electro-neutral in both cases and no membrane potential develops.

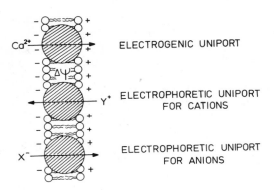

Fig. 20. Non-coupled uniport transmembrane movement of Ca^{2+}. The Ca^{2+} transfer is electrogenic, generating a difference in membrane potential ($\Delta\Psi$). This $\Delta\Psi$ can drive cations (y^+) and anions (x^-) electrophoretically against their chemical gradient.

and K^+ for the same binding sites (51,52). The ions could not be removed from the SR membranes by dilution with 0.25 M sucrose, unless Ca^{2+} (or other cations) were present which would exchange for Mg^{2+} and K^+. This exchange with Ca^{2+} took place if the external Ca^{2+} concentrations were raised sufficiently, i.e., about 50% of the Mg^{2+} taken up was displaced by Ca^{2+}, when the external ratio of free Ca^{2+} to free Mg^{2+} was about 0.6 (Fig. 22). We argue on the basis of these results that the SR membranes have binding sites for cations (about 350 meq/mg of protein) and that if the binding sites are on the internal side of the membrane, then the membrane must be relatively permeable to the cations under the experimental conditions employed.

Sarcoplasmic reticulum vesicles instantaneously loaded with Mg^{2+} in a buffered medium containing 3,8 mM free Mg^{2+}, retained about 300 meq of Mg^{2+}/mg of protein. If we then added ATP to the medium and again tested the effectiveness of Ca^{2+} in displacing Mg^{2+} from the SR vesicles, we found that displacement of 50% of the Mg^{2+} originally retained by SR was achieved by Ca^{2+} concentrations 1000-fold lower than those necessary in the absence of ATP (Fig. 22). It is evident that ATP enhances the displacement of Mg^{2+} from binding sites in the SR membranes in exchange for Ca^{2+} which must substitute for Mg^{2+} at the binding sites. However, on the basis of these results one cannot distinguish between a mechanism in which the ATP directly increases the affinity of the binding sites for Ca^{2+} and another in which ATP selectively translocates the Ca^{2+} across the membrane, thus increasing the intravesicular Ca^{2+} activity sufficiently for Ca^{2+} to displace Mg^{2+} (or K^+, H^+, etc) from the membrane binding sites. All recent evidence suggests that the latter mechanism is the correct one (47,55,56,73,78).

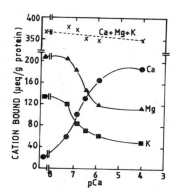

Fig. 21. Accumulation of Ca^{2+} by SR vesicles previously "loaded" with Mg^{2+} and K$^+$. Accumulation of Ca^{2+} occurs in exchange for Mg^{2+} and K$^+$, so that the total meq of charge in the SR membrane remains constant. Samples containing 10 mg of SR protein were added to a medium at 23°C containing 3.8 mM MgCl$_2$, 110 mM KCl, 10 mM imidazole at pH 6.9, 1.0 mM EGTA and CaCl$_2$ to give the final pCa values indicated in the abcissa. After adding 1.0 mM ATP, the suspensions were immediately centrifuged for 20 min. at 105,400 $\underline{g}$ and the pellets were washed once with 10 ml of 0.25 M sucrose. After Carvalho and Leo (51).

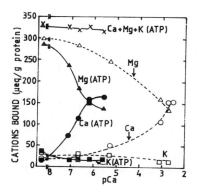

Fig. 22. Effect of ATP on the release of Mg^{2+} by Ca^{2+} from SR vesicles. Experimental conditions were similar to those described for Fig. 21, except that the KCl was 10 mM. Solid and dashed lines represent experiment performed in the presence and absence of ATP, respectively. After Carvalho and Leo (51).

The number of binding sites available for the binding of Ca^{2+}, Mg^{2+} and K^+ depends on the concentration of H^+ in the medium, since this cation strongly competes with the other cations for the binding sites in the membranes (51,52). At the lower pH values, the binding sites are protonated, and we observed that below a pH value of about 6.2, some of the Ca^{2+} transported exchanged for H^+, instead of Mg^{2+} and K^+ (51). These results have been confirmed recently by Dr. Madeira in our laboratory who finds that at pH 6.0, there is a large ejection of protons in exchange for Ca^{2+} transported (58).

Recently, Zimniak and Racker (27) utilized reconstituted SR vesicles to measure the membrane potential, which develops during Ca^{2+} transport, by a voltage clamp technique using K^+-valinomycin to generate a constant transmembrane potential. These workers also measured the membrane potential of SR vesicles more directly by using the fluorescent probe 8-anilino-1-naphthalenesulfonic acid (ANS). They conclude that the Ca^{2+}-ATPase mediated transport of Ca^{2+} is electrogenic, generating a membrane potential of about +60 mV (positive inside the vesicles). In view of the results we reported earlier showing that there is exchange of transported Ca^{2+} for Mg^{2+}, K^+ and H^+, this potential in normal SR membranes must necessarily be transient since it would be collapsed by the efflux of Mg^{2+} and K^+ (51). This idea is also supported by the recent results of Beeler et al (97) who could not detect the formation of a membrane potential during Ca^{2+} transport by SR. However, Zimniak and Racker (27) chose for their experiments reconstituted SR vesicles which are much more impermeable to cations and anions than normal SR vesicles (53,54). Recently, Madeira (56) was able to show that SR vesicles do in fact generate a transient membrane potential coincident in time with the transport of Ca^{2+}.

Formation of a Proton Gradient and a Membrane Potential During Ca^{2+} Transport

Careful measurements of the flux of protons across the SR membrane during Ca^{2+} transport have been carried out recently by Dr. Madeira in our laboratory (56-58). Addition of ATP to SR vesicles, in the presence of external Ca^{2+} causes an efflux of H^+ which precedes the transport of Ca^{2+}. Furthermore, following the efflux of H^+, there occurs the development of a membrane potential which is not synchronized with the formation of the proton gradient, but coincides with the Ca^{2+} transport event (Fig. 23).

The proton gradient and membrane potential are transient if small amounts of Ca^{2+} are present to be transported. If large amounts of Ca^{2+} (in excess of about 150 nmol/mg of protein) are transported, then there is a significant back diffusion of Ca^{2+} which continuously activates the Ca^{2+}-ATPase. In the latter case, the proton gradient, and probably the membrane potential, are

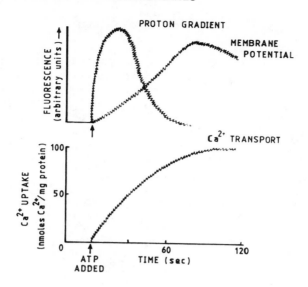

Fig. 23. Time course of Ca^{2+} transport, formation of a proton gradient and a membrane potential in SR vesicles. Data replotted from reference 56. Proton gradient formation was followed by measuring the changes in the fluorescence of 9-amino-6-chloro-2--methoxyacridine and the membrane potential was followed by measuring the changes in 3,3'-dipentyloxadicarbocyanine during Ca^{2+} uptake. See reference 56 for experimental details.

sustained over long periods of time because the transport system continues to recycle Ca^{2+} (56,57).

The SR membrane is relatively impermeable to H$^+$ (58), so that the energy of the proton gradient which is generated by ATP can be utilized to transport Ca^{2+}, although the mechanism of this coupling is not clear. About 30 nmol of H$^+$ per mg of SR protein are ejected, and this could, in theory, produce a large proton gradient, but the ΔpH measured is only about 0.5 because apparently the interior of the vesicles is strongly buffered (58).

If we assume that it is the proton motive force that sustains the transport of Ca^{2+}, according to Mitchell (49) the total protonic potential difference ($\Delta\bar{\mu}_{H^+}$) is given by the sum of the electric potential difference, $\Delta\Psi$, ($\Delta\Psi = nF\Delta E$) and a thermodynamic potential difference that is equal to $-Z\Delta pH$ ($Z = 2.303$ RT/F and ΔpH is the pH difference between both sides of the membrane. Thus,

$$\Delta\bar{\mu}_{H^+} = \Delta\Psi + Z\Delta pH \qquad\qquad [3]$$

At 25°C the value of Z is about 60 mV when the potential are given in mV.

Thus, the proton motive force appears partly as a potential difference and partly as a pH gradient as is the case for mitochondria, chloroplasts (49,50) and bacteria (80,81). The potential difference developed by SR after adding ATP seems to coincide with the uptake of Ca^{2+}, so that the entry of Ca^{2+} is electrogenic, generating a potential which is positive inside the vesicles. This potential is then collapsed by the outflux of Mg^{2+} and K^+, so that the original proton motive force was partly converted into a Ca^{2+} motive force, which in turn can drive Mg^{2+} and K^+ against their chemical gradients. It is possible that other cations and anions can be similarly driven. These events have been summarized by Madeira (56) as follows:

$$
\begin{array}{ccccc}
\text{ATP} & & \text{Ca}_i & & \text{Mg}^{2+}{}_i,\ \text{K}^+{}_i \\
\Big) \xrightarrow{(1)} \Delta\text{pH} & & \Big) \xrightarrow{(2)} \Delta\Psi & & \Big(\\
\text{ADP + Pi} & & \text{Ca}_o & & \text{Mg}^{2+}{}_o,\ \text{K}^+{}_o
\end{array}
$$

This interpretation presents some difficulties. Since there is no great change in pH (ΔpH) upon addition of ATP (58), a large membrane potential would be expected to develop coincident with the pumping of protons to the exterior. It is probable that the technique does not detect this early membrane potential and that the alteration in potential, positive inside, which develops during the entry of Ca^{2+}, really corresponds to a collapse of the electric potential developed during the proton efflux. The SR membrane is permeable to anions, including Cl^- (97-99), which was the predominant anion in the medium in these experiments. It is also likely that the membrane is relatively permeable to Mg^{2+} and K^+ (51,59). Therefore, even if a membrane potential develops because of the electrogenic pumping of protons by the Ca^{2+}-ATPase, such potential would be immediately collapsed by the passive electrophoretic movement of anions and cations either through pores or specific porters in the membrane. At present, any scheme will have to account for an early formation of a ΔpH, a possible $\Delta\Psi$ and a movement of Ca^{2+} in opposite direction to the movements of Mg^{2+} and K^+.

The strong buffering capacity of the SR membranes could be predicted from our previous results in which we measured the H^+ binding by the SR membranes (51,52). We found that dissociable groups exist in the SR membranes which have a binding capacity of about 150 nmol/mg of protein, and their average pK value is about 6.6 in the physiological range of pH values of 6-8. Furthermore, the H^+ binding sites also bind Ca^{2+}, Mg^{2+} and K^+, but display somewhat lower affinity for these cations than for H^+ (Table II).

TABLE II

AVERAGE pK_M VALUES FOR THE INTERACTION
BETWEEN RABBIT SKELETAL MUSCLE SARCO-
PLASMIC RETICULUM AND VARIOUS CATIONS (52)

Cation	H^+	Zn^{2+}	Ca^{2+}	Mg^{2+}	Na^+	K^+
pK_M	6.6	5.2	4.7	4.2	1.3	1.3

Therefore, the concentration of free Ca^{2+} and Mg^{2+} in the SR
vesicles are expected to be buffered in the same sense that the
vesicles buffer the pH. Attempts at distinguishing between internal
and external cation binding sites in SR vesicles were made in our
laboratory (59). The results showed an internal Ca^{2+} binding of
about 15 nmol/mg of protein (Fig. 24) under conditions in which a
large fraction of the binding sites were occupied with Mg^{2+}, K^+ and
H^+, so that the actual internal cation binding capacity is much
higher, and can serve to create a strong buffering effect for Ca^{2+}
and Mg^{2+} in the 10^{-4} M range and for H^+ in the pH range of 6-8 (52).

The SR membrane is reported to be impermeable to Ca^{2+} and H^+
(58,81). The results represented in Fig. 25 can be interpreted to
mean that the membranes are in fact relatively impermeable to Ca^{2+},
but may be permeable to Mg^{2+}. Thus, incubation of the SR vesicles

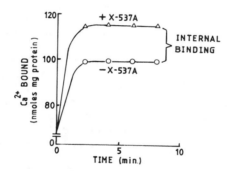

Fig. 24. Binding of Ca^{2+} in the absence and in the presence of
X-537A. In the absence of X-537A, the Ca^{2+} does not penetrate the
vesicles within the short periods of incubation, so that the Ca^{2+}
retained represents external binding. Upon addition of X-537A (20 μM),
the additional Ca^{2+} retained represents binding at the internal
binding sites. The SR (10 mg/mg) was suspended at 3°C in media
containing 100 mM KCl, 2 mM $MgCl_2$, 20 mM $CaCl_2$ and 20 mM Tris-maleate
at pH of 6.9. At various times, the media were diluted 20 fold with
0.25 M sucrose, and samples (0.5 mg of protein) were filtered by
Millipore and Ca^{2+} retained in the filters was measured by atomic
absorption spectrophotometry (59).

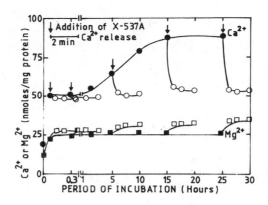

Fig. 25. Passive loading and release of Ca^{2+} and Mg^{2+} by SR vesicles (10 mg/ml). The medium contained 20 mM $CaCl_2$, 2 mM $MgCl_2$ and 100 mM KCl was buffered at pH 6.9 with 20 mM Tris-maleate. After various periods of incubation at 3^oC samples containing 0.5 mg of protein were removed before and after adding 20 μM X-537A and were diluted 20 fold, and were filtered by Millipore filters (0.45 μ pore diameter). Ca^{2+} and Mg^{2+} retained in the filter were measured by atomic absorption spectrophotometry. After Vale and Carvalho (59).

in a medium which contains Ca^{2+} and Mg^{2+}, in the absence of ATP, readily retains the maximal amount of Mg^{2+}, but the maximal amount of Ca^{2+} retained is attained only after about 15 hours of incubation (Fig. 25). During the first 2-3 hours of incubation, X-537A, an ionophore which makes the membrane permeable to Ca^{2+} and Mg^{2+}, does not release Ca^{2+} when the SR is placed in a medium low in Ca^{2+}, which suggests that all Ca^{2+} retained in this first period of incubation is bound to the external surface of the membrane. After 5 hours of incubation, X-537A releases the fraction of Ca^{2+} accumulated during the period beyond the initial 2-3 hours of incubation, which suggests that this Ca^{2+} had been retained inside the SR vesicles. The X-537A also causes accumulation of Mg^{2+} (and probably K^+ which was also present in the medium, but was not measured) in exchange for the released Ca^{2+} (Fig. 25).

Is Ca^{2+} Accumulated Free or Bound ?

The presence of calsequestrin and high affinity Ca^{2+}-binding protein inside the SR vesicles provide fixed binding sites which serve to sequester the Ca^{2+} once it is transported (32). Furthermore, the Ca^{2+}-ATPase also binds significant amounts of Ca^{2+} (66). These binding sites are non-specific and have low affinity, since dissociation constant is of the order of 10^{-5} M, but have a cation

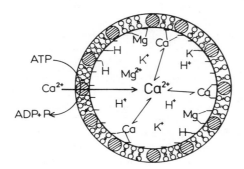

Fig. 26. Schematic representation of the binding of cations in the interior of the SR vesicles. Ca^{2+} is first transported across the SR membrane and then displaces H^+, K^+ and Mg^{2+} at the binding sites.

binding capacity which could account for all the Ca^{2+} transported. We have estimated that if all Ca^{2+} transported by the vesicles remained free, the concentration of Ca^{2+} in SR would be about 20 mM (51), which is sufficient to saturate the binding sites of low affinity. Therefore, I believe that most Ca^{2+} transported exchanges for other cations (Mg^{2+}, K^+ and H^+) at the internal binding sites of the membrane (Fig. 26).

GENERALIZATIONS AND RESEMBLANCES BETWEEN THE Ca^{2+}-ATPase AND THE Na^+-K^+-ATPase

It appears that the sarcoplasmic reticulum membrane utilizes ATP primarily to form a proton motive force ($\bar{\mu}_{H^+}$) which can drive the formation of a Ca^{2+} gradient (56-58). The charge balance of this system probably is maintained primarily by Mg^{2+} and K^+ which are driven electrophoretically out of the SR vesicles. The proton gradient appears to be the primary event in this transport process, but its magnitude is low, although a large quantity of protons are translocated to the outside of the vesicles (58). Therefore, if a chemiosmotic process, similar to that which is operative in mitochondria (49), functions in SR membranes, it is expected that a membrane potential should develop, according to equation 3, as is in fact observed (56,58). A difficulty which arises presently is that the time course of the development of the membrane potential does not coincide with the formation of the proton gradient, but rather coincides with the transport of Ca^{2+}. Thus, the transport of Ca^{2+} is electrogenic and generates the membrane potential which electrophoretically drives Mg^{2+}, K^+ and probably anions.

The postulate that Mg^{2+} and K^+ move out of SR vesicles electrophoretically does not specify whether the cations   cross the membrane through a pore system or in the form of a complex formed with some membrane "carrier". A protein to act as a diffusing carrier would have to reorientate in the membrane, and any hydrophilic portions exposed to the surfaces would have to move through the hydrophobic interior of the membrane. Energetically, this is an improbable event, but the proteins may refold to form more hydrophobic outer surfaces at their ends during the diffusion process. One should be able to test whether a "carrier" diffuses by studying its behavior at different temperatures. Its activity should drop abruptly below the transition temperature of the membrane lipid in which it is inserted. On the other hand a pore system should be relatively insensitive to temperature.

An attractive alternative is that, in the case of SR membrane, one   part of the Ca^{2+}-ATPase forms a pore through the hydrophobic interior of the membrane as suggested in Fig. 16 (45,46). It is not clear whether the pore utilized by Ca^{2+} is the same through which Mg^{2+} and K^+ pass. An important difference in the movements of ions through these pores is that two types of movements should be distinguished. The movement of Ca^{2+} directly catalyzed by the Ca^{2+}-ATPase is achieved and controlled by the molecular interaction of the enzyme or transport system, perhaps   through conformational changes associated with phosphorylation and dephosphorylation of the enzyme. On the other hand, there should also be movements of Mg^{2+} and K^+ driven electrophoretically by the membrane potential, as illustrated in Fig. 20, which should be of a simpler nature.

The notion that the "carriers" in many cases are "pores" formed by proteins that span the entire thickness of the membrane is also supported for other systems where such proteins have been identified (48). An example which has been extensively studied is that of the Na^+-K^+-ATPase (Fig. 27) which shows some similarities with the Ca^{2+}-ATPase of SR (82-84).

The Na^+-K^+-ATPase

There are some similarities between the Ca^{2+}-ATPase of sarcoplasmic reticulum and the Na^+-K^+-ATPase found in most plasma membranes. Thus, Mg^{2+} is required for activity of the Na^+-K^+-ATPase, the enzyme molecule is an intrinsic protein, embedded in the lipid structure of the membrane and, when isolated, it requires phospholipid for its activity, very much like the Ca^{2+}-ATPase (82). The Na^+-K^+-ATPase is composed of at least two polypeptides with molecular weights of 100,000 and 50,000 (83,84).The larger polypeptide has a relatively large proportion of non-polar amino acid residues and it is reversibly phosphorylated and dephosphorylated at a β-carboxyl of an aspartyl residue, as is also the case for the Ca^{2+}-ATPase of

SR (82,83). The smaller polypeptide is a glycoprotein which is an essential component of the ATPase since antibodies against it inhibit the enzyme. Furthermore, the two polypeptides are located close together since they can be cross-linked (85). The Ca^{2+} pump and the Na^+-K^+ pump systems form ion gradients, and utilize ion gradients to generate ATP (82). Moreover, both ATPase systems form a phosphorylated intermediate (55,82). The Na^+-K^+-ATPase is responsible for transport of Na^+ out of the cell and K^+ in, and the transport of the ions is tightly coupled to ATP hydrolysis (82). In the red blood cell 3 Na^+ are transported out for each 2 K^+ transported (82). Both Na^+ and K^+ are necessary for the pump to operate. Furthermore, Na^+, ATP and Mg^{2+} must be presented to the inside of the membrane and K^+ to the outside for the pump to function (82,85), whereas ouabain inhibits the system when presented to the outside of the membrane and Ca^{2+} inhibits when presented to the inside (82). Fig. 27 summarizes these principal concepts relevant to the Na^+-K^+-ATPase of most plasma membranes which have been studied.

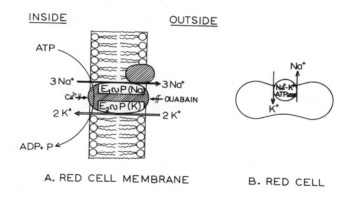

Fig. 27. A. Model for Na^+ and K^+ transport by the Na^+-K^+-ATPase. See text for details. The 100,000 subunit of the ATPase extends the entire thickness of the membrane. During transport of Na^+ and K^+, the first step is the formation of a phosphorylated intermediate $E_1{\sim}P$ which binds Na^+ in the inside of the cell and requires Mg^{2+}. Then a conformational change transforms the $E_1{\sim}P$ into $E_2{\sim}P$ which has higher affinity for K^+ than for Na^+. The K^+ is translocated to the inside with the hydrolysis of $E_2{\sim}P$. Some of these steps have been verified experimentally in red cell ghosts. Ouabain inhibits the transport when added from the outside, and Ca^{2+} has a similar effect when added from the inside. B. Red cell showing high concentration of Na^+ out and high concentration of K^+ in. The Na^+ and K^+ gradients can also synthesize ATP.

Other details are also present in the legend of Fig. 27. The
Na^+-K^+-ATPase maintains Na^+ and K^+ gradients across the membrane of
most cells, and the process is electrogenic (82). The gradient of
Na^+ (ΔNa^+) and the membrane potential ($\Delta\Psi$) which develop constitute
a store of energy ($\Delta\bar{\mu}_{Na}+$) which can be utilized to generate and
maintain gradients of metabolites across the plasma membrane (49).

UTILIZATION OF ION GRADIENTS TO DRIVE MOVEMENTS
OF OTHER SUBSTANCES ACROSS CELL MEMBRANES

Formation of Proton Gradients by
Mitochondria, Chloroplasts and Bacteria

Mitchell (49,50,86) has pointed out that the electrochemical
proton gradient ($\Delta\bar{\mu}_H+$) constitutes the energy storage of most
membranes which can be utilized to drive the transport of many ions
and metabolites. The three best known systems in which a proton
electrochemical potential develops are mitochondria (49), chloroplasts (87) and photosynthetic bacteria, Halobacterium halobium (80).
The common characteristics of these three membrane systems is that
they are capable of generating a proton gradient and a membrane
potential, i.e., $\Delta\bar{\mu}_H+$, and utilize this form of energy store to
either synthesize ATP or transport ions and metabolites (49).

In the case of mitochondria (and in bacteria such as E. coli)
the energy for the formation of the electrochemical potential comes
from the oxidation of substrates (49,80,81,88,90). In the case of
mitochondria the electrons flow in a zig-zag manner through the
electron transport chain located in the inner mitochondrial membrane
(88). The electrons flow from NADH with a standard redox potential
of -0.32 V (or another substrate with more positive redox potential)
to the flavoproteins, and then through the other components (iron-
-sulphur proteins, quinones and cytochromes) until the electrons
are transferred to O_2 by cytochrome oxidase where the redox
potential is +0.82. Thus, the change in redox potential between
NADH and oxigen is 1.14 V, representing a change in free energy of
about 220 kJ/NADH, which is more than enough to eventually generate
3 mol of ATP. However, in an early step, before the synthesis of
ATP, the energy is preserved as an electrochemical proton gradient.

The zig-zag arrangement of the electron and hydrogen transport
system is important for the vectorial transfer of protons, but such
arrangement, or even the presence of specific hydrogen-carrying
components, is not essential for generating a proton gradient in
the Halobacterium halobium, since it contains a single protein,
bacteriorodopsin, inserted in the lipid bilayer (80,81). This
protein is the proton pump itself, and it derives the energy for
pumping protons directly from light (80).

The proton pumping by mitochondria and bacteria causes an accumulation of protons outside, whereas chloroplasts pump protons in (87,88). In both cases, the membranes are impermeable to protons, so that an electrochemical potential develops due to the difference in pH and membrane potential which results (49). Discharging of this potential occurs when protons flow in the reverse direction through the ATPase, to synthesize ATP (Fig. 28). The potential can also be utilized to transport other substances as will be discussed.

The ATPase molecule in mitochondria, chloroplasts and bacteria, is similar in its basic structure. It is located asymmetrically in the membrane and contains a component (F_1) which spans the entire lipid bilayer and another (F_0) located more superficially on the membrane (88). In mitochondria and bacteria the F_1-F_0 complex which forms the ATPase is oriented so that knobs (F_1) about 85 Å in diameter protrude from the inner surface of the membrane. In chloroplasts, the equivalent ATPase, designated CF_1-F_0 complex, is oriented

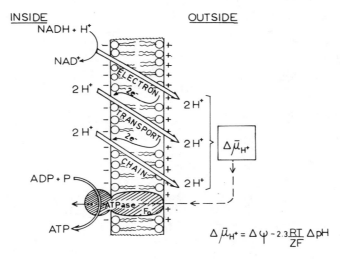

$$\Delta\bar{\mu}_{H^+} = \Delta\psi - 2.3\frac{RT}{ZF}\Delta pH$$

Fig. 28. Generation of a proton motive force ($\Delta\bar{\mu}_{H^+}$) across the inner mitochondrial membrane by the electron transport chain, and synthesis of ATP during the back flow of electrons through the ATPase which spans the thickness of the membrane. F_0 represents the hydrophobic part of the ATPase molecule which is buried in the lipid. The F_1 component protrudes from the inner surface of the membrane. Bacteria have similar electron transport systems for generating $\Delta\bar{\mu}_{H^+}$ and ATPases for synthesizing ATP. Chloroplasts and photosynthetic bacteria utilize light for generating $\Delta\bar{\mu}_{H^+}$ and a similar ATPase system for synthesizing ATP.

in the opposite direction, with the knobs (CF_1) protruding from the outer surface of the membrane. It will be recalled that the proton gradient is also in opposite directions in the two membrane types (49,87,88).

Because of the difference in concentration and in electric potential, a proton which is expelled across the membrane experiences a force tending to draw it back across the membrane. The movement of the protons in response to this force can be made to do work which can be translated into the synthesis of ATP according to the equation:

$$ADP^{3-} + H_2PO_4^- + 2H_1^+ \rightleftharpoons ATP^{4-} + H_2O + 2H_2^+$$

Where H_1^+ and H_2^+ represent protons before and after they have crossed the membrane down their electrochemical gradient. Note that the reaction is reversible so that the ATPase can generate a proton motive force if ATP is added. This resembles the situtations which we discussed for the Ca^{2+}-ATPase of sarcoplasmic reticulum and the Na^+-K^+-ATPase of most plasma membranes, except that the mechanism is quite different. A basic difference is that in the case of chloroplasts, mitochondria and bacteria, ATP is formed and hydrolysed without the formation of a phosphorylated intermediate (E~P) which is essential for the energy transduction by the Ca^{2+}-ATPase and Na^+-K^+-ATPase (55,83,88).

Solute Movement Driven by
Electrochemical Gradients of Protons

The impermeability of the cell membrane to H^+ and to most cations makes it an ideal system to store electrochemical gradients of protons or of other cations. Once an electrochemical gradient of ions is generated across the membrane, it can be utilized to drive the transport of other ions and metabolites against their concentration gradients. This aspect has been extensively studied for Na^+, amino acid, and sugar transport in bacteria (89,90) and for the transport by mitochondria of metabolites utilized in the Krebs cycle (49,90-92,95).

The uphill movement of the solutes transported is coupled to the relaxation of the ion gradients in such a way that the energy of the entire system decreases, but most of it is preserved in the form of new electrochemical   gradients. As discussed earlier, Mitchell (see reference 49 for review) postulated that this is accomplished by symport and antiport movement of the solutes. In the case of symport, the substrate and the ion from the ion gradient move in the same direction, and in the case of antiport, they move in opposite directions, across the membrane. This concept implies the obligatory interdependence of ion and solute movements coupled through a specific membrane component ("carrier") which facilitates the translocation.

The Case of Mitochondria

The inner mitochondrial membrane has "carriers" for ADP, ATP, inorganic phosphate and for several metabolites of the Krebs cycle mentioned earlier (49,91,95). ATP^{4-}, with four negative charges is synthesized in the mitochondria and diffuses across the mitochondrial membrane in exchange for ADP^{3-} with three negative charges. The carrier that facilitates this antiport exchange is inhibited by atractylocide and the exchange is driven electrophoretically by the membrane potential difference (49,92,95), since at physiological pH there is a difference in charge between ATP^{4-} and ADP^{3-}. In addition to ADP^{3-}, inorganic phosphate (HPO_4^{2-}) also moves into the mitochondria catalysed by another carrier which promotes an electroneutral exchange between HPO_4^{2-} and $2OH^-$ (91). The gradient of OH^- is in the opposite direction of that of H^+. The transport of Ca^{2+} by mitochondria is thought to be by electrophoresis through a "carrier" which acts as uniport, but this is controversial (49,93, 95,100). In the absence of carriers, there may still occur the movement of some ions if the membrane is leaky, as illustrated for K^+ and Cl^- (Fig. 29).

Note that the $\Delta\bar{\mu}_{H^+}$ creates gradients of other ions (ATP^{4-}, ADP^{3-}, HPO_4^{2-}, Ca^{2+}, etc.) which can themselves drive the transport of other substances. Thus, the mitochondria has electroneutral antiports for exchange of HPO_4^{2-} for the dicarboxylic acid malate and for the exchange malate/α-ketoglutarate, etc. (49,91). In Fig. 29 I present a summary of some of these concepts.

The Case of Bacteria

The photosynthetic bacteria (Halobacterium halobium) provide a very valuable tool to study the nature of membrane transport and for coupling of transport to the electrochemical gradients generated by the cell membrane (80,81,89,90).

When the bacteria are grown at low O_2 concentration in the light, they synthesize a protein, bacteriorhodopsin (a protein similar to rhodopsin) which forms distinct patches in the cell membrane. Up to 50% of the total surface membrane may be covered by these "purple patches" (80,81,89) and pieces of these membrane

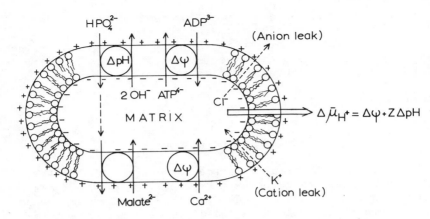

Fig. 29. Solute movements in mitochondria driven by the
electrochemical gradient of protons ($\bar{\mu}_{H^+}$). The pumping of protons
out by the mitochondrial membrane creates a $\bar{\mu}_{H^+}$ composed of a
and a pH. These forces can then be utilized to transport other
substances through "carriers" which function as uniports, symports
or antiports. Cation and anion "leaks" occur at low rates. There
is controversy as to whether Ca^{2+} is transported by an uniport or
a symport and it is difficult to distinguish between a $HPO_4^{2-}/2OH^-$
antiport and a $HPO_4^{2-}/2H^+$ symport (49,95,100).

patches can be isolated by osmotic shock, giving purple membrane
fragments which are in the form of vesicles, containing about 75%
protein and 25% lipid by weight (89).

Illumination of these vesicles causes the extrusion of H^+ and
the generation of a membrane potential, as observed also in the
intact bacterial cell (80,89). Since the only protein that these
membranes contain is the bacteriorhodopsin, it must be the proton
pump. The reaction for the H^+ pumping has been worked out in some
detail, and it can be summarized as follow.

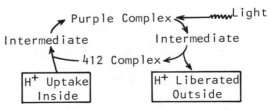

Thus, H^+ is picked up on the inner surface of the membrane and
is liberated on the outer surface.

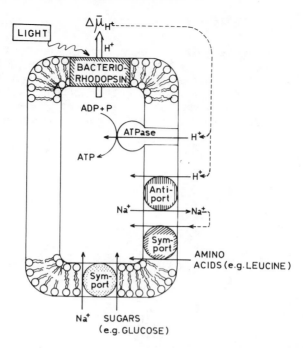

Fig. 30. Formation of an electrochemical gradient of protons ($\Delta\bar{\mu}_{H^+}$) by the photosynthetic bacteria <u>Halobacterium halobium</u>. The $\Delta\bar{\mu}_{H^+}$ is then utilized to transport Na^+ by an antiport. The electrochemical gradient of Na^+ then drives the transport of some amino acids and sugars by specific symport systems. (89).

The extrusion of protons is accompanied by some efflux of counter-ions (e.q. Cl^-) and influx of co-ions (e.q. K^+), but the movement of these ions is slower than that of the proton, which accounts for the electrogenic nature of the proton pump, i.e., there is always a gap between the protons pumped and the ions passively transported.

The $\Delta\bar{\mu}_{H^+}$ which develops in the intact bacterial cell is used by synthesize ATP through the ATPase system (80,89) and to pump Na^+ <u>via</u> a H^+/Na^+ antiporter, and, as a result, Na^+ is extruded (Fig. 30). It should be noted that these cells do not have a Na^+-K^+-ATPase so that the function of this enzyme in other cells is fulfilled in photosynthetic bacteria by the $\Delta\bar{\mu}_{H^+}$ through a specific antiporter (carrier) for H^+/Na^+ exchange (89). The Na^+ gradient which is generated can also drive the transport of several amino acids through specific symports (80,81,88,89,90).

THE GENERAL CONCEPT

The general concept which has emerged in the last ten years, especially with the advent of the chemiosmotic hypothesis (49,86), is that a gradient of solute and of electrical potential is generated during coupling between electron transport and oxidative phosphorylation. For the transport systems recognized to operate as ATPases (Ca^{2+}-ATPase and Na^+-K^+-ATPase), the formation of the

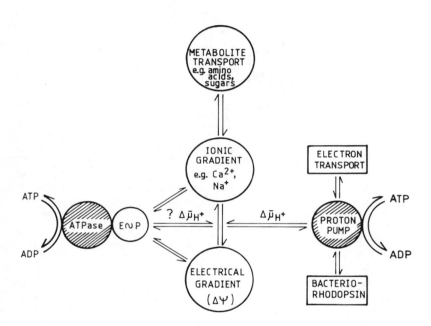

Fig. 31. Principal pathways of energy transduction by cell membranes. The proton pump in mitochondria and chloroplasts is an electron transport chain, whereas in bacteria it is bacterio-rhodopsin. At least in sarcoplasmic reticulum, the Ca^{2+}-ATPase generates a proton gradient and a membrane potential. The electro-chemical potential ($\Delta\bar{\mu}_{H^+}$) can then drive the formation of other ion gradients which in turn drive the transport of the various meta-bolites. The electrical gradient may also drive the transport of ions and other metabolites. In the case of the ATPases, the energy is transiently stored in a phosphorylated intermediate (E~P) which has not been found for the proton pump of mitochondria, chloro-plasts or bacteria.

electrochemical potential is energized by the transfer of the terminal phosphoryl groups from ATP to a protein (ATPase) and, subsequently, to water to form inorganic phosphate (48,49,55,82). In Fig. 31, I outline the principal pathways of energy transduction in cell membranes.

The chemiosmotic theory (49,86) gives a reasonable explanation for the vectorial transfer of protons in mitochondria, chloroplasts and bacteria responsible for developing the electrochemical potential ($\Delta\bar{\mu}_H+$), but it is not clear how the cleavage of ATP to give ADP and Pi drives transport through the intermediate phosphorylation of the ATPase. The reversal process, in which ATP is synthesized by the migration of solutes down their electrochemical gradient, must involve a reaction which is the reverse of that which hydrolyses ATP and forms solute gradients.

ACKNOWLEDGEMENTS

I am grateful to Prof. V. Madeira for making avaiable information not yet published. This work was supported by a grant from NATO (Research Grant Nº 1513) and by the Instituto Nacional de Investigação Científica, Portuguese Ministry of Education.

BIBLIOGRAPHY

1. Gorter, E. and F. Grendel (1925). J. Exp. Med. 41: 439.

2. Dutton, A., E. D. Rees and S. J. Singer (1976). Proc. Natl. Acad. Sci. 73: 1532.

3. Singer, S. J. and G. L. Nicolson (1972). Science 175: 720.

4. Glaser, M. and S. J. Singer (1971). Biochemistry 10: 1780.

5. Pullman, M. E., H. S. Penefsky, A. Data and E. Racker (1960). J. Biol. Chem. 235: 3322.

6. MacLennan, D. H. and P. T. S. Wong (1971). Proc. Natl. Acad. Sci. U.S. 68: 1231.

7. Singer, S. J. (1975). In: Cell Membranes, Weissmann, G. and R. Claiborn, Editors, HP Publishing Co., Inc. New York, Chapter 4, p. 35.

8. Fowler, V. and D. Branton (1977). Science 268: 23.

9. Luzzati, V. (1968). In: Biological Membranes. Physical Facts and Functions, Ed. D. Chapman, Academic Press, London, p. 71.

10. Lenaz, G. (1979). Subcell. Biochem. 6: 233.

11. Lenaz, G. (1977). In: Membrane Proteins and their Interactions

with Lipids, Ed. Capaldi, R., Marcel Dekker, Inc., New York, p.47.

12. Chapman, D. (1973). In: Biological Membranes, Editor Chapman D. and D. F. H. Wallach, Vol. 2, Acad. Press, London, p. 91.

13. Reinert, J. and J. M. Steim (1970). Science 168: 1580.

14. Verkleij, A. J., B. De Kuyff, P. H. Ververgaert, J. F. Tocanne, and L. L. M. van Deenen (1974). Biochim. Biophys. Acta 339: 432.

15. Carvalho, A. P. and V. M. C. Madeira (1974). In: Biomembranes, Lipids, Proteins and Receptors, Burton, R. M. and L. Packer, Editors, BI-Science Publications Division, Webster Groves, Missouri.

16. Madeira, V. M. C. and A. P. Carvalho (1974). Biochem. Biophys. Res. Comm. 58: 897.

17. Carvalho, C. A. M. (1979). Ph. D. Thesis, Faculty of Science and Technology, University of Coimbra, Portugal.

18. Madeira, V. M. C. and M. C. Antunes-Madeira (1975). Can. J. Biochem. 54: 516.

19. Raison, J. K. (1973). Bioenergetics 4: 285.

20. Singer, S. J. (1974). Ann. Rev. Biochem. 43: 805.

21. Nobel, P. S. (1974). Plants (Berlin) 115: 369.

22. Bashford, C. L., S. J. Harrison, G. K. Radda and Q. Mehdi (1975). Biochem. J. 146: 473.

23. Houslay, M. D., T. R. Hesketh, G. A. Smith, G. B. Warren and J. C. Metcalfe (1976). Biochim. Biophys. Acta 436: 495.

24. Kumamoto, J., J. K. Raison and J. M. Lyons (1971). J. Theor. Biol. 31: 47.

25. Lee, A. G., N. S. M. Birdsall, J. C. Metcalfe, P. A. Toon and G. B. Warren (1974). Biochemistry 13: 3699.

26. Jacobson, K. and D. Papahadjopoulos (1975). Biochemistry 14: 152

27. Zimniak, P. and E. Racker (1978). J. Biol. Chem. 253: 4631.

28. Knowles, A. F. and E. Racker (1975). J. Biol. Chem. 250: 3538.

29. Warren, G. B., P. A. Toon, N. S. M. Birsdall, A. G. Lee and J. C. Metcalfe (1974) FEBS Letters 41: 122.

30. MacLennan, D. H. (1970). J. Biol. Chem. 245: 4508.

31. Baskin, R. J. (1977). In: Membrane Proteins and their Interactions with Lipids, Editor Capaldi, R. Marcel Dekker, Inc., New York, p.151.

32. MacLennan, D. H., T. J. Ostwald and P. S. Stewart (1974). Ann. N. Y. Acad. Sci. 227: 527.

33. Saito, A., C. Wang and S. Fleischer (1979). J. Cell Biol. 79:601.

34. Scales, D. and G. Inesi (1976). Biophys. J. 16: 735.

35. Inesi, G. and D. Scales (1974). Biochemistry 13: 3298.

36. Ikemoto, N., F. A. Sreter and J. Gergely (1971). Arch. Biochem. Biophys. 147: 571.

37. Madeira, V. M. C. (1977). Biochim Biophys. Acta 464: 583.

38. Vale, M. G. P. (1977). Biochim. Biophys. Acta 471: 39.

39. Hidalgo, C. and N. Hikemoto (1977). J. Biol. Chem. 252: 8446.

40. Hasselbach, W., A. Migala and B. Agostini (1975). Z. Naturforsch 30c: 600.

41. Devaux, P. and H. M. McConnell (1971). Ann. N. Y. Acad. Sci. 222: 733.

42. Rothman, J. E. and E. A. Dawidowicz (1976). Biochemistry 14: 2809.

43. Rothman, J. E. and J. Lenard (1977). Science 195: 743.

44. Shamoo, A. E., T. L. Scott and T. E. Ryan (1977). J. Supramol. Struct. 6: 345.

45. Shamoo, A. E. and T. E. Ryan (1975). Ann. N. Y. Acad. Sci. 264: 61.

46. Abramson, J. J. and A. E. Shamoo (1978). J. Membrane Biol. 44: 233.

47. Vale, M. G. P., V. R. O. Castro and A. P. Carvalho (1976). Biochem. J. 156: 239.

48. Christensen, H. N. (1975). Biological Transport, 2nd Edition, W. A. Benjamin, Inc., London.

49. Mitchell, P. (1979). Eur. J. Biochem. 95: 1.

50. Mitchell, P. (1967). Adv. Enzymol. 29: 33.

51. Carvalho, A. P. and B. Leo (1967). J. Gen. Physiol. 50: 1327.

52. Carvalho, A. P. (1966). J. Cellular Physiol. 67: 73.

53. Meissner, G. and D. McKinley (1976). J. Membrane Biol. 30: 79.

54. Kometani, T. and M. Kasai (1978). J. Membrane Biol. 41: 295.

55. Hasselbach, W. (1978). Biochim. Biophys. Acta 515: 23.

56. Madeira, V. M. C. (1978). Arch. Biochem. Biophys. 185: 316.

57. Madeira, V. M. C. (1979). Arch. Biochem. Biophys. 193: 22.

58. Madeira, V. M. C. (1979). Arch. Biochem. Biophys. In Press.

59. Vale, M. G. P. and A. P. Carvalho (1975). Biochim. Biophys. Acta 413: 202.

60. Davson, H. (1961). In: Symposium on the Plasma Membrane,
    Fishman, A. P. Editor, New York Heart Association, Inc.,
    p. 1022.

61. Danielli, J. F. and N. Harvey (1935). J. Cellular Physiol. 5:
    483.

62. Danielli, J. F. and D. H. Davson (1935). J. Cellular Physiol.
    5: 495.

63. Robertson, J. D. (1966). In: Intercellular Transport, Academic
    Press, New York, p.1.

64. Stoecknenius, W. and D. Engelman (1969). J. Cell Biol. 42: 613.

65. Marchesi, V. T. and H. Furthmayer (1976). Ann. Rev. Biochem.
    45: 667.

66. Meissner, G. and S. Fleischer (1974). In: Calcium Binding
    Proteins, Drabikowsski, W. and E. Carafoli, Editors,
    Elsevier Scientific Publishing Company, Amsterdam.

67. Zwall, R. F. A., R. A. Demell, B. Roelofsen and L. L. M. van
    Deenen (1976). Trends Biochem. Sci. 1: 112.

68. Hesketh, T. R., G. A. Smith, M. D. Houslay, K. A. McGill,
    N. J. M. Birdsall, J. C. Metcalfe and J. B. Warren (1976).
    Biochemistry, 15: 4145.

69. Moore, B. M., B. R. Lentz and G. Meissner (1978). Biochemistry
    17: 5248.

70. Blazyk, J. F. and J. M. Steim (1972). Biochim. Biophys. Acta
    226: 737.

71. Kleeman, W. and H. M. McConnell (1976). Biochim. Biophys. Acta
    419: 206.

72. Thorley-Lawson, D. A. and N. M. Green (1973). Eur. J. Biochem.
    40: 403.

73. Tada, M., T. Yamamoto and Y. Tonomura (1978). Physiol. Rev. 58: 1.

74. Martonosi, A. (1971). In: Biomembranes, Vol.1, Edited by
    Manson, L. A., Plenum Press, New York, 191.

75. De Meis, L. and R. K. Tume (1977). Biochemistry 16: 4455.

76. Martonosi, A., T. L. Chyn and A. Schibeci (1978). Ann. N. Y.
    Acad. Sci. 307: 148.

77. Froehlich, J. P. and E. W. Taylor (1976). J. Biol. Chem. 251:
    2307.

78. MacLennan, D. H. and P. C. Holland (1976). In: The Enzymes of
    Biological Membranes, Vol. 3, Edited by Martonosi, A.,
    John Wiley and Sons, New York, p.221.

79. Kanazawa, T. and P. D. Boyer (1973). J. Biol. Chem. 248: 3163.

80. Oesterhelt, D. (1976). Angewandte Chemie 15: 17.

81. Eisenbach, M. and S. R. Caplan (1977). Trends Biochem. Sci. 2: 245.

82. Dahl, J. L. and L. E. Hokin (1974). Ann. Rev. Biochem. 43: 327.

83. Barnett, R. E. (1977). In: Membrane Proteins and their Interactions with Lipids, Editor Capaldi, R., Marcel Dekker, Inc., New York, p. 189.

84. Post, R. L. and S. Kume (1973). J. Biol. Chem. 248: 6993.

85. Kyte (1972). J. Biol. Chem. 247: 7642.

86. Mitchell, P. (1961). Nature 191: 144.

87. Avron, M. (1978). FEBS Letters 96: 225.

88. Racker, E. (1976). Mechanisms in Bioenergetics, Academic Press, New York.

89. MacDonald, R. E. and J. Lanyi (1977). Fed. Proc. 36: 1828.

90. Kaback, H. R. (1976). J. Cellular Physiol. 89: 575.

91. Lehninger, A. (1975). Biochemistry, 2nd Edition, Worth Publishers, Inc., New York.

92. LaNoue, K., S. Mizani and M. Klingenberg (1978). J. Biol. Chem. 253: 191.

93. Reynafarje, B. and A. L. Lehninger (1977). Biochim. Biophys. Res. Comm. 77: 1273.

94. De Meis, L. and A. L. Vianna (1979). Ann. Rev. Biochem. 48: 275.

95. LaNoue, K. F. and A. C. Schoolwerth (1979). Ann. Rev. Biochem. 48: 471.

96. Op den Kamp, J. A. F. (1979). Ann. Rev. Biochem. 48: 47.

97. Beeler, T., J. T. Russell and A. Martonosi (1979). Eur. J. Biochem. 95: 579.

98. Duggan, P. F. and A. Martonosi (1970). J. Gen. Physiol. 56: 147.

99. Meissner, G. and D. McKinley (1976). J. Membrane Biol. 30: 79.

100. Carafoli, E. (1979). FEBS Letters 104. 1.

101. Gómez-Fernandez, F. M. Goñi, D. Bah, C. Restall and D. Chapman (1979). FEBS Letters 98: 224.

102. Madden, T. D., D. Chapman and P. J. Quinn (1979). Nature 279: 538.

103. Chapman, D., J. C. Gómez-Fernandez and F. M. Goñi (1979). FEBS Letters 98: 211.

BIOPHYSICAL ASPECTS OF MEMBRANE PERMEABILITY

J.J.P. De LIMA, Ph.D.

Faculty of Medicine, University of Coimbra, Coimbra
Portugal

Many biological compartments, although exchanging mass continuously with the environment, maintain their chemical identities.
This occurs because the exchanges which take place across the barriers that surround the biological systems are qualitatively and quantitatively controlled. Such control is achieved through a balanced
use of multiple barrier mechanisms like diffusion, specific permeability and transport of ions against electrochemical potentials.

Physical models have been purposed to the study of either artificial or biological membranes. Such models particularly those
based on the sieving of size and charge of molecules or on the permeation of substances dissolving in the membrane phase, have been
very important to establish the general principles and to understand
the actual phenomena related with membrane permeability.

The transport phenomena of substances across membranes are primarily divided into two complementary groups of phenomena: the passive and the active. In the first group are included all the phenomena produced by classical diffusion forces such as gradients of
chemical potential, of pressure, or of electric potential.

In these terms diffusional fluxes produced by concentration differences across membranes, solvent drug effects, coupling between
fluxes, facilitated diffusion, exchange diffusion, etc., belong to
the first group.

In the active phenomena, metabolic energy is utilized to transport molecules against potential gradients.

In this lecture we shall review some important physical characteristics of the passive membrane mechanisms.

I. THE FLUX EQUATIONS

We define flux as the mass of a solute which per second crosses the unit area normal to the direction of transport.

A flux of solute particles can always be written as a product

1. $$J = C\overline{v}$$

where J is flux, C the concentration and $\overline{v}$ the mean velocity of the particles.

The mean velocity $\overline{v}$ is related to the driving force by the equation

2. $$\overline{v} = u'f$$

u' is the mobility of the particles and f is the driving force.

In the case of translational free diffusion of neutral particles the driving force per mole is the negative gradient of the chemical potential μ. Then the driving force per particle along the x direction is

3. $$f = -\frac{1}{L}\frac{d\mu}{dx}$$

where L is the Avogadro's number.

The flux is then

4. $$J = -\frac{Cu'}{L}\frac{d\mu}{dx}$$

the diffusion flux occurs from the higher to the lower chemical potential.

The chemical potential and the activity of a solution are related by the equation

5. $$\mu = \mu_0 + RT \, \ln a$$

The gradient of the chemical potential along the x direction is

$$\frac{d\mu}{dx} = RT \frac{1}{a}\frac{da}{dx}$$

For dilute solutions we can equalize activity with concentration and

$$\frac{d\mu}{dx} = RT \frac{1}{C} \frac{dC}{dx}$$

Then eq. 4 becomes

6.
$$J = - \frac{u'RT}{L} \frac{dC}{dx}$$

This is the first Fick's law for free diffusion usually written in the form

7.
$$J = -D \frac{dC}{dx}$$

D is the diffusion constant and the equation $D = \frac{u'RT}{L}$ is the Einstein relationship. The diffusion constant D is generally measured in cm^2/s.

Assuming that the solute molecules are spheres moving in a viscous medium such that the driving force is balanced by the frictional force, Stoke's law can be used to relate D with r, the radius of the spheres, and with η the viscosity by equation

8.
$$D = \frac{RT}{La} \quad \text{with}$$

$$a = 6\pi\eta r$$

Generally eq. 8 is a poor approximation of the actual situation.

Knowing the values of η for water and for media roughly analogous to biological membranes such as vegetable oils it is possible to grossly compare the diffusion in these two cases using eq. 8. For the same molecular size the value of D for water is at least 10^2 times greater than for the vegetable oils.

It is important to extend our study to the charged particles. Let us use eq. 1 for the case of charged particles.

We are interested in the charge which goes per second through the unit area normal to the direction of the movement, i.e. current density

9.
$$\Phi = \rho \bar{v}$$

where Φ is the flux of charge or current density, ρ is the density of charge and $\bar{v}$ is the mean velocity of the ions.

If C is the molar concentration of the ions then

10. $\rho = CFZ$

The mean velocity is related to the electric mobility u and electric field E by the equation

11. $\bar{v} = u E$

Since the electric field E is the negative gradient of the electric potential

12. $\bar{v} = -u \dfrac{dV}{dx}$

Using eqs. 9, 10 and 12 it comes

13. $\Phi = -u C \dfrac{d(VFZ)}{dx}$

where (VFZ) is the electric potential energy per mole.

Eq. 13 is formally identical to eq. 4, i.e. both equations include concentration times mobility times a gradient of potential energy. However, these two equations are expressed in different units because u' is dimensionally different from u.

If across a phase of thickness dx both an electric potential gradient and a chemical potential gradient act on a positive ion then the current density resulting from the added driving forces is

14. $\Phi = -C(\dfrac{u'}{L} \dfrac{d\mu}{dx} FZ + u \dfrac{dV}{dx} FZ)$

Note that the diffusion term has been converted into current density. It can be shown that $u' = u/|Z|e$, then

15. $\Phi = -(\dfrac{uZ}{|Z|} RT \dfrac{dC}{dx} + uCF|Z| \dfrac{dV}{dx})$

in C/m^2 sec. This is a variation of the Nernst-Planck equation of great interest in the study of ionic flows through membranes. Eq. 15 applies to ions of both signs. As it is expected the diffusion current term depends on the sign of the ion but the electric field term does not since electric current is in the field direction for either positive or negative ions.

Generally we are interested in the solution of this equation when we consider the flux through a membrane. In order to have this solution we must know the values of C across the membrane, the variation of the electric potential inside the membrane and the partition coefficients, i.e. the ratio between the concentrations of the ions at the surface of the membrane and at the bulk of the solution for both sides of the membrane.

Let us assume that the potential gradient across the membrane
is constant – constant field model – and that the partition coefficients are constant over the surfaces and equal for both the surfaces, i.e.

$$C_{1\,surf} = \beta C_{1\,bulk} \qquad (side\ 1)$$

16.

$$C_{2\,surf} = \beta C_{2\,bulk} \qquad (side\ 2)$$

With these assumptions the Nernst-Planck equation gives by integration

17.
$$\Phi_i = \frac{\beta u F}{\Delta x} \Delta V \; \frac{C_1 - C_2\ e^{-\frac{F}{RT}\Delta V}}{1 - e^{-\frac{F}{RT}\Delta V}}$$

This equation represents the flux of an ionic species i across
a membrane of thickness Δx through which exists a potential difference $\Delta V = V_2 - V_1$.

Equation 17 deserves some attention.

When $\Delta V \to 0$ this equation becomes

18.
$$\Phi = \frac{\beta u R T}{\Delta x} (C_1 - C_2) = \beta D \frac{\Delta C}{\Delta x}$$

Eq.18 is formally identical to the integration of Fick's law
for the limits C_1 and C_2. This equation applies to 1) the diffusional transport of uncharged molecules across a membrane and 2) the
diffusional transport of ions when the transmembrane potential is
null.

In these two situations the flux is directly proportional to
the concentration gradient across the membrane. In eq. 18 C_1 and C_2
refer to the concentrations inside the membrane at the left and
right membrane-solution interfaces. It was also assumed that there
was no net flux of water (solvent) across the membrane. If there
were a net flux of water a solute flow coupled to the water flow
should be taken into account. Assuming a net water flux J_w in moles/
/cm^2 sec and writing $\overline{V}_w$ for the partial molar volume of water the
volume flux associated with the flux of water is

19.
$$J_v = J_w \overline{V}_w$$

Then the flux of solute coupled to the water flux is

20.
$$J_s = J_v \overline{C}$$

where $\overline{C}$ is the average concentration across the membrane.

If a reflection coefficient σ is defined as the fraction of the solute molecules which happen to have such an orientation or position in the stream line of solvent that they are reflected back without passing through the membrane then the flux of solute coupled to the flux of water becomes

21.
$$J_s = J_v (1 - \sigma) C$$

If the net flux of a positive monovalent ion species across a membrane which is permeable to the ion is zero, eq. 17 becomes

$$\Phi = 0 = \frac{\beta\mu F}{\Delta x} \Delta V \frac{C_1 - C_2 \ e^{-\frac{F}{RT}\Delta V}}{1 - e^{-\frac{F}{RT}\Delta V}}$$

or
$$C_1 = C_2 \ e^{-\frac{F}{RT}\Delta V}$$

and
$$\Delta V = \frac{RT}{F} \ln \frac{C_2}{C_1}$$

which is the Nernst equation when applied to positive monovalent ions. The general form of Nernst equation is

22.
$$\Delta V = \frac{RT}{ZF} \ln \frac{C_2}{C_1}$$

This equation gives the electric potential difference which must be generated in order to maintain the concentration ratio C_2/C_1.

Eq. 22 when applied to the concentrations of the ions in extra- and intra-cellular compartments does not satisfy for some particular ions, for example the Na^+ in the nervous cell, although for K^+ and Cl^- it gives approximate results.

Returning to eq. 17 let us define the permeability coefficient P_i, for the ion species i, as

23.
$$P_i = \frac{u_i \beta RT}{\Delta x F}$$

and write the current density corresponding to a flux of these ions

24.
$$\Phi_i = P_i \frac{F^2 \Delta V}{RT} \frac{C_1 - C_2 \ e^{-\frac{F}{RT}\Delta V}}{1 - e^{-\frac{F}{RT}\Delta V}}$$

Supposing that across a membrane fluxes of Na^+, Cl^- and K^+ are occurring (for example in the axon plasma membrane) we can write the last equation for the three ions, i.e.

$$\Phi(K^+) = P_{(K^+)} \frac{F^2 \Delta V}{RT} \frac{C(K^+)_1 - C(K^+)_2 \, e^{-\frac{F}{RT} \Delta V}}{1 - e^{-\frac{F}{RT} \Delta V}}$$

25.
$$\Phi(Na^+) = P_{(Na^+)} \frac{F^2 \Delta V}{RT} \frac{C(Na^+)_1 - C(Na^+)_2 \, e^{-\frac{F}{RT} \Delta V}}{1 - e^{-\frac{F}{RT} \Delta V}}$$

$$\Phi(Cl^-) = P_{(Cl^-)} \frac{F^2 \Delta V}{RT} \frac{C(Cl^-)_2 - C(Cl^-)_1 \, e^{-\frac{F}{RT} \Delta V}}{1 - e^{-\frac{F}{RT} \Delta V}}$$

If no electrical current is passing through the membrane although equilibrium does not occur for the individual ions

26.
$$\Phi_{K^+} + \Phi_{Na^+} + \Phi_{Cl^-} = 0$$

Substituting the values of the current densities and solving for ΔV it comes

27.
$$\Delta V = \frac{RT}{F} \ln \frac{C(Na^+)_2 + \alpha_k C(K^+)_2 + \alpha_{Cl} C(Cl^-)_1}{C(Na^+)_1 + \alpha_k C(K^+)_1 + \alpha_{Cl} C(Cl^-)_2}$$

in which
$$\alpha_k = \frac{P(K^+)}{P(Na^+)} \quad \text{and} \quad \alpha_{Cl} = \frac{P(Cl^-)}{P(Na^+)}$$

Eq. 27 is known as the Goldman equation and has been used to calculate the transmembrane potentials when the concentration of Na^+, K^+ and Cl^- are known as well as the permeability coefficients which are supposed to be independent of the ion concentration.

By means of eq. 17 and using a double labelling with radioisotopes it is possible to characterize a diffusional transport.

Suppose two large compartments separated by a membrane having Na^{22} ions in compartment 1 and Na^{24} ions in compartment 2. Either the concentration of Na^{22} in compartment 2 or the concentration of Na^{24} in compartment 1 are negligible since we are dealing with large compartments. Using eq. 17 we can write for the unidirectional fluxes

28.
$$\Phi_{Na^{22}} = \frac{\beta u F}{\Delta x} \Delta V \frac{C(Na^{22})}{1 - e^{-\frac{F}{RT} \Delta V}}$$

$$\Phi_{Na^{24}} = \frac{\beta uF}{\Delta x} \Delta V \frac{-C(Na^{24})e^{-\frac{F}{RT}\Delta V}}{1 - e^{-\frac{F}{RT}\Delta V}}$$

then

29.

$$\frac{\Phi Na^{22}}{\Phi Na^{24}} = \frac{C(Na^{22})}{C(Na^{24})} e^{\frac{F}{RT}\Delta V}$$

This equation - flux ratio equation - gives the ratio between the flux of ions from compartment 1 to 2 and the flux of ions from 2 to 1.

When this equation is obeyed the flux is very likely diffusional in nature.

II. WATER TRANSPORT

Let us now consider the osmotic flow of water. A schematic set up to study this flow is shown below

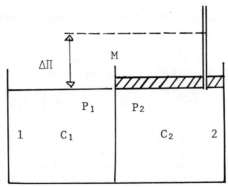

Different concentrations of an aqueous solution are separated by membrane M which is permeable to water but impermeable to the solute molecules. Suppose $C_2 > C_1$ and $P_1 = P_2$ at the beginning of the experiment.

The system will tend to a state where the chemical potential of permeant ions is the same at both sides of the membrane. This equilibrium has to be achieved at the expenses of a flow of water through the membrane. An osmotic flow of water from reservoir 1 to reservoir 2 is expected if $C_2 > C_1$. For dilute solutions the osmotic flow of water will be shown to be proportional to the difference of concentration between the two compartments.

The flow of water will be opposed by the hydrostatic pressure between the compartments which is built up. When equilibrium is reached the pressure difference across the membrane is the difference in osmotic pressure between solutions 2 and 1.

If compartment 1 contained pure water the pressure difference at the equilibrium was the osmotic pressure of solution 2.

We can say that hydrostatic pressure builds up a water flux which compensates the osmotic flow. A difference in hydrostatic pressure is obviously another way of creating a flux of water across the membrane. If $P_1 > P_2$ a flux of water from 1 to 2 is obtained which is proportional to $P_1 - P_2$.

Let us use the chemical potential to quantitate the osmotic flow of water.

The chemical potential of an ideal solution of a non-electrolyte of a species i can be written

30. $$\mu_i = \mu_i(T) + \overline{V}_i\, P + RT\, lnX_i$$

where $\overline{V}_i$ is the partial molar volume of species i, P is the hydrostatic pressure and $\mu_i(T)$ depends only on temperature.

In a dilute aqueous solution for solute of species i

31. $$X_i \simeq C_i\, \overline{V}_w$$

where $\overline{V}_w$ is the partial molar volume of water. Then eq. 30 becomes

32. $$\mu_i = \mu_i^o(T) + \overline{V}_i\, P + RT\, ln\, C_i$$

where

$$\mu_i^o(T) = \mu_i(T) + RT\, ln\, \overline{V}_w$$

is standard chemical potential.

For water the chemical potential from eq. 30 is

33. $$\mu_w = \mu_w(T) + \overline{V}_w P + RT\, ln\, X_w$$

The molar fraction of water is

34. $$X_w = \frac{n_w}{n_w + \sum_s n_s} = 1 - \frac{\sum_s n_s}{n_w + \sum_s n_s}$$

where s refers to solute species.

Taking into account that for dilute solutions $n_w \gg \sum_s n_s$ and $n_w \simeq \dfrac{V}{\overline{V}_w}$ it comes

35.
$$X_w \simeq 1 - \overline{V}_w \frac{\sum_s n_s}{V}$$

$$\simeq 1 - \overline{V}_w \sum_s C_s$$

and
$$ln\, X_w \simeq ln(1 - \overline{V}_w \sum C_s) \simeq -\overline{V}_w \sum C_s$$

then

36.
$$\mu_w = \mu_w^o(T) + \overline{V}_w(P - RT \sum_s C_s)$$

The term $RT \sum_s C_s$ is the osmotic pressure of the solution. The equation

37.
$$\Pi = RT \sum_s C_s$$

is Van't Hoffs law for dilute solutions. The equation for the chemical potential of water can now be written

38.
$$\mu_w = \mu_w^o(T) + \overline{V}_w(P - \Pi)$$

The driving force for the flux of water will be then

39.
$$\frac{d}{dx} \mu_w = \frac{d}{dx} \{\overline{V}_w(P - \Pi)\}$$

The flux of water is

40.
$$\Phi_w = -u_w' \, \overline{V}_w \frac{d}{dx} (P - \Pi)$$

Integrating this equation and for $P = 0$

41.
$$\Phi_w = -L_{PD}\Delta\Pi$$

L_{PD} is the coefficient of osmotic flow.

For $\Pi = 0$

42.
$$\Phi_w = L_P\Delta P$$

L_P is the filtration coefficient.

For a true semipermeable membrane

$$L_P = -L_{PD}$$

If the membrane is also permeable to the solute then L_P differs from $-L_{PD}$ and the ratio

43.
$$\sigma = - \frac{L_{PD}}{L_P}$$

is the reflection coefficient.

The reflection coefficient is equal to unit for a true semipermeable membrane and less than unit for membranes permeable to the solute.

A more general equation can then be written

44.
$$\Phi_w = L_P (\Delta P - \sigma \Delta \Pi)$$

III. DONNAN EQUILIBRIUM

Let us now consider the case of an idealized membrane model with perfect selective permeability to different ion species — the Donnan membrane. When such a membrane is used to separate two solutions a potential difference is developed across the membrane.

Suppose that equal concentrations of NaCl are added to both sides of the membrane and that a quantity of sodium proteinate is added to side 1. Assume that the membrane is freely permeable to Na^+ and Cl^- but impermeable to the large protein ions P^{zp-}.

Then the concentration of Na^+ is greater in side 1 than in side 2 and Na^+ will tend to diffuse across the membrane to side 2. Also Cl^- will tend to diffuse from side 1 to side 2 to satisfy electroneutrality. This ion transport will occur until diffusion and electric forces are balanced. At the equilibrium the transmembrane potential is called the Donnan potential.

For the permeable ion species we can write

45.
$$\Phi_{Donnan} = \frac{RT}{F} \ln \frac{C(Na^+)_2}{C(Na^+)_1}$$

$$= \frac{RT}{F} \ln \frac{C(Cl^-)_1}{C(Cl^-)_2}$$

Hence

46.
$$\frac{C(Na^+)_2}{C(Na^+)_1} = \frac{C(Cl^-)_1}{C(Cl^-)_2}$$

which is Gibbs-Donnan equation relating ion concentration of two ions both at equilibrium.

A further condition which must apply to each side of the system is the electrical neutrality, thus on side 1

47.
$$C(Na^+)_1 = C(Cl^-)_1 + Z_p(P)_1$$

where Z_p is the valence of the ion proteinate, and

48.
$$C(Na^+)_2 = C(Cl^-)_2 \qquad \text{on side 2}$$

Using eqs. 46, 47 and 48

49.
$$C(Na^+)_2 = \frac{C(Na^+)_1 \{C(Na^+)_1 - Z_p C(P)_1\}}{C(Na^+)_2}$$

or

50.
$$C(Na^+)_1^2 - Z_p C(P^-)_1 C(Na^+)_1 - C(Na^+)_2^2 = 0$$

This is a quadratic equation in $C(Na^+)_1$ which has the solution

51.
$$C(Na^+)_1 = \frac{Z_p C(P)_1 + \{Z_p^2 C(P)_1^2 + 4C(Na^+)_2^2\}^{1/2}}{2}$$

Therefore

52.
$$\Phi_{Donnan} = \frac{-RT}{F} \ln \frac{C(Na^+)_1}{C(Na^+)_2}$$

$$= \frac{-RT}{F} \ln \{\frac{Z_p C(P)_1 + \{Z_p^2 C(P)_1^2 + 4C(Na^+)_2^2\}^{1/2}}{2C(Na^+)_2}\}$$

If $C(P)_1 = 0$ the Donnan potential becomes zero, i.e. $\Phi_{Donnan} = 0$.

This model leads to the conclusion that when $C(P)_1 \neq 0$ a standing transmembrane potential is built up that will rest without expenditure of energy.

If the osmotic flow of water has been canceled by exerting a pressure $\Delta\Pi$ between compartments 1 and 2 let us call n and P the initial concentrations of NaCl and proteinate respectively. Then the equilibrium concentrations will be

53. $C(Cl^-)_1 = n - x$ $C(Cl^-)_2 = n + x$

54. $C(Na^+)_1 = n - x + ZP$ $C(Na^+)_2 = n + x$

Equ. 46 is also

46.a. $(n + x)^2 = (n - x)(n - x + ZP)$

which gives

55. $(n - x) < (n + x) < (n - x + ZP)$

since $(n + x)$ is the geometric mean of $(n - x)$ and $(n - x + ZP)$. Then

56. $C(Cl^-)_2 > C(Cl^-)_1$ and $C(Na^+)_1 > C(Na^+)_2$

on the other hand

57. $C(Cl^-)_1 + C(Na^+)_1 > C(Cl^-)_2 + C(Na^+)_2$

This can easily be proved using eq. 46.a .

Then

58. $C(Cl^-)_1 + C(Na^+)_1 + C(P)_1 > C(Cl^-)_2 + C(Na^+)$

We conclude from equation 57 that the ionic concentration of the dispersing medium of the proteinate ions is greater than the ionic concentration in reservoir 2.

From equation 58 we can write for the osmotic pressure difference between compartments 1 and 2

59.
    $\Delta\Pi = RT \{C(Cl^-)_1 + C(Na^+)_1 + C(P)_1 - C(Cl^-)_2 - C(Na^+)_2\}$

From eq. 57 we easily see that $\Delta\Pi$ is greater than the osmotic pressure of the proteinate alone, i.e. at the same concentration in the absence of small ions added to the solution.

IV. FACILITATED DIFFUSION

The permeation of a large amount of molecular species shows departures from the diffusional laws studied above.

This is for example the case of the entry of sugars into red cells. However, these permeants have in common with the processes studied that an equilibrium is reached when the concentration is the same in both sides of the membrane. We have already seen that in a true diffusional pro ess the equation $\Phi = K\Delta C$ is verified, i.e.

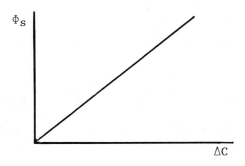

a straight line is obtained in a plot of Φ_s vs. ΔC.

In the case of the sugars and the red cells the plot Φ_s vs. ΔC gives a curve which looks like the one below

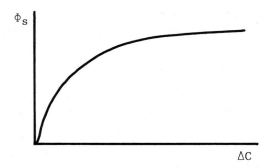

However, a double reciprocal plot of sugar entry against sugar concentration is a straight line showing a Michaellis-Menten type of reaction, i.e.

60.
$$\Phi_s = \frac{C\Phi_m}{C + K_m}$$

Such membrane processes called facilitated diffusion processes depend on a saturable mechanism and show some characteristics of the enzymatic reaction such as inhibition, competition, higher rate of penetration at the beginning than in diffusional processes, etc.

The facilitated diffusion processes do not occur against electrochemical gradients;on the contrary,they take place on existing gradients of the permeant solutes and invariably lead to the dissipation of these gradients.

When the movement of a permeant molecule down its electrochemical potential gradient occurs simultaneously with the movement in the opposite direction of a structurally similar molecule the process is called counter-flow or counter-current.

Let us study a model of facilitated diffusion. In the picture below

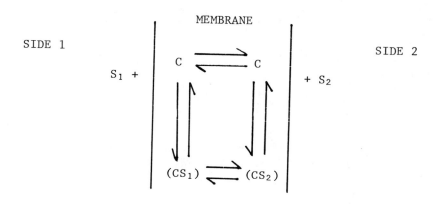

C is the carrier concentration, S_1 and S_2 the concentration of permeant molecules at sides 1 and 2 and (CS_1) and (CS_2) the complex carrier-permeant at sides 1 and 2.

It is assumed that:

1. The system and its components are at equilibrium at both faces.

2. The total carrier concentration (carrier + complex) is constant through the membrane.

3. Carrier and complex movements across the membrane are diffusional.

4. The movement of the carrier complex is the rate limiting step.

Then the flux of complex across the membrane is given by

61. $\Phi_{comp} = B\{(CS_1) - (CS_2)\}$

on the other hand

62.
$$\frac{C_1 S_1}{(CS_1)} = \frac{C_1 S_2}{(CS_2)} = K_m$$

and

63.
$$C_1 + (CS_1) = C_2 + (CS_2) = C_T$$

Using eqs. 61, 62 and 63, we obtain for the flux of complex across the membrane

64.
$$\Phi_{comp} = K_m \left(\frac{S_1}{S_1 + K_m} - \frac{S_2}{S_2 + K_m} \right)$$

and since in the steady state there is no accumulation of solute in the membrane

$$\Phi_{comp} = \Phi_s$$

or

65.
$$\Phi_s = K \left(\frac{S_1}{S_1 + K_m} - \frac{S_2}{S_2 + K_m} \right)$$

which is the flux of permeant through the membrane.

If
$$K_m \gg S_1 , S_2$$

66.
$$\Phi_s \simeq \frac{K}{K_m} (S_1 - S_2)$$

This is formally identical to the equation for a simple diffusional process through the membrane.

If
$$K_m \ll S_1 , S_2$$

$$\Phi_s = 0$$

There is no net flux of permeant even when there exists a concentration gradient, $S_1 \gg S_2$ for example.

The ratio between unidirectional flows Φ_{12} and Φ_{21} is

67.
$$\frac{\Phi_{12}}{\Phi_{21}} = \frac{S_1}{S_1 + K_m} \frac{S_2 + K_m}{S_2}$$

For the first case $K_m \gg S_1, S_2$

$$\frac{\Phi_{12}}{\Phi_{21}} = \frac{S_1}{S_2}$$

which still is a diffusional relationship.

For the second case $K_m << S_1, S_2$

$$\frac{\Phi_{12}}{\Phi_{21}} = 1$$

The unidirectional flows cancel each other.

V. EXCHANGE DIFFUSION

Using radioactive tracers it has been observed in systems in a steady state that a 1:1 exchange of substrate molecules across a cell membrane can occur without measurable net flow.

This has been described as exchange diffusion a passive transport mechanism based on the scheme below

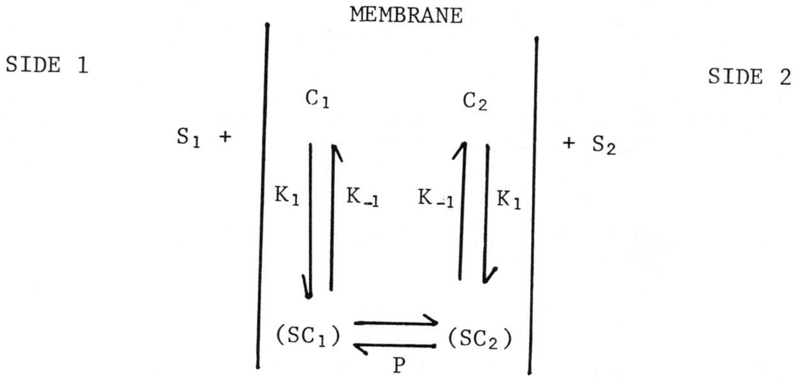

MEMBRANE

SIDE 1

C_1 $\qquad$ C_2

S_1 +

K_1 K_{-1} K_{-1} K_1

(SC_1) $\rightleftarrows$ (SC_2)

P

SIDE 2

+ S_2

The uncombined carrier C has a very low mobility in the membrane phase.

In the steady state

68. $\qquad \frac{dC_1}{dt} = K_{-1}(SC_1) - K_1 C_1 S_1 = 0 \qquad$ and

69. $\frac{d(SC_1)}{dt} = K_1 C_1 S_1 - K_{-1}(SC_1) - P\{(SC_1) - (SC_2)\} = 0$

combining eqs. 68 and 69 and

$$(SC_1) = (SC)_2$$

But $$\Phi_S = P \{(SC_1) - (SC_2)\}$$

then $$\Phi_S = 0$$ as expected.

The unidirectional fluxes measurable with radioisotopes are

$$\Phi_{12} = P(SC_1)$$

70.

$$\Phi^{21} = P(SC_2)$$

Assuming the complex at equilibrium at both sides of the membrane

$$(SC_1) = K_1 C_1 S_1$$

71.

$$(SC_2) = K_2 C_2 S_2$$

entering with

$$C_T = (SC_1) + (SC_2) + C_1 + C_2$$

and eq. 71 in eq. 70 it comes

72. $$\Phi_{12} = \Phi_{21} = PK_1 C_T \frac{S_1 S_2}{2K_1 S_1 S_2 + S_1 + S_2}$$

If $S_2 = 0$ $\therefore$ $\Phi_{12} = 0$. No unidirectional flux occurs if the substrate concentration is null in the compartment which receives the flux.

Eq. 72 can also describe counter-flow mechanisms.

REFERENCES

ADELMAN, Jr.,W.J. (ed.) (1971). Biophysics and physiology of excitable membranes - Van Nostrand-Reinhold.

BUNNER, F. and KLENSELLER, A. (ed.) (1971). Current topics in membranes and transport. Academic Press.

DAVIES, M. (1973). Functions of biological membranes. Outline series in Biology - Chapman and Hall.

PLONSEY, R. (1969). Bioelectric Phenomena. Mac Graw-Hill Series in Bioengineering.

STEIN, W.D. (1967). The movement of molecules across membranes. Academic Press.

VILLARS, F.M.H. and BENEDEK, G.B. (1974). Physics - vol. 2 - Statistical Physics, Addison-Wesley.

CEREBRAL ENDOTHELIUM, BLOOD-BRAIN-BARRIER AND THE ASTROCYTE MEMBRANE

K. Dorovini-Zis, J. J. Anders and M. W. Brightman

Laboratory of Neuropathology and Neuroanatomical Sciences
National Institute of Neurological and Communicative
    Diseases and Stroke
National Institutes of Health, Bethesda, Maryland 20205

The manner in which protein crosses from blood to the extracellular clefts of the brain, when the barrier to such passage has been disrupted, has not been fully elucidated. The barrier, which maintains a sharp gradient between the high concentration of protein within the blood and the very low amount in the extracellular fluid of the cerebral parenchyma, is endothelial. The occlusion of the extracellular clefts between adjacent endothelial cells by successive belts of tight junctions together with the absence of vesicular transfer ensure that proteins do not cross the cerebral vessel (Reese and Karnovsky, 1967). The degree of occlusion is complete with regard to protein and substances as small as ionic lanthanium (La^{3+}) (Bouldin and Krigman, 1975), which has a diameter of about 0.9 nm.

The junctions remain structurally intact when hyperosmotic fixative containing 2% NaCl is perfused through the heart. The cytoplasm of endothelial and epithelial cells of the brain are more electron dense than usual, the organelles more crowded, and the extracellular clefts distended, yet the tight junctions appear, in thin, plastic sections, to be unaltered (Brightman and Reese, 1969). However, when hyperosmotic non-electrolytes are applied directly to the brain surface or infused into the carotid artery before fixation, there is indirect evidence that the junctions are rendered permeable to protein such as horseradish peroxidase (HRP), even though their pentalaminar configuration is

65

unaltered (Brightman et al., 1973). Thus, the extracellular
pools normally inaccessible to protein now contain HRP,
indicating that the once impermeable junctions had opened
sufficiently to allow HRP (MW 40,000), about 5 nm in diameter, to
pass. The substance used in these experiments was 2.2 M urea.
Because urea is a denaturant, it has been proposed that, in
addition to deformation of the junctions following shrinkage of
the endothelial cells bathed by the hyperosmotic urea, this
molecule may also reversibly denature the protein of the tight
junction strands. The strands would thus become discontinuous
and therefore permeable to protein without evincing any
alteration in thin sections (Brightman et al., 1974). The
possible role of calyciform vacuoles, which took up HRP following
urea exposure, in the transport of protein across the endothelium
was unknown (Brightman et al., 1973).

In addition to hyperosmotic shock, a number of other events
lead to the escape of blood-borne HRP from cerebral blood into
the parenchymal fluid. Trauma (Beggs and Waggener, 1976;
Povlishock, 1979), hypertension (Robinson and Brightman, 1976;
Westergaard et al., 1977; Nag et al, 1977), seizures (Petito et
al., 1977), exposure to serotonin (Westergaard, 1975),
hyperglycemia (Shivers, 1979) and hypervolemia (Horton and
Hedley-White, 1978) are accompanied by extravasation of
blood-borne peroxidase into the brain substance. These
investigators failed to detect a penetration of HRP through the
endothelial junctions and, instead, have noted an increase in
endocytotic vesicles. The greater number of vesicles, labeled
with HRP or unlabeled, are regarded as moving from luminal to
abluminal surface of the endothelium, so transferring the protein
from blood to brain. The most convincing evidence of passage in
membrane bounded vacuoles has been provided by the serial
sectioning of endothelium after concussive damage (Beggs and
Waggener, 1976).

Colloidal lanthanum, which is less than 2 nM in diameter,
has been dissolved in aldehyde fixative, which is then perfused
through the heart of rats after administration of hyperosmotic
mannitol or hypertensive agents. This smaller tracer appears to
penetrate successive tight junctions under these conditions
(Nagy, 1979a, b). This inference was based on the presence of
colloid within single interjunctional pools at some distance from
the luminal surface rather than on a succession of filled pools
viewed in serial sections. We have been re-examining by
sequential sectioning the effects of a hyperosmotic
non-electrolyte, arabinose, which at a threshold level of 1.4M,
opens the barrier to Evans blue-albumin (Rapoport, 1972). The
tracer used here is the smallest one yet available: ionic
lanthanum.

A second aspect of cellular influence on the composition of the extracellular fluid of the brain is a cell which does not itself form a continuous barrier to passive, extracellular flow. This cell, the astrocyte, though it does not form a continuous cellular barrier but is, instead, circumventable by extracellular protein (Brightman, 1968), ensheaths over 90% of the vessel wall in the CNS. The ubiquitous astrocyte can indeed modify the composition of perineuronal fluid with respect to potassium (Kuffler and Nicolls, 1966) and probably other substances. It is, therefore, appropriate to consider the structure of the astrocytic membrane which is involved in maintaining the constancy of the cerebral microenvironment.

BLOOD-BRAIN BARRIER TO IONIC LANTHANUM

In contrast to the tight junctions between adjacent epithelial cells of the choroid plexus which are penetrated by ionic lanthanum (Castel, et al., 1974) those of the cerebral endothelium are impermeable (Bouldin and Krigman, 1975). When we confirmed these results, it became apparent that, if we were to find exuded La which is indescernible by light microscopy, HRP had to be used simultaneously as a marker. The necessity of using HRP together with La^{3+} is the randomness of barrier opening. Regardless of the type of stimuli, listed previously, all barrier openings share one aspect: they are spotty; only isolated segments of different vessels are rendered permeable so that exudates are formed sporadically at many sites, all of them unpredictable in location.

By priming rats with HRP injected into a femoral vein before or after the introcarotid infusion of 3 to 5 nM lanthanum chloride, we were able to choose areas of lanthanum escape by the localization of HRP exudates. The simultaneous use of these two tracers have the disadvantage of dense HRP reaction product obscuring a light deposit of La^{3+} in some specimens. By short incubation periods, however, the density of reaction product should be diminished so as to enable the distinction between the particulate form of ionic lanthanum and HRP reaction product.

A threshold concentration of 1.4 M arabinose dissolved in 2.9 ml. of saline is infused over a period of 30 seconds into one internal carotid artery in adult rats that had been injected intravenously with 0.25 mg. HRP/gm. body weight. A volume of 0.6 ml. of the HRP solution was infused either before or after the lanthanum infusion. One ml. of 3 to 5 mM lanthanum chloride is infused into the same carotid artery 15 to 30 seconds following the administration of arabinose. The animals were fixed by perfusion of aldehydes through the aorta 5 minutes after the La^{3+} infusion. Chopped sections from all regions of the brain were incubated for peroxidatic activity. Only those regions containing HRP exudates were processed for electronmicroscopy.

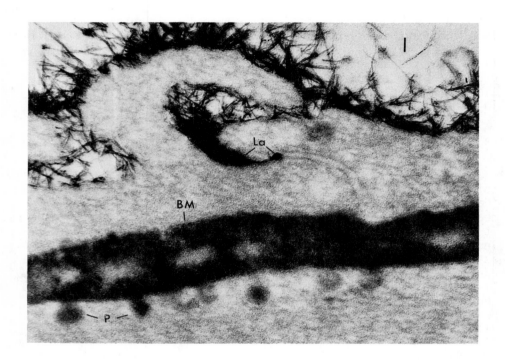

Fig. 1   Lanthanum (La) penetrates interjunctional pools between
          two adjacent endothelial cells. Needle-shaped La^{3+}
          deposits attach to the plasma membrane on the luminal
          side. The basement membrane (BM) and abluminal pits (p)
          contain HRP. 1 - lumen. X136,000.

        Within 2 minutes after the infusion of the arabinose, HRP
was exuded from blood vessels throughout the brain. These protein
exudates were most numerous in the temporal and parietal regions of
the cerebral cortex and in the brain stem. As with hyperosmotic
(2.2M) urea infused into the internal carotid artery of rabbits,
the exudates of HRP formed around segments of arterioles and capillaries primarily. The number of junctional clefts were most
numerous in arterioles.

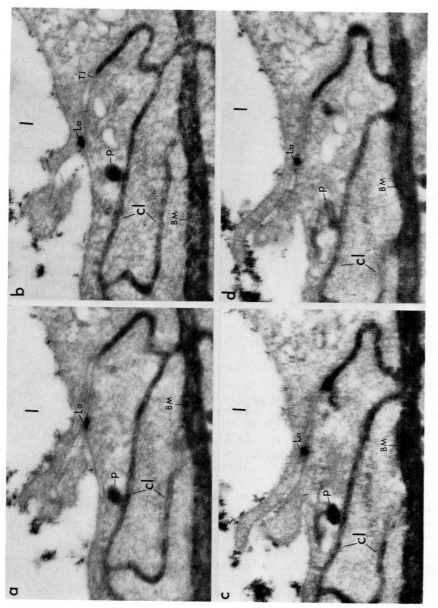

Fig. 1. Cerebral arteriole. Serial sections. a-d: HRP fills intercellular clefts (cl), basement membrane (BM) and pits (p). Small lanthanum deposits (La) in the same clefts that HRP enters from the abluminal side up to a tight junction (tj). l – lumen. fig. b. X80,000.

Considerably less La^{3+} passed into the parenchymal clefts than did HRP, as viewed electron-microscopically. The lanthanum was extravasated from the same vessel or from adjacent vessels across which HRP had migrated (Fig. 1). Ionic lanthanum appeared as needle-shaped deposits, a continuous, very dense electron mass or as a granular aggregate -- all three states being observable in the same section. The most common type of deposit was the needle or fusiform one.

In a few vessels, La^{3+} penetrated three or more successive tight junctions as manifested by its entry into the extracellular pools between the junctions (Figs. 2, 3). In serial sections, La^{3+} could be followed as a deposit in 3 or more of these pools but usually not all of them, from luminal to abluminal surface. However, a continuous row of pools containing HRP could occasionally be discerned in a few junctions. Rarely, all of the pools contained La in a single, thin plastic section and La could be followed from the luminal pool to the abluminal one and thence the basal lamina. The filling of the basal lamina was uneven. An extremely dense, continuous column of deposit could end abruptly leaving the remainder of the lamina with only a stippling of La^{3+}. Nevertheless, the granular form could not be confused with lead deposit inasmuch as the sections were not stained with either lead or uranyl acetate. It is as though the binding to the basal lamina in these regions was variable with segmental leaching or deposit during succeeding washes in buffer, alcohol or organic solvent. The leaching may have taken place even though 3-5 mM lanthanum chloride had been added to the osmium and buffer solutions.

The same cleft between contiguous endothelial cells that is penetrated by ionic lanthanum may also be entered by peroxidase. Usually, the two fronts are separated by a tight junction or by an interjunctional pool. This separation implies two events: (a) each tracer entered the cleft from a different source -- either luminal or abluminal and (b) neither tracer penetrated the entire row of successive junctions. Most frequently, the La^{3+} entered from the luminal side of the cleft, whereas the HRP did so from the abluminal side, that side facing the basal lamina (Figs. 1d, 2). We do not know how the much larger substance, HRP (MW 40,000, with a diameter of about 5 nM) crossed the endothelium. There are four possible routes by which the protein traversed the vessel wall: passive movement through open tight junctions, passive flow across a damaged, "torn" endothelial cell, active vesicular transport, and active canalicular transfer.

Unlike the experiments with hyperosmotic urea, HRP did not penetrate all interjunctional pools from luminal to abluminal surface in any single, thin section of endothelium. Several pools were penetrated and this entry might signify passage through all junctions but at different levels of the cleft. It would, however,

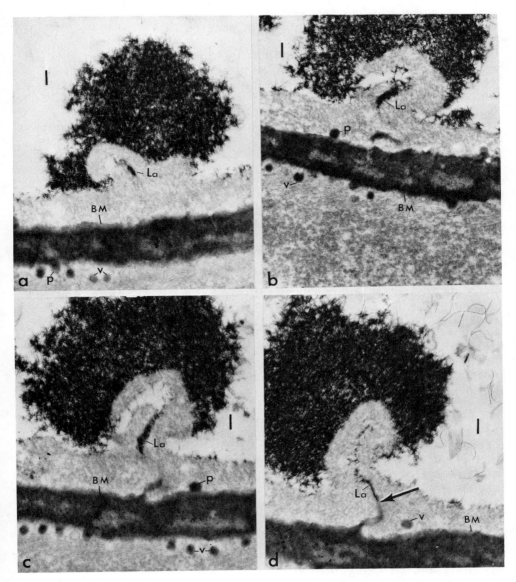

Fig. 3. Serial sections of cerebral arteriole. a-d.: lanthanum
(La) enters an extracellular cleft from the lumen (l).
HRP, already deposited in the basement membrane (BM), has
penetrated the same intercellular cleft from the opposite
side (b-d). The two tracers meet in d at arrow. Abluminal
pits (p) and vesicles (v) contain HRP. Some vesicles may
be pits with a communicating neck in another plane of
section. X50,000.

be considerably easier to regard the junctions as having been
rendered permeable had the peroxidase entered all of the interjunctional pools visible in a single section.

The second route - discontinuities in the endothelium - is a
possibility that has yet to be demonstrated unequivocally. The
flooding of endothelial cytoplasm by freely dispersed peroxidase
indicates that the endothelial cell membrane has been damaged
(Brightman, 1965). An intact and, therefore, semi-permeable
membrane would not allow the free entry of protein. The inundation
of some endothelial cells, however, does not result in the escape
of protein into the perivascular clefts. In almost all instances,
the freely dispersed protein remains within the endothelial cell
with no discernible reaction product in the subjacent basal lamina.
Either the binding capacity of the cytoplasm is considerable so
that very large amounts of circulating HRP are necessary before
the protein spills out of the cells, or the abluminal portion of
the cell membrane is still intact (Brightman, 1977). An actual
tear in the endothelium has not been found. Nevertheless, after
exposure to hyperosmotic arabinose, the endothelium might be
rendered susceptible to disruption by the hydrostatic pressure
and high flow rates during perfusion of balanced salt solution and
aldehyde fixatives. If breaks in the endothelium are created at
that time, there would be little time for peroxidase to form
characteristic exudates. For one thing, the rush of fixative would
rapidly dilute the HRP being flushed past the break. Although
still elusive, a few, small ruptures of the endothelium might
account for the escape of protein without accompanying red blood
cells.

A third mechanism, proposed by a number of investigators, is
vesicular transport. A number of unrelated stimuli, listed in the
introductory part of this account, all result in the exudation of
peroxidase from cerebral vessels by way of active vesicular transfer rather than by the passive flow through permeable junctions,
according to these authors. The mechanism here is the formation
of pits by the luminal plasma membrane of the endothelium, and
their pinching off to form vesicles containing whatever luminal
contents that had been entrapped within the omega-shaped pits.
The vesicles then move rapidly across the endothelium to fuse with
the abluminal plasma membrane and so eject their contents into
the perivascular space.

An experiment that does not support this type of transfer is
one where hyperosmotic arabinose is infused as usual and, within
minutes, the brain fixed with aldehydes. Two to three hours after
fixation, a solution of peroxidase is perfused through the heart.
Exudates of HRP surround cerebral vessels in a pattern similar to
that following administration of the protein in the brain that had
been exposed to the arabinose (Brightman, 1977). The HRP did not

penetrate successive tight junctions between endothelial cells; however, a few short clefts between endothelial cells appeared to have become separated and contained HRP. Since formation and migration of vesicles must have been completely halted by 2 to 3 hours of fixation in glutaraldehyde, vesicular transfer could not have accounted for the escape of protein. It was hypothesized that parajunctional channels were actively formed and remained open at their luminal and abluminal ends long enough to be fixed in an open condition.

Two alternative explanations are consistent with this result. In the highly attenuated regions of capillaries, where the thickness of the endothelium may be no greater than the diameter of a single pit, a single pit, opening onto the luminal and abluminal face of the endothelium may act as a channel. The second alternative is the formation of longer channels by the confluence of vesicles. In the capillaries of skeletal muscle, transendothelial channels form by vesicle fusion (Simionescu et al., 1975). Such channels, as just discussed, may be one vesicle wide or several vesicles long (Brightman, 1977). Lossinsky et al., (1979) have described such channels in cerebral endothelium. However, anything less than the depiction of either a channel with both a luminal and abluminal opening or a continuous column of reaction product extending from luminal to abluminal surface, is insufficient evidence for a role in transfer. Ideally, the transport should just have begun so that the abluminal end of such a column would extend as a focal "puff" of reaction product in an otherwise empty basal lamina. Once the basal lamina is completely infiltrated with HRP, there is no way of ascertaining the source of the protein, whether it be from vesicle, channel, tear or permeable junction. We have yet to encounter a channel that would satisfy these conditions.

The insistence that the channel be visualizable from its luminal end all the way to its abluminal opening is not a captious one. The cerebral endothelium of the hagfish is tunneled by many channels that either extend from a luminal opening to a point near the opposite, abluminal surface or from an abluminal opening to a point near the luminal surface. A channel that was open at both ends in the same section was not described, and all of these vessels have a blood-brain barrier to HRP (Bundgaard et al., 1979). Thus, an endothelium with zonular tight junctions, though honeycombed by channels that almost extend across the endothelium, stands as a barrier to protein. We reiterate that channels, either one vesicle in diameter or the length of a vesicular chain, and open at both ends simultaneously have not been found in our specimens. The question of whether the passage of peroxidase across cerebral endothelium bathed by hyperosmotic arabinose solutions is passive by way of permeable junctions or tears, or active via parajunctional channels is still unresolved.

The Astrocyte Membrane

Although most of the surface of cerebral vessels is ensheathed by astrocytes, these cells do not act as a barrier to the extra-cellular movement of protein (Brightman, 1968). Instead of forming tight junctions, the cell membranes of contiguous astrocytes are united by gap junctions (Brightman and Reese, 1969). These junctions are not zonular and HRP can flow around them. The astrocytes, however, have been purported to influence the composition of extra-cellular fluid within the central nervous system (Kuffler and Nicholls, 1966). This influence might, in part, be exerted through the astrocytic cell membrane and a consideration of its internal structure under different conditions will now be presented.

The inside of cell membranes can be visualized by the following method. Small pieces of aldehyde-fixed tissue are cryoprotected by immersion in 25% glycerol, frozen at liquid nitrogen temperature and cracked under a high vacuum. The fracture plane runs through the middle, hydrophobic portion of cell membrane and the artifi-cially produced faces: an inner or protoplasmic (P) one and an external (E) one, are then replicated by depositing, under vacuum, a thin film of platinum and carbon. The vacuum is broken, the tissue is dissolved in a strong oxidant and the freed replica is mounted on a grid for electron microscopic examination.

Astrocytes, so prepared, display aggregates of small particles called assemblies (Landis and Reese, 1974) within their plasma membranes. Each assembly consists of subunit particles, 5-7nM wide, which stud the inner or P face leaving complementary pits on the opposite E face (Fig. 4a). The assemblies within the astro-cytes' cell membrane are especially numerous, but are not peculiar to this cell. Orthogonal aggregates of particles, which are identical in appearance to astrocyte assemblies, also occupy the plasma membranes of Muller cells in the retina (Fig. 4b) (Reale and Luciano, 1974), ependyma cells (Brightman et al., 1975; Privat, 1977), satellite cells in autonomic and spinal ganglia (Pannese et al., 1977; Elfvin and Forsman, 1978), hepatocytes (Kreutziger, 1968), epithelial cells of the intestine (Staehelin, 1972) and trachea (Inoue and Hogg, 1977), light cells of the kidney collecting tubules (Humbert et al., 1975; Ellisman and

---

Fig. 4.   Replicas of the inner or P face of freeze-cleaved cell
           membranes. Assemblies (arrow) are interspersed among
           background particles (lines) within the membrane.

    a.   Cell membrane of astrocyte from glia limitans (subpial)
          Rat. X 120,000.
    b.   Cell membrane of Müller cell. Retina of goldfish
          X 114,000.

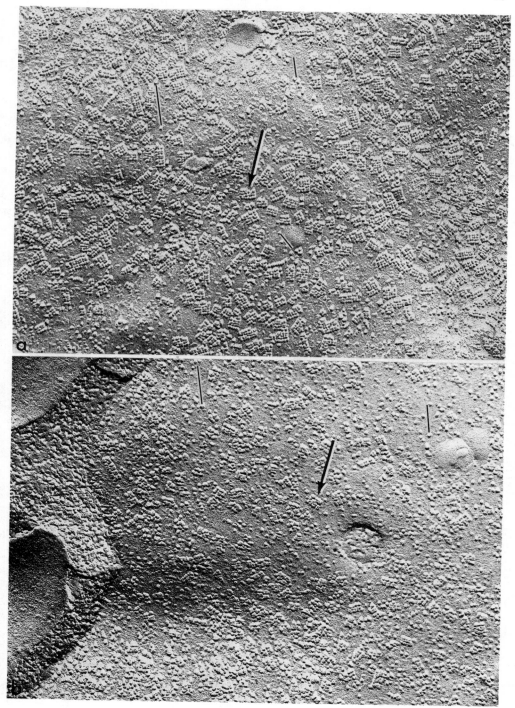

Rash, 1977). The astrocytic membrane is unusual in having many more of the assemblies per unit area of membrane except for the parietal cells of the stomach, where the assemblies also appear to be densely packed (Bordi and Perrelet, 1978).

The assemblies are composed of protein. Astrocytes derived from 5-7 day old rats have been kept in vitro and exposed to cycloheximide, an inhibitor of protein synthesis. Within 3 hours of exposure, the assemblies disappeared although background particles and particles belonging to gap junctions were unaffected in the same fracture face (Anders and Pagnavelli, 1979). The assemblies, at least in the astrocytes of young rats, consist of protein with what is apparently a high turnover rate.

The assemblies reflect the degree of differentiation of astro-cytes and appear first in glial cells of rat fetuses between 19 and 20 days of age and do not reach the numbers characteristic of adult animals until approximately the 40th day postpartum (Anders and Brightman, 1979). The astrocytic membrane thus matures by a continual addition of assembly subunits and background particles. Initially, most assemblies consist of four subunit particles to which more subunits accrue with time until the assemblies form larger squares and rectangles.

The numbers and area of membrane occupied by assemblies differ consistently from region to region. It had been noted that astro-cytes lining fluid compartments, i.e. subpial and perivascular cells, contain more assemblies than do those astrocytes that are satellite to neurons (Landis and Reese, 1974). Assemblies within the subpial or glia limitans astrocytes have a mean area of 0.0010 per um^2 of membrane face with a range of 0.0004 um^2 to 0.0024 um^2. The number of assemblies in the glia limitans of the medulla (469-595 um^2) is consistently greater than that of the cerebral cortex (185-495 um^2) (Anders and Brightman, 1979). In all regions examined, the subpial end-feet were most densely packed with assemblies which decreased in number in the underlying astrocytic processes. The consistently greater number of assemblies in the glia limitans affords a base-line for future comparisons after exposing glial cultures to various agents.

A striking change in the arrangement of assemblies is brought about in reactive astrocytes. A subtle gliosis, one confined to a discrete area, has been induced subpially by transplanting frag-ments of superior cervicle ganglion to the brain surface of young, 6 to 10 day old rats (Rosenstein and Brightman, 1978). The manginal astrocytes responded by emitting excrescences into the cerebro-spinal fluid, while the underlying astrocytic processes formed parallel sheets. The result was a thickened glia limitans in which the deeper, parallel layers contained more assemblies than the deeper layers of non-reactive astrocytes in the glia limitans. Within the excrescences, assemblies were no more numerous than in "resting" marginal astrocytes, but the assemblies now became aligned linearly as long trains. The trains were often arranged as parallel rows along the circumference of the excrescences. The functional import of this alignment or of the assemblies themselves is unknown. It is conceivable that the alignment may be imposed by the decreased radius of curvature of a narrow excrescence, yet the flat perivascular astrocyte of normal rats likewise contain rows of assemblies, albeit far fewer. If the radius were a determinant, than it should be just as likely for some subunits to form square assemblies in addition to linear ones. However, only linear arrays appear to be formed. These experiments have established the numbers, area and configuration of assemblies in selected astrocytes so that changes in any of these parameters should be recognizable after exposure to different agents. Such changes might provide clues as to whether the assemblies are involved in modulating the composition of the extracellular fluid in the brain and, perhaps. other organs as well.

REFERENCES

1. Anders, J.J. and Brightman, M.W. (1979) J. Neurocytol. (In press).
2. Anders, J.J. and Pagnanelli, D.M. (1979) Anat. Rec. 193:470.
3. Beggs, I.L. and Waggener, J.D. (1976) Lab. Invest. 34:428-439.
4. Bordi, C. and Perrelet, A. (1978) Anat. Rec. 192: 297-304.
5. Bouldin, T.W. and Krigman, M.R. (1975). Brain Res. 99: 444-448.
6. Brightman, M.W. (1965) J. Cell. Biol. 26: 99-123.
7. Brightman, M.W. (1967) Progr. Brain Res. 29: 19-37
8. Brightman, M.W. (1977) Morphology of blood-brain interfaces. In: The Ocular and Cerebrospinal Fluids (ed. by Bito, L.X., Davson, H. and Fenstermacher, J.D.), pp. 1-25.
9. Brightman, M.W., Hori, M., Rapoport, S.I., Reese, T.S. and Westergaard, E. (1973) J. Comp. Neurol. 152 317-326.
10. Brightman, M.W., Prescott, L. and Reese, T.S. (1975) In: Brain-Endocrine Interaction II. The Ventricular System (ed. by Knigge, K.M., Scott, D.E., Kobayashi, H. and Ishii, S.), pp. 146-165, Basel, Karger.
11. Brightman, M.W., and Reese, T.S. (1969) J. Cell. Biol. 40: 648-677.
12. Brightman M.W. and Robinson, J.S. (1976) In: Head Injuries (ed. by McLaurin, R.L.) pp. 107-113. Grune and Stratton, Inc.
13. Bundgaard, M. Cserr, H., and Murray, M. (1979) Cell Tissue Res. 198: 65-77.

14. Castel, M., Sahar, A. and Erlij, D. (1974) Brain Res. 67: 178-184.
15. Elfvin, L.G. and Forsman, C. (1978) J. Ultrastruct. Res. 63: 26-274.
16. Ellisman, M.H. and Rash, J.E. (1977) Brain Res. 137: 197-206.
17. Harned, H.S. and Owen, B.B. (1958) The Physical Chemistry of Electrolyte Solutions, pp. 164, 700, 702, 3rd ed., Reinhold Publ. Co., New York.
18. Heuser, J.E., Reese, T.S. and Landis, D.M.D. (1974) J. Neurcytol. 3: 109-131.
19. Horton, J.C. and Hedley-White, E.T. (1978) J. Neuropath. Exper. Neurol. 37:630.
20. Humbert, F., Pricam, C., Perrelet, A. and Orci, L. (1975) J. Ultrastruct. Res. 52: 13-20.
21. Inoue, S. and Hogg, J.C. (1977) J. Ultrastruct. Res. 61: 89-99.
22. Kreutziger, G.O. (1968) In: Proceedings of the 26th Meeting of the Electron Microscope Society of America, p. 234. Claitors Publishing Division, Baton Rouge.
23. Kuffler, S.W. and Nicholls, J.G. (1966) Ergeb. Physiol. 57: 1-90.
24. Landis, D.M.D. and Reese, T.S. (1974) J. Cell Biol. 60: 316-320.
25. Lossinsky, A.S., Garcia, J.H., Iwanowski, L. and Lightfoote, W.E., Jr. (1979) Acta Neuropath. (Berl.) 47: 105-110.
26. Machen, T., Erlij, D. and Wooding, F.B.P. (1972) J. Cell Biol. 54: 302-312.
27. Nag, S., Robertson, D.M. and Dinsdale, H.B. (1977) Lab. Invest. 36: 150-160.
28. Nagy, Z., Pappius, H.M., Mathieson, F., and Huttner, I. (1979a) J. Comp. Neurol. 185: 569-578.
29. Nagy, Z., Mathieson, G. and Huttner, I. (1979b) J. Comp. Neurol. 185: 579-586.
30. Pannese, E., Luciano, L., Iurato, S. and Reale, E. (1977) J. Ultrastruct. Res. 60: 169-180.
31. Petito, C.K., Schaefer, J.A. and Plum, F. (1977) Brain Res. 127: 251-267.
32. Privat, A. (1977) Neurosci. 2: 447-457.
33. Rapoport, S.I. (1976) Blood-Brain Barrier in Physiology and Medicine, pp. 146, 148. Raven Press, New York.
34. Rapoport, S.I., Hori, M. and Klatzo, I. (1972) Am. J. Physiol. 223: 323-331.
35. Reale, E. and Luciano, L. (1974) Albrecht von Graefes Archiv fur klinische und experimentelle Ophthalmologie 192: 73-87.
36. Reese, T.S. and Karnovsky, M. (1967) J. Cell Biol. 34: 207-217.
37. Rosenstein, J.M. and Brightman, M.W. (1978) Nature (London) 275: 83-85.
38. Shivers, R. (1979) Brain Res. 170: 509-522.
39. Simionescu, N., Simionescu, M. and Palade, G.E. (1975) J. Cell Biol. 64: 586-607.

40. Smith, D.S., Baerwald, R.J. and Hart, M.A. (1975) Tissue and
     Cell, 7: 369-382.
41. Staehelin, L.A. (1972) Proc. Nat. Acad. Sci. (USA) 69: 1318-
     1321.
42. Westergaard, E. (1975) Acta Neuropath. 32: 27-42.
43. Westergaard, E., van Deurs, B. and Brondsted, H.E. (1977)
     Acta Neuropath. (Berlin) 37: 141-152.
44. Whittembury, G. and Rawlins, F.A. (1971) Pflugers Arch. ges.
     Physiol. 330: 302-309.
45. Wolff, J. (1963) Z. Zellforsch. 60: 409-431.
46. Wolff, J., and Nemecek, St. (1968) Experientia 24: 930.

CEREBROVASCULAR PERMEABILITY IN THE NORMAL BRAIN AND FOLLOWING OSMOTIC OPENING OF THE BLOOD-BRAIN BARRIER

Stanley I. Rapoport, M.D., Laboratory of Neurosciences

National Institute on Aging, Gerontology Research Center

Baltimore City Hospitals, Baltimore, Maryland 21224

SUMMARY

Cerebrovascular permeability of nonelectrolytes and organic electrolytes is directly proportional to the octanol/water partition coefficient of these substances, as was determined by a new method of compartmental analysis which is sufficiently sensitive to examine permeability coefficients as low as 10^{-8} cm sec^{-1} (i.e., sucrose permeability) or as high as 10^{-4} cm sec^{-1} (i.e., antipyrine and caffeine permeabilities). In the latter case, cerebral blood flow must be taken into account to correct for extraction of tracer during its passage through the brain. The compartmental analysis method was employed in conscious rats, when radiotracer was injected i.v. as a bolus and tracer entry into the brain was analyzed in terms of a permeability coefficient and cerebral distribution volume. The proportionality between cerebrovascular permeability and octanol/water partition coefficient suggests that substances enter the brain by dissolving in the lipoid membranes of the continuous cerebrovascular endothelium (blood-brain barrier) and not by passing through aqueous pores within the endothelium. In order to overcome permeability limitations to intravascular water-soluble compounds, furthermore, it is possible to open the blood-brain barrier by infusing, into the carotid artery, a hypertonic solution of a water-soluble solute such as arabinose. Physiological and ultrastructural evidence indicates that osmotic opening of the blood-brain barrier is mediated by widening of tight junctions between cerebrovascular endothelial cells. In the rat, osmotic barrier opening occurs abruptly at a threshold arabinose concentration of 1.6 molal, and at an infusion time of 20 sec. ^{14}C-sucrose permeability is increased 10-20 fold by osmotic treatment, but the increase disappears

within about 1 hr. Brain edema and stimulation of cerebral glucose
consumption follow osmotic treatment, and also disappear without
resultant evidence of long-term brain damage. Osmotic barrier
opening has proven useful for allowing normally-excluded substances
into the brain.

INTRODUCTION

The blood-brain barrier at the cerebral vasculature (Fig. 1,
left) is composed of a continuous layer of endothelial cells that
are connected by tight junctions (zonulae occludentes), close intercellular connections that prevent intercellular diffusion of
water-soluble nonelectrolytes, ions and proteins. Vesicular transport furthermore is minimal at the cerebrovascular endothelium.
Thus, the layer as a whole has properties of an extended lipoid
cell membrane, and is permselective for lipid-soluble as compared
to water-soluble substances (Reese and Karnovsky, 1967; Rapoport,
1976a).

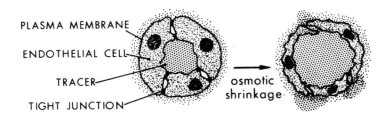

PLASMA MEMBRANE

ENDOTHELIAL CELL

TRACER

TIGHT JUNCTION

osmotic
shrinkage

Figure 1. Model for normal cerebral capillary (left) and for
osmotic barrier opening by widening of interendothelial tight
junctions. It is suggested that, when endothelial cells shrink
in a hypertonic environment, their membranes stress tight junctions and make them permeable to intravascular tracer. From
Rapoport (1976a).

The selective permeability of the barrier to lipid-soluble
drugs qualitatively explains different rates of drug passage from
plasma to spinal fluid and brain, and may account for observed cor-
relations between therapeutic effectiveness of centrally acting
drugs and lipid solubility (Brodie et al., 1960). For example,
the central effectiveness of a series of barbiturates, hydantoins

and imides increases with lipid solubility (Millichap, 1963; Rapoport, 1976a; Rapoport, 1980).

Lipid-soluble agents rapidly equilibrate between brain and blood. It is not difficult therefore to estimate their brain concentrations from their plasma levels, once a steady state brain/plasma measurement has been made in an animal model. On the other hand, the intensity and time course of a central response to a poorly permeant, more water-soluble drug may not be related simply to the plasma level, because of restricted blood-brain exchange and limited intracerebral distribution (Rapoport, 1976a; Davis et al., 1978). For such drugs, it is important to know which factors quantitatively determine their rates of entry into and their distribution within brain tissue.

We approached this question by first establishing an empirical relation between cerebrovascular permeability and the octanol/water partition coefficient for different substances, and then by considering how drugs distribute within the brain parenchyma. I have presented an extended model of blood-brain exchange that explicitly takes into account transfer at the cerebral capillary, loss of material from brain to cerebrospinal fluid, and intracellular sequestration, binding or metabolism (Rapoport, 1980). In the following discussion, however, I shall consider a simplified two-compartment model that has been used to experimentally examine blood-brain barrier permeability and intracerebral drug distribution in short-term studies in conscious rats.

CURRENT METHODS TO MEASURE CEREBROVASCULAR PERMEABILITY AND BLOOD-BRAIN EXCHANGE

Current techniques to measure cerebrovascular transfer in animal experiments are useful for substances that enter the brain rapidly, but not at a moderate or slow rate. Excluding the method of compartmental analysis, four major techniques are presently employed -- the Indicator Dilution technique, the Single-Injection External Registration technique, the Brain Uptake Index technique and the Concentration Profile Analysis technique (Rapoport, 1976a; Crone, 1963; Raichle et al., 1976; Oldendorf, 1971; Patlak and Fenstermacher, 1975). These techniques have several limitations. None provides accurate permeability coefficients, P, of poorly-penetrating compounds ($P = 10^{-8}$ to 10^{-7} cm sec^{-1}) such as peptides, L-glucose, mannitol, sucrose or methotrexate, or of rapidly penetrating compounds ($P \approx 10^{-4}$ cm sec^{-1}) like antipyrine and caffeine. All apply to the brain as a whole but not to specific brain regions. They require that cerebral blood flow be known, and are inaccurate if pathological or altered physiological conditions cause flow to change (Ohno et al., 1978).

CEREBROVASCULAR PERMEABILITY AND LIPID SOLUBILITY IN CONSCIOUS
ANIMALS

The method of compartmental analysis was used to measure
cerebrovascular permeability and cerebral distribution volume of a
number of different substances in conscious rats (Ohno et al., 1978;
Rapoport et al., 1978, 1979). Conscious rather than anesthetized
animals were used to be certain of consistent regional cerebral
blood flows. Flow must be known in order to calculate regional
cerebrovascular permeability of lipid-soluble substances.

A radiotracer was injected i.v. as a bolus. Femoral artery
plasma radioactivity was measured and fit by least squares with the

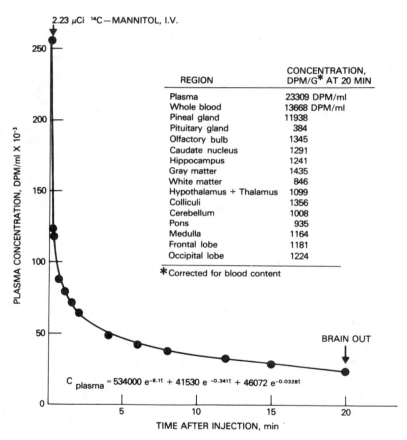

2.23 µCi ¹⁴C—MANNITOL, I.V.

REGION	CONCENTRATION, DPM/G* AT 20 MIN
Plasma	23309 DPM/ml
Whole blood	13668 DPM/ml
Pineal gland	11938
Pituitary gland	384
Olfactory bulb	1345
Caudate nucleus	1291
Hippocampus	1241
Gray matter	1435
White matter	846
Hypothalamus + Thalamus	1099
Colliculi	1356
Cerebellum	1008
Pons	935
Medulla	1164
Frontal lobe	1181
Occipital lobe	1224

*Corrected for blood content

$C_{plasma} = 534000\, e^{-8.1t} + 41530\, e^{-0.341t} + 46072\, e^{-0.0328t}$

Figure 2. Plasma concentration of ¹⁴C-mannitol following
intravenous injection, and regional brain concentration 20-min
after injection. The curve is a fit of Eq. 1 to the data points,
with t in min. From Ohno et al. (1978).

following equation, where C_{art} dpm/ml = concentration of unbound tracer in plasma, α_i (dpm/ml) and α_i (sec^{-1}) are constants, t = time (sec) and n = 3-4 (Knott and Shraeger, 1972; Ohno et al., 1978, Rapoport et al., 1979).

$$C_{art} = \sum_i^n A_i e^{-\alpha_i t} \tag{1}$$

Fig. 2 illustrates a typical plasma curve following an i.v. injection of ^{14}C-mannitol, and gives constants for the best fit of Eq. 1 to the data (Ohno et al., 1978).

In the absence of cerebral binding, intracellular sequestration or brain metabolism (factors taken into account in another publication (Rapoport, 1980)), brain uptake is given as follows, where C_{brain} dpm/g = parenchymal (extravascular) concentration, P cm sec^{-1} = cerebrovascular permeability, A = 240 cm^2/cm^3 (or cm^{-1}) (capillary surface area) (Crone, 1963), $C_{br.\ cap.}$ dpm/ml = mean concentration in cerebral capillaries, and V = cerebral distribution volume of tracer,

$$dC_{brain}/dt = PA\ (\overline{C}_{br.\ cap.} - C_{brain}/V) \tag{2}$$

$\overline{C}_{br.\ cap.}$ is related as follows to the measured arterial plasma concentration and measured regional cerebral blood flow F (sec^{-1}) (Patlak and Fenstermacher, 1975),

$$\overline{C}_{br.\ cap.} = \frac{F}{PA}\ (C_{art} - C_{brain}/V)\ (1 - e^{-PA/F}) + C_{brain}/V \tag{3}$$

$\overline{C}_{br.\ cap.}$ approximates C_{art} if PA << F, i.e., if little tracer is extracted from the capillary, but is less than C_{art} if extraction is high because permeability is large. Substituting Eq. 3 into Eq. 2 gives, where $M = F\ (1 - e^{-PA/F})$,

$$dC_{brain}/dt = M\ (C_{art} - C_{brain}/V) \tag{4}$$

Thus, brain accumulation is proportional to the concentration difference between arterial plasma and brain, multiplied by a factor M which is less than PA to the extent that tracer is extracted during its passage through the cerebral capillary. Substituting Eq. 1 into Eq. 4, and integrating to time T of decapitation, gives $C_{brain}(T)$ in terms of two unknowns M (or PA) and V,

$$C_{brain}(T) = \sum_i^n \frac{MA_i}{M/V - \alpha_i}\ (e^{-\alpha_i T} - e^{-MT/V}) \tag{5}$$

PA alone can be obtained simply from experiments that are limited to short times after i.v. injection of tracer, when $C_{brain}/V \ll C_{art}$. In this case back diffusion from brain to plasma is negligible in Eq. 4 and that equation is integrated to give,

$$PA = -F \ln_e (1 - C_{brain}(T)/F\int_o^T C_{art} dt) \tag{6}$$

For poorly penetrating substances, furthermore, $C_{brain}(T)/\int_o^T C_{art} dt \approx 0$. Eq. 6 then becomes simplified to give PA in terms of measured brain concentration at T and the integrated arterial plasma concentration,

$$PA = \frac{C_{brain}}{\int_o^T C_{art} dt} \tag{7}$$

Table 1 presents blood flows F and blood volumes in different brain regions of conscious rats (Ohno et al., 1978, 1979). F was used in Eqs. 5 and 6. Intravascular radioactivity was calculated as: Regional Blood Volume (ml/g) x Whole Blood Concentration (dpm/ml). C_{brain} was calculated as net tissue radioactivity minus intravascular radioactivity. $\int_o^T C_{art}$ was obtained, when necessary, by integrating the plasma concentration curve.

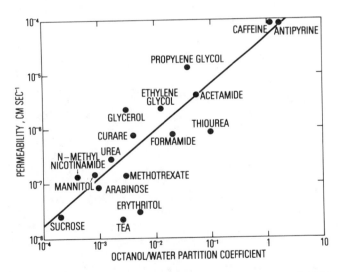

Figure 3. Relation between cerebrovascular permeability and octanol/water partition coefficient for different substances. Data are from Rapoport et al (1979).

Table 1. Regional cerebral blood volume and blood flow in
conscious rats. Data are from Ohno et al. (1978, 1979).

Brain region	Blood volume ml g^{-1} x 100	Blood flow (F) sec^{-1}
Olfactory bulb	4.68 ! 0.23 (4)[a]	0.017 ! 0.0016 (6)
Caudate nucleus	1.24 $\pm$ 0.25	0.030 $\pm$ 0.0031
Hippocampus	1.61 $\pm$ 0.16	0.023 $\pm$ 0.0027
Frontal lobe	2.09 $\pm$ 0.04	0.028 $\pm$ 0.0048
Occipital lobe	2.42 $\pm$ 0.26	0.030 $\pm$ 0.0049
Thalamus + Hypothalamus	1.79 $\pm$ 0.10	0.025 $\pm$ 0.0028
Superior colliculus	} 2.01 $\pm$ 0.020	0.028 $\pm$ 0.0028
Inferior colliculus		0.034 $\pm$ 0.0042
Cerebellum	3.46 $\pm$ 0.26	0.017 $\pm$ 0.0019
Pons	2.56 $\pm$ 0.27	0.021 $\pm$ 0.0020
Medulla	3.53 $\pm$ 0.70	0.020 $\pm$ 0.0022
Gray matter, parietal	2.70 $\pm$ 0.40	0.040 $\pm$ 0.0061
White matter	1.14 $\pm$ 0.22	0.019 $\pm$ 0.0023

[a]Mean $\pm$ S.E.M. (number of animals).

Eq. 5 or 6 was fit to data for different nonelectrolytes and
organic electrolytes, so as to estimate individual values of PA and
V. Fig. 3 illustrates that P, which was calculated by dividing PA
by A = 240 cm^{-1} (Crone, 1963), is directly related to the
octanol/water partition coefficient. The relation indicates that
substances penetrate the blood-brain barrier mainly because of
their lipid solubility, although deviations from the regression
line show that permeability is determined as well by such factors
as size, steric and electronic configuration and interaction with
the cell membrane (Rapoport et al., 1979).

Membrane permeability should depend directly on the oil/water
partition coefficient if transfer occurs by simple diffusion through
an aporous lipoid membrane (Collander, 1937; Davson and Danielli,
1943). The relation in Fig. 3, which is consistent with this theory,
occurs as well at lipoid membranes of single cells. Furthermore,
cerebrovascular permeability of different agents is quantitatively
like that at membranes of single cells and at aporous bimolecular

lipid membranes. These facts suggest that intravascular drugs
enter the brain by dissolving in and diffusing through lipoid
endothelial cell membranes of cerebral capillaries, without passing
through aqueous membrane pores or interendothelial tight junctions
(Rapoport, 1976a; Ohno et al., 1978; Rapoport, et al., 1979).

OSMOTIC OPENING OF THE BLOOD-BRAIN BARRIER

The known relations between central effectiveness of drugs in
a homologous series and lipid solubility (e.g., Rapoport, 1976a)
have stimulated efforts to synthesize lipid-soluble drugs that can
easily enter the brain. In some cases, however, as with methotrexate and its esters, the lipid-soluble derivatives have not proved
more effective against brain tumors than the poorly-permeable water-
soluble parent compound (Johns et al., 1973). In other cases, critical brain enzymes that are genetically absent, yet might be effective when allowed into the brain, cannot be altered enough to allow
them to diffuse through the blood-brain barrier (Barranger et al.,
1979). One possible approach to therapy of brain disease in these
cases is to reversibly modify cerebrovascular permeability, so as
to allow the water-soluble parent compound into the brain.

The cerebrovascular endothelium can be made permeable to normally excluded proteins and solutes by infusing a hypertonic solution of a poorly lipid-soluble solute into the internal carotid
artery. In this section, I will present physiological and ultrastructural evidence that indicates that the permeability increment
is caused by osmotic shrinkage of endothelial cells and widening of
tight junctions.

Tight junctions between cells are networks of fibrillar strands
that limit intercellular diffusion. In epithelial tissues, osmotic
or hydrostatic pressure stresses can alter structure and permeability of these junctions by physically deforming them (Ussing 1971;
reviewed by Rapoport 1976). A model which can account for osmotic
opening of the blood-brain barrier, based partially on these observations, is illustrated in Fig. 1. Its premise is that tight junctions between cerebrovascular endothelia are also distorted and made
permeable when endothelial cells shrink in hypertonic solutions.

The model is consistent with the following evidence: (a) osmotic thresholds (minimal osmolal concentrations), both for opening
of the blood-brain barrier and for shrinkage of single cells, increase with increasing solute lipid solubility, (b) osmotic barrier
opening is reversible, (c) osmotic opening produces observable transfer of intravascular protein (exogenous horseradish peroxidase) between cerebrovascular endothelial cells and not through them (M. W.
Brightman, K. Zis and S.I. Rapoport, this Symposium), (d) osmotic

opening may be graded with respect to the size of penetrating molecule. Reversible graded barrier opening that follows the rules of
osmotic cell shrinkage would not be expected if endothelial cells
were irreversibly damaged, or if vesicular transport were stimulated
so as to increase barrier permeability.

TEST OF MODEL FOR OSMOTIC BARRIER OPENING

Overton (1895) and Collander (1937) showed that single plant
or animal cells shrank reversibly when placed in a hypertonic solution of a lipid-insoluble solute. Shrinkage by equiosmolal solutions of non-electrolytes which were slightly lipid-soluble declin-
ed when lipid solubility increased. Cell membranes appeared impermeable to lipid-insoluble solutes, allowing water but not the
solutes to pass, and slightly permeable to somewhat lipid-soluble
solutes. It seemed reasonable to suppose that cerebrovascular endothelial cells also would shrink in hypertonic solutions as a function
of solute lipid solubility, and that tight junctions between the
cells might widen as illustrated in Fig. 1.

To test this hypothesis, hypertonic solutions of solutes with
different lipid solubilities were applied to the arachnoid surface
of the rabbit or cat brain for 10 min and were then removed
(Rapoport 1970; Rapoport et al. 1972). Barrier opening was studied
by evaluating the pH response at the arachnoid surface to an intravenous injection of $NaHCO_3$ (a measure of barrier integrity to ions),
or by determining the minimal osmolal concentration (threshold osmolality) that produced extravasation of blood-borne Evans' blue-
albumin from pial vessels. In the latter experiments, reversibility
of opening was determined by injecting Evans' blue intravenously 30
min after, rather than before, a threshold osmolality had opened the
barrier at the arachnoid surface.

The results are summarized in Table 2, where test substances
are ranked according to their octanol/water partition coefficient,
a measure of lipid solubility. Osmolal thresholds at the barrier
site (presumably at the vascular endothelium) were estimated by
taking into account differences in diffusion at the pia-arachnoid
membranes.

The data in the table support the interpretation that hypertonic solutions open the barrier by shrinking endothelial cells, as
illustrated in Fig. 1. Electrolytes, and non-electrolytes less
lipid-soluble than propionamide, opened the barrier reversibly.
More lipid-soluble solutes acted irreversibly, probably by destroying endothelial cell membranes. The table also shows that osmolal
thresholds of the reversibly acting solutions increased with increasing lipid solubility, as expected from the inverse relation between lipid solubility and shrinkage of single cells by hypertonic
solutions (Overton 1895; Collander 1937).

Table 2. Effect of topically applied concentrated solutions on
          blood-brain barrier in the rabbit.

Substance	Octanol/water partition	Reversibility of opening	Threshold osmolality at barrier[a]
LiCl	–	Yes	0.87
Na_2SO_4	–	Yes	0.82
NaCl	–	Yes	1.0
Sucrose	0.0002	Yes	1.1
Glucose	0.0005	Yes	1.0
Urea	0.0016	Yes	1.7
Glycerol	0.003	Yes	2.1
Lactamide	0.005	Yes	–
Ethylene glycol	0.012	No	–
Methyl urea	0.016	Yes	2.2
Formamide	0.02	Yes	2.9
Propylene glycol	0.039	No	–
Acetamide	0.055	Yes	3.5
Propionamide	0.16	Yes	3.2
Cyanamide	0.16	No	–
Methanol	0.20	No	–
Ethanol	0.48	No	–
Methyl carbamate	0.50	No	–
Ethyl carbamate	0.71	No	–

[a] Thresholds relative to NaCl threshold = 1.
A solution was applied to a cortical region for 10 min, then removed.
Intravascular Evans' blue-albumin was used as a barrier tracer. The
osmolal threshold for barrier opening was calculated from the surface osmolality by taking into account diffusion through the pia-
arachnoid. Reversibility of opening indicates that the barrier
closed 30 min after arachnoidal application of a threshold concentration of a particular solute. Solutes are ranked according to
their octanol/water partition coefficients. Data are from Rapoport
et al. (1972).

The topical observations in Table 2 were extended to vessels within the brain by infusing hypertonic solutions into the carotid artery of different species (Fig. 4) (Thompson 1970; Rapoport et al. 1972; Studer et al. 1974; Rapoport 1976a). Patterns of reversible and irreversible opening held at intracerebral vessels just as they did at the pial vasculature. Intracarotid infusion of hypertonic solutions of lactamide or urea opened the barrier reversibly on the hemisphere homolateral to infusion, whereas hypertonic solutions of propylene glycol or ethanol acted irreversibly.

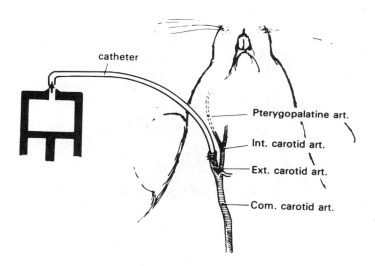

Figure 4. Brain perfusion via a catheterized external carotid artery in the rat. From Rapoport (1978).

ULTRASTRUCTURAL STUDIES, REVERSIBILITY AND THRESHOLDS FOR
OSMOTIC BARRIER OPENING

Electron microscopic studies in rats and rabbits confirmed that hypertonic solutions of water-soluble solutes, whether infused into the carotid artery or applied to the brain surface, increased cerebrovascular permeability by opening interendothelial tight junctions. Carotid artery infusion of 2M to 3M urea, of Hypaque 50 (a hypertonic contrast medium employed in cerebral angiography), and of 1.6 molal arabinose or mannitol, allowed intravascular horseradish peroxidase into the brain via interendothelial tight junctions

(Fig. 5) Brightman et al. 1973; Sterrett et al. 1976; Nagy et al. 1979; M. Brightman, K. Zis and S.I. Rapoport, in Brightman, this Symposium). Reaction product did not flood vascular endothelial cells and pinocytosis was not stimulated.

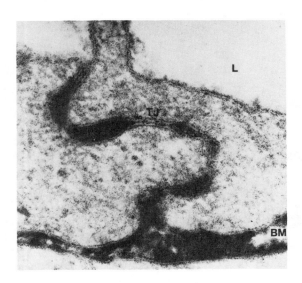

Figure 5. Opening of tight junctions between cerebrovascular endothelial cells to horseradish peroxidase tracer after intracarotid infusion of 3 M-urea in the rabbit. Peroxidase was administered intravenously before infusion, and the animal was killed 90 sec after infusion. The tracer was washed from the capillary lumen (L) during fixation. Reaction product is present along the interface between endothelial cells, in the gaps between tight junctions (TJ) and in the basement membrane (BM) (X 88 000). From Brightman et al. 1973.

       Hypertonic arabinose infusion appears to increase the number of endothelial pinocytotic vesicles that contain reaction product of horseradish peroxidase. Transendothelial vesicular transport is not stimulated, however, because the vesicles are found in brains that have been infused in situ with concentrated glutaraldehyde before the intravascular administration of horseradish peroxidase. Glutaraldehyde fixation stops vesicular transport (Westergaard & Brightman 1973). It remains possible that the vesicles contribute to channels that are 'frozen' in situ by glutaraldehyde fixation. (cf. Sterrett et al. 1976; Simionescu et al. 1975).

Different extents of tight junctional widening could account for the observed gradation of opening with respect to the size of test molecule (Table 3) (Rapoport, 1970, Thompson 1970; Studer et al., 1974). For example, carotid infusion in the rat of a 1.2 molal sucrose solution opens the barrier to ^{22}Na but not to the larger ^{125}I-labeled albumin molecule, whereas a 4.2 molal sucrose solution opens the barrier to both tracers.

Table 3. Brain spaces of tracers injected intravenously in rats after infusion of different solutions into internal carotid artery.

Infusate	^{125}I-labelled albumin space X 10^2		^{22}Na space X 10^2	
	30 min[a]	4 h	30 min	4 h
Control	1.73	1.73	10.8	10.8
Isotonic saline	1.61	1.75	11.0	11.5
Sucrose, 4.2 mol/kg	2.15[b]	1.66	19.7[b]	11.6
Sucrose, 1.2 mol/kg	1.72	1.81	17.0[b]	11.2

[a]Time after infusion.
[b]Significantly different from control (P < 0.05).
The brain space is the ratio of brain concentration to blood concentration. Data are from Studer et al. (1974).

In order to further apply the osmotic method to studies of brain pharmacology, we thought it useful to quantitatively define critical thresholds of infusion time and infusate concentration that are required to open the blood-brain barrier, as well as the time course and reversibility of such opening. We used the method of compartmental analysis (see above) to study cerebrovascular permeability of ^{14}C-sucrose in control and experimental animals (Rapoport et al. 1978, 1980). In the rat, significant barrier opening was produced by 30 sec of infusion, into the carotid circulation via the external carotid artery (Fig. 4), of 1.6 molal but not of 1.4 molal arabinose solution. A 1.8 molal solution had no marked further effect (Fig. 6). Thus the concentration threshold for barrier opening was very sharp, between 1.4 and 1.6 molal arabinose.

The infusion duration threshold also was abrupt. At an arabinose concentration of 1.6 molal, 20 sec but not 10 sec of carotid infusion significantly increased cerebrovascular permeability to ^{14}C-sucrose, by a factor of about 20 above normal permeability. A minimum time threshold of 10 to 20 sec could explain why X-ray contrast agents do not produce brain damage when used clinically in carotid angiography, despite the facts that their osmolality approaches

1.6 osmol and they can open the barrier in animals when infused into the carotid artery for 30 sec. In carotid angiography, however, they are infused for 5 sec or less, far below the infusion time threshold for osmotic opening (Nomura, 1970; Rapoport, et al., 1974).

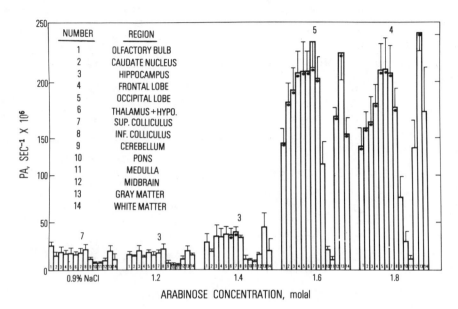

Figure 6. Cerebrovascular permeability-area product (PA) for ^{14}C-sucrose, at right hemisphere regions, to concentration of arabinose infusate. Arabinose or isotonic saline solution was infused into the right carotid artery (Fig. 4) for 30 sec. PA was measured by injecting ^{14}C-sucrose i.v. 5 min thereafter, and killing the animals 10 min after tracer injection (Eq. 7). Bars are means ± S.E.M., and number of experiments at a given concentration are noted. Asterisk (*) signifies significant difference (p < 0.05) from regional PA following isotonic saline infusion (left side of figure). From Rapoport et al. (1980).

Infusion of isotonic saline solution for 30 sec, at the same rate (0.12 ml/sec) and under the same conditions as 1.6 molal arabinose infusion, had no effect on cerebrovascular permeability to ^{14}C-sucrose. Thus, carotid hypertension during the infusion procedure did not produce a barrier effect (Fig. 7, below). Hypertensive barrier breakdown will occur if carotid artery pressure is elevated in the rat to 150-160 mm Hg (Rapoport, 1976b), whereas a mean pressure of only 125 mm Hg is produced during carotid infusion at a rate of 0.12 ml/sec in the rat (Rapoport et al., 1980).

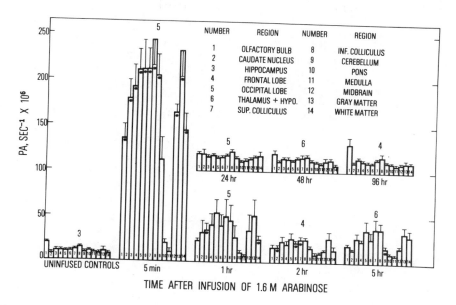

Figure 7. Reversibility of osmotic barrier opening. 1.6 molal arabinose solution was infused into the right external carotid artery for 30 sec, and ^{14}C-sucrose was injected at designated times thereafter. Animals were killed 10 min after tracer was injected, and the cerebrovascular permeability-area product, PA, was calculated by Eq. 7. Bars are means ± S.E.M., and number of experiments are noted. Asterisk (*) signifies significant difference (p < 0.05) from regional PA in uninfused controls. From Rapoport et al. (1980).

With the compartmental method of measuring cerebrovascular permeability to ^{14}C-sucrose, we were able to quantitatively describe the time course of the osmotic effect and to demonstrate its reversibility (Rapoport et al. 1980). As illustrated by Fig. 7, the maximum increase in the product of cerebrovascular permeability and capillary surface area (PA) occurred within the first 15 min following carotid infusion of 1.6 molal arabinose solution, but permeability was approximately normal at 1 hr. Regional PA following isotonic saline infusion did not differ significantly (p > 0.05) from respective regional PA in uninfused animals. The data in Table 3 also indicate that the osmotic effect is reversible.

Reversible barrier opening without neurological sequelae or obvious brain damage or edema can be produced in rhesus monkeys and baboons that are infused, via a catheterized lingual artery, with 3 molal urea or 2.5 molal lactamide solution, and in rats infused with 1.8 molal arabinose solution (Fig. 4). Measurable, long-term brain damage associated with the osmotic procedure is prevented if the cerebral circulation is not permanently compromised, if cerebral oxygenation is maintained to counteract effects of possible apnea or bradycardia due to hypertonic infusion, if filtered solutions of purified solutes are used for infusion, and if carotid hypertension is prevented (Rapoport & Thompson 1973; Rapoport 1967a,b; Rapoport et al. 1980; MacKenzie et al. 1976; Pickard et al. 1977; Chiueh et al. 1978).

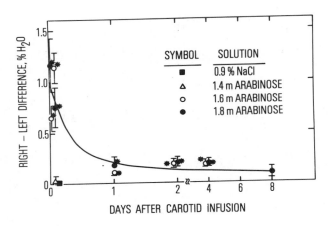

Figure 8. Difference in % water between right and left hemispheres, following right-sided carotid infusion of hypertonic arabinose and isotonic saline solutions. Points are means ± S.E.M. (10 animals). Asterisk (*) designates significant value (p < 0.05).

Transient cerebral changes do occur if osmotic barrier opening is produced in conscious rats. Regional cerebral glucose consumption is stimulated, as measured by the 2-deoxy-D-glucose technique (Pappius et al. 1979). Blood flow may be reduced, which indicates that the normal coupling between blood flow and metabolism is disrupted. Finally, brain water transiently increases by 1-1.5% on the osmotically-perfused hemisphere (Fig. 8). The basis for this vasogenic edema, as well as its mode of resolution, has been discussed in detail elsewhere (Rapoport 1978).

The cerebral changes that are associated with osmotic barrier opening are transient, and disappear within hours after osmotic treatment. The absence of long-term brain damage indicates that the osmotic method may be useful for studying central effects of drugs that normally are excluded from the brain, and as an adjunct to chemotherapy of central nervous system disease (Barranger et al. 1979; Neuwelt et al. 1979). E.A. Neuwelt and colleagues (unpublished observation) have demonstrated recently that osmotic barrier opening can be accomplished in man, with an aim to treat metastatic brain tumors, without producing evidence of long-term neurological sequellae.

REFERENCES

Barranger, J.A., Rapoport, S.I., Fredericks, W.R., Pentchev, P.G., MacDermot, K.D., Steusing, J.K. and Brady, R.O. (1979) Modification of the blood-brain barrier: Increased concentration and fate of enzymes entering the brain. Proc. Natl. Acad. Sci. USA 76:481-485.

Brightman, M.W., Hori, M., Rapoport, S.I., Reese, T.S. and Westergaard, E. (1973). Osmotic opening of tight junctions in cerebral endothelium. J. Comp. Neurol. 152:317-326.

Brodie, B.B., Kurz, H. and Schanker, L.S. (1960). The importance of dissociation constant and lipid solubility in influencing the passage of drugs into the cerebrospinal fluid. J. Pharmacol. Exp. Ther. 130:20-25.

Chiueh, C.C., Sun, C.L.,Kopin, I.J., Fredericks, W.R. and Rapoport, S.I. (1978). Entry of ^{3}H-norepinephrine, ^{125}I-albumin and Evans blue from blood into brain following unilateral osmotic opening of the blood-brain barrier. Brain Res. 145:291-301.

Collander, R. (1937). The permeability of plant protoplasts to nonelectrolytes. Trans. Faraday Soc. 33:985-990.

Crone, C. (1963). The permeability of capillaries in various organs as determined by use of the "indicator diffusion" method. Acta Physiol. Scand. 58:292-305.

Davis, J.M., Erickson, S. and Dekirminjian, H.   (1978).   Plasma
    levels of antipsychotic drugs and clinical response.   In
    Psychopharmacology: A Generation of Progress (Ed. Lipton,
    M.A., DiMascio, A., Killam, K.F.) Raven Press, New York.
    pp. 905-915.

Davson, H. and Danielli, J.F.   (1943).   The Permeability of Natural
    Membranes. Cambridge University Press, London, pp. 80-117.

Johns, D.G., Farquhar, D., Wolpert, M.K., Chabner, B.A. and Loo,
    T.L. (1973).   Dialkyl esters of methotrexate and 3'5'-
    dichloromethotrexate synthesis and interaction with aldehyde
    oxidase and dihydrofolate reductase.   Drug. Metab. Dispos.
    1, 580-589.

Knott, G.D. and Shraeger, R.I.   (1972).   On-line modeling by curve
    fitting.   In Computer Graphics: Proc. SIGGRAPH Computers in
    Medicine Symp., 6.   ACM:SIGGRAPH Notices, No. 4, p. 138-151.

MacKenzie, E.T., McCulloch, J., O'Keane, M., Pickard, J.D. and
    Harper, A.M. (1976) Cerebral circulation and norepinephrine:
    relevance of the blood-brain barrier.   Am. J. Physiol.   231:
    483-488.

Millichap, J.G. (1963) Anticonvulsant drugs.   In Physiological
    Pharmacology (Ed. Root, W.S., Hofmann, F.G.) Academic Press,
    New York, Vol. 2, pp. 97-173.

Nagy, Z., Pappius, H.M., Mathieson, G. and Huttner, I.   (1979)
    Opening of tight junctions in cerebral endothelium.   1.
    Effect of hyperosmolar mannitol infused through the internal
    carotid artery.   J. Comp. Neurol.   185:569-578.

Neuwelt, E.A., Maravilla, K.R., Frenkel, E.P., Rapoport, S.I.,
    Hill, S.A., Barnett, P.A. (1979) Osmotic blood-brain barrier
    disruption: Computerized tomographic monitoring of chemo-
    therapeutic agent delivery.   J. Clin. Invest., 64:684-688.

Nomura, T. (1970) Atlas of Cerebral Angiography.   Igaku Shoin,
    Tokyo, p. 322.

Ohno, K., Pettigrew, K.D. and Rapoport, S.I. (1978) Lower limits
    of cerebrovascular permeability to nonelectrolytes in the
    conscious rat.   Am. J. Physiol.   235:H299-H307.

Ohno, K., Pettigrew, K.D. and Rapoport, S.I.   (1979) Local
    cerebral blood flow in the conscious rat as measured with
    ^{14}C-antipyrine, ^{14}C-iodoantipyrine and ^{3}H-nicotine.   Stroke,
    10:62-67.

Oldendorf, W.H. (1971) Brain uptake of radiolabeled amino acids, amines and hexoses after arterial injection. Am. J. Physiol. 221:1629-1639.

Overton, E. (1895) Über die osmotischen Eigenschaften der lebenden Pflanzen und Tierzelle. Vierteljahresschr. Naturforsch, Ges. Zür, 40:159-201.

Pappius, H.M., Savaki, H.E., Fieschi, C., Rapoport, S.I. and Sokoloff, L. (1979) Osmotic opening of the blood-brain barrier and local cerebral glucose utilization. Ann. Neurol. 5:211-219.

Patlak, C.S. and Fenstermacher, J.D. (1975) Measurements of dog blood-brain transfer constants by ventriculocisternal perfusion. Am. J. Physiol. 229:877-884.

Pickard, J.D., Durity, F., Welsh, F.A., Langfitt, T.W., Harper, A.M. and MacKenzie, E.T. (1977) Osmotic opening of the blood-brain barrier: value in pharmacological studies on the cerebral circulation. Brain Res. 122:170-176.

Raichle, M.E., Eichling, J.O., Straatmann, M.G., Welch, M.J., Larson, K.B. and Ter-Pogossian, M.M. (1976) Blood-brain barrier permeability of ^{11}C-labeled alcohols and ^{15}O-labeled water. Am. J. Physiol. 230:543-552.

Rapoport, S.I. (1970) Effect of concentrated solutions on blood-brain barrier. Am. J. Physiol. 219:270-274.

Rapoport, S.I. (1976) Opening of the blood-brain barrier by acute hypertension. Exp. Neurol. 52:467-479.

Rapoport, S.I. (1976) Blood-Brain Barrier in Physiology and Medicine. Raven Press, New York.

Rapoport, S.I. (1978) A mathematical model for vasogenic brain edema. J. Theor. Biol. 74:439-467.

Rapoport, S.I. (1980) Factors which can be used to quantitatively predict drug entry into and distribution within the brain. In Influence of Age on the Pharmacology of Psychoactive Drugs. (Ed. Raskin, A.) Raven Press, New York. (in press)

Rapoport, S.I., Fredericks, W.R., Ohno, K. and Pettigrew, K.D. (1980) Quantitative aspects of reversible osmotic opening of the blood-brain barrier. Am. J. Physiol. (in press).

Rapoport, S.I., Hori, M. and Klatzo, I. (1972) Testing of a hypo-
    thesis for osmotic opening of the blood-brain barrier. Am.
    J. Physiol. 223:323-331.

Rapoport, S.I., Ohno, K., Fredericks, W.R. and Pettigrew, K.D.
    (1978) Regional cerebrovascular permeability to ^{14}C-sucrose
    after osmotic opening of the blood-brain barrier. Brain Res.
    150:653-657.

Rapoport, S.I., Ohno, K. and Pettigrew, K.D. (1979) Drug entry
    into the brain. Brain Res. 172:354-359.

Rapoport, S.I. and Thompson, H.K. (1973) Osmotic opening of the
    blood-brain barrier in the monkey without associated neuro-
    logical deficits. Science. 180:971.

Rapoport, S.I., Thompson, H.K. and Bidinger, J.M. (1974) Equi-
    osmolal opening of the blood-brain barrier in the rabbit by
    different contrast agents. Acta Radiol. (Diagn. 15:21-32.

Reese, T.S. and Karnovsky, M.J. (1967) Fine structural localiza-
    tion of a blood-brain barrier to exogenous peroxidase.
    J. Cell Biol. 34:207-217.

Simionescu, N., Simionescu, M. and Palade, G.E. (1975) Per-
    meability of muscle capillaries to small heme-peptides.
    Evidence for the existence of patent transendothelial
    channels. J. Cell Biol. 64:586-607.

Sterrett, P.R., Bradley, I.M., Kitten, G.T., Janssen, H.F. and
    Holloway, K.S. (1976) Cerebrovasculature permeability
    changes following experimental cerebral angiography. A
    light-and electronmicroscopic study. J. Neurol. Sci.
    30:385-403.

Studer, R.K., Welch, D.M. and Siegel, B.A. (1974) Transient
    alteration of the blood-brain barrier: effect of hypertonic
    solutions administered via carotid artery injection. Exp.
    Neurol. 44:266-273.

Thompson, A.M. (1970) Hyperosmotic effects of brain uptake of non-
    electrolytes, in Capillary Permeability (Crone, C. and Lassen,
    N.A., eds.) (Alfred Benzon Symp. 2) Munksgaard, Copenhagen,
    pp. 459-467.

Ussing, H.H. (1971) Introductory remarks. Philos. Trans. R. Soc.
    Lond. (Biol.) Sci. 262:85-90.

Westergaard, E. and Brightman, M.W. (1973) Transport of proteins
    across normal cerebral arterioles. J. Comp. Neurol. 153:
    17-44.

SITES AND FUNCTIONS OF THE BLOOD-RETINAL BARRIERS

Jose Cunha-Vas, M.D., Ph.D.
Department of Ophthalmology, University of Coimbra,
Coimbra, Portugal
Department of Ophthalmology, University of Illinois Eye
and Ear Infirmary, Chicago, USA

Studies on the blood-brain relationship have yielded evidence that the rates of exchange and the concentrations in the brain at steady state for many substances are quite different from those in other organs. These differences reflect a distinct set of permeability characteristics at the blood-brain interface, thus originating the concept of a blood-brain barrier (BBB).

Although the term BBB implies an impermeable barrier between blood and brain, it must be permeable to some solutes in blood because some drugs (such as barbiturates) have an instantaneous effect on brain function and because the brain is metabolically active and must receive its substrates from blood. The BBB is more correctly thought as selectively permeable rather than impermeable.

As regards the posterior segment of the eye and, particularly, the retina, two early studies (appearing in 1913 and 1947 by Schnaudigel (1) and Palm (2) respectively) repeated the classical work of Goldmann (3) in the brain, showing that trypan blue injected intravenously induced a blue staining of all tissues with the exception of the brain and retina. These two studies, however, had little impact on the ophthalmic literature and, until 1965, most textbooks considered the permeability of the retinal vessels to be comparable to that of other vessels on the body.

It was only in 1965 that the effect of histamine on the permeability of the ocular vessels was examined by Ashton and Cunha-Vaz (4) using the technique of vascular labeling of Majno and Palade (5). Histamine markedly increased the vascular permeability of the various ocular tissues except for the retina. This behavior of the retinal vessels, in clear contrast to almost every other vessel of the body,

was similar only to that of the cerebral vessels, a finding which
pointed to the existence of a barrier in the retina similar to the
BBB. Subsequent research has confirmed the existence of a blood
-retinal barrier (BRB).

The introduction of the concept of the BRB into the ophthalmic
literature excited much interest, as evidenced by a series of reports studying its basic mechanisms (6). This interest was supported
by the development and widespread use of fundus fluorescein angiography (7), a clinical method that has documented the importance of
the BRB in retinal disease. Angiography, a qualitative technique,
has recently been extended by the use of quantitative vitreous fluorophotometry, which can assess the degree of breakdown of the BRB
(8, 9). Abnormal functioning of the BRB is now widely accepted as
one of the most important factors in development of retinal vascular
disease and macular pathology, two of the most significant causes
of blindness (10).

Finally, although the anatomical location of the BRB and many
of its transfer characteristics are now better understood, the teleology of this unique system is not at all clear. Certain advantages
to retinal function are apparent, but their relative importance is
quite unknown. An attempt will be made here to define certain of the
unique structural features of the BRB, to establish its selective
permeability, and, finally, to speculate upon its teleology and its
possible role in retinal disease.

I. THE BLOOD-OCULAR BARRIERS (BLOOD-AQUEOUS BARRIER AND BLOOD-RETI-
NAL BARRIER)

The situation regarding the sites, mechanisms,and physiological
significance of solute exchanges between blood and intraocular fluids
and between the intraocular fluids and surrounding intraocular tissues is better understood if we consider two main barrier systems
in the eye (fig. 1). One, regulating exchanges between blood and the
intraocular fluids and involving a variety of structures, concerns
primarily the ciliary body and is called the blood-acqueous barrier
(BAB). Here, inward movements from the blood into the eye predominate.
Aqueous humor is secreted into the posterior chamber by the ciliary
processes from where it flows through the pupil into the anterior
chamber and leaves the eye by bulk flow at the chamber angle by the
trabecular or uveoscleral routes. There are diffusional solute exchanges between aqueous humor and surrounding tissues, the posterior
chamber, and the vitreous compartment (11, 13).

The other,particularly tight, where outward movement from the
eye into the blood appears to predominate and where penetration into
the eye of only a few important metabolic products is allowed, is
called the blood-retinal barrier (BRB). It is responsible for home-

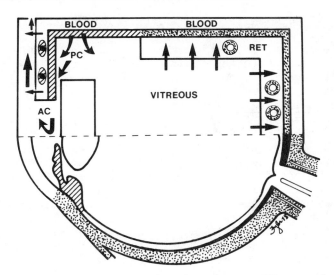

Fig. 1. Diagram of the blood-ocular barriers. RET - retina;   PC -
- posterior chamber; AC - anterior chamber. (From ref. 10).

ostasis of the neuroretina. In the posterior segment it is the only
well-defined barrier situation.

The concept of a blood-vitreous barrier is vague, has no morphological basis, and is, on the whole, untenable. Such a barrier
is entirely absent in the anterior region of the vitreous where a
situation of passive diffusion is present between the anterior and
posterior segments of the eye. There are, therefore, no significant
selective barriers to molecular markers between the vitreous and the
posterior chamber on the one hand, and between the vitreous and the
extracellular space of the retina on the other hand. The vitreous
humor, appears therefore, to be located between two barriers - the
BAB anteriorly, and the BRB posteriorly.

At the level of the optic nerve a situation of barrier is present between the blood and the extracellular space bathing the neural tissue, but it appears to bear close resemblance to the BBB. Of
particular interest is the observation that in the optic nerve head,
like in the brain, there is a small region where a barrier situation
is lacking (14). Here, tracers originating from the peripapillary
choriocapillaries may diffuse into the optic nerve head. It is puz-
zling why the optic nerve head, interposed between the BRB anteriorly
and the BBB posteriorly, does lack a barrier. It may explain, however, reported observations on a certain degree of fluid flow at
this level.

II. SITES OF THE BLOOD-RETINAL BARRIER

It should be kept in mind that the retina has two areas of direct relationship with the blood - namely at the level of the retinal vessels and at the chorioepithelial interface.

A. Retinal vessels. The first electron microscopic studies of
the brain and retina failed to show any differences between these
vessels and those of the rest of the body that have a continuous endothelium (15). It was in 1966 that Shakib and Cunha-Vaz (15) found
that the interendothelial junctions of the retinal vessels were different from those in other vessels of the body. They were shown to
represent particularly extensive "zonulae occludentes" which sealed
the intercellular spaces, apparently surrounding completely the endothelial interface cells (fig. 2). It has been shown that tissues
in which the intercellular spaces incorporate extensive and belt
like areas of close contact offer high resistance to the passage of
ions (Table 1). Furthermore, the amount of cross-linking in the

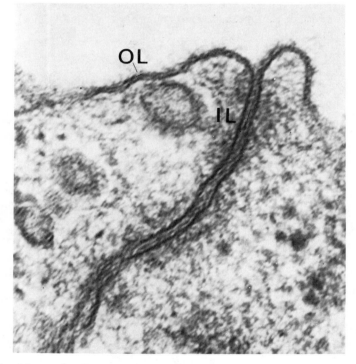

Fig. 2. Small retinal vessel showing a tight junction. An extensive
zonula occludens is visible all along the junction. The outer leaf-
lets (OL) of the lateral cell membranes of the adjoining endothelial
cells fuse into an intermediate line (IL). Uranyl acetate and lead
citrate stained section x 124,000.

Table 1. Nomenclature, characteristics, and examples of major types of cell junctions

Type	Subtype	Other name	Major function	Characteristics	Examples
Adherens	1)Zonula and fascia adherentes		Mechanical attachment	150-250A interspace between apposed plasma membranes	Cardiac muscle cells
	2)Macula adherens	Desmosome	Cell-to-cell adhesion	1)250-350A interspace 2)Condensed proteinaceous material in intercellular matrix 3)Fibrillar plaques in subjacent cytoplasm	Stratified squamous epithelia
Occludens	1)Zonula occludens	"Nonleaky" tight junction	Restriction of intercellular diffusion	1)Belt-like zone of membrane union 2)Usually 140A in total thickness in region of two 75A plasma membranes 3)Fibrillar network links adjacent plasma membranes (stable)	Endothelial cells of brain and retinal capillaries; retinal pigment epithelium
	2)Macula and fascia occludentes	"Leaky" tight junction	Discontinuities may represent "pores" for by-pass diffusion	1)Focal membrane-to-membrane areas of union 2)Short fibrillar network (labile)	Muscle capillary endothelium
Gap junctions	Small subunit Large subunit	Nexus	Cell-to-cell communication	1)20-40A wide gap between apposed membranes 2)Hexagonally arrayed subunits contain exchange channels	Cardiac muscle; hepatocytes

areas of cellular contact appears to be responsible for their capability to withstand stress (16). It is noteworthy that the tight junctions of the retinal vessels were shown to be very stable, much more so than the iridial vessels. When the eye was submitted to paracentesis or when histamine was applied directly to the retina, the junctional complexes remained closed and intraluminal particles were always arrested at the side of the endothelial cell facing the lumen. By contrast, local application of histamine or lowering of the ocular pressure by paracentesis opened up the interendothelial junctions of the iris vessels, allowing particles to pass easily through the interendothelial spaces. These studies led Cunha-Vaz et al. (17) to propose that the endothelial cells along with their junctional complexes are the main site of the BRB, at least for substances like thorium dioxide, trypan blue, and fluorescein (figs. 3 and 4).

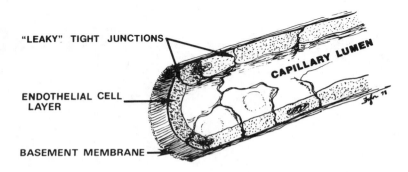

Fig. 3. Diagram of the ultrastructural characteristics of an iris capillary.

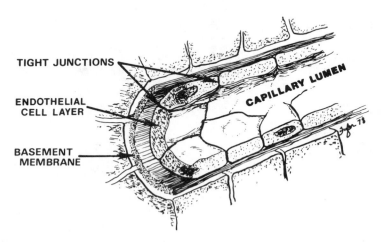

Fig. 4. Diagram of the ultrastructural characteristics of a retinal capillary.

These findings have since been confirmed in the brain and retina using peroxidase as a tracer (18, 19) and with microperoxidase
(20), which has a molecular diameter of approximately 2 nm. The
tight junctions of the retinal and cerebral vessels appear to be
particularly stable, showing characteristics of "non-leaky" tight
junctions (Table 2). Whereas general capillary permeability is based
upon molecular size, BRB permeability is based upon quite different
criteria. General capillaries to allow all small molecules to diffuse through clefts between endothelial cells and through fenestrae.
In addition, capillary cell cytoplasm contains numerous pinocytotic
vesicles, presumably moving large molecules across the capillary
wall. In the retina these routes of nonspecific exchange are not
present. The endothelial cells are fused to each other by "non-leaky"
tight junctions, no fenestrae are seen, and pinocytosis is virtually
absent. Furthermore, tight junctions of the "non-leaky" type, preventing non-selective exchange, establish steep gradients across
the membrane where they are located and are usually associated with
active transport mechanisms in the cell membrane. It is of particular
interest that active transport of organic anions has been shown to
occur in the retinal vessels (13).

Additionally, the endothelial cells of the retinal and brain
vessels appear to be histochemically different from other vascular
endothelial cells of the body. The endothelium of the retinal and
brain capillaries appears to be uniquely rich in alkaline phospha-
tase activity (21, 22), monoamine oxidase (MAO) and DOPA-decarboxi-
lase (23).

B. Chorioretinal interface. 1. Choriocapillaris. The capillaries of the choroidal layer have structural characteristics which
are entirely different from those of the retinal vessels. Their endothelium displays numerous fenestrations which occur preferentially
in the region of the vessel wall that abuts on Bruch's membrane.
Electron microscopic studies using a variety of tracer have shown
that the vessels of the choroid, like those of the ciliary body stroma, are permeable to macromolecules (17, 19, 24). Trypan blue, fluorescein and similar substances permeate freely this vascular layer
of the choroid. In summary, the choriocapillaris does not appear to
have much significance as regards barrier function.

2. Bruch's membrane. This membrane, located between the choriocapillaris and the pigment epithelium of the retina, does not obstruct the passage of fluorescein nor of tracers like horseradish
peroxidase or ferritin (19). Bruch's membrane, like most other vascular basement membranes, acts as a diffusion barrier only to molecules of large molecular size.

3. Retinal pigment epithelium. The retinal pigment epithelium
is the first cellular layer which opposes the penetration into the
retina of any substance originating from the choroid. Light micros-

copic studies indicated that the penetration of carbon, trypan blue
and fluorescein from the choroid into the retina stops at the level
of the retinal pigment epithelium (25). Finally, electron microscopy
(19, 26, 27) showed that adjacent pigment epithelial cells are united
by extensive "zonulae occludentes" very similar to the ones previously described between the endothelial cells of the retinal vessels
(fig. 5). These junctional complexes present all the morphological
and permeability characteristics of the tight junctions of the "non-
-leaky" type. Ion flux and microelectrode experiments performed on
isolated frog pigment epithelium demonstrated that the plasma membrane at the apex and the base of the epithelial cells has a high
permeability to K+, an "intracellular ion", and a relatively low
permeability to Na+ and Cl (28), which are "extracellular ions".

   In conclusion, the intercellular spaces in the retinal pigment
epithelium are firmly closed, most molecular movements being forced
to take through the more selective transcellular route.

   C. Glia and extracellular space. The glial cells of the brain,
notably the astrocytes, due to their intimate contact with the capillaries, were for a time regarded as responsible for the barrier
effect. This concept was a consequence of electron microscopical
observations reporting that the glial processes invested completely
the capillaries and that there was little extracellular space avai-

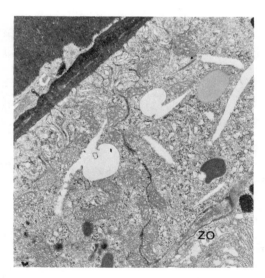

Fig. 5. Retinal pigment epithelium. Intravenous administration of
horseradish peroxidase. The peroxidase stops at an extensive area of
union between the apposed cellular membranes (ZO - zonula occludens).
(Uranyl acetate and lead citrate, x 25,800). (From ref. 10). (Reduced
45% for reproduction.)

lable (29). However, refinements in electron microscopic technique, the use of tracers, and a series of physiological studies showed that these assumptions were not true (30, 31). In a variety of experimental situations, particularly when tracer particles have access to the extracellular space of the retina by circumventing the barrier (e.g., after intravitreal injection), tracer particles were found to move freely in the extracellular space and were not restricted by the inner and outer limiting membranes.

A very clear demonstration that the glia does not play a major role in barrier phenomena was offered by electron microscopic studies of the rabbit retina. In this animal, the retinal vessels lie on the surface of the retina, in the vitreous, free from any direct glial contact (fig. 6), but a BRB remains present (17).

In conclusion, the extracellular space of the retina is functional and cannot be responsible for the barrier effect. It is possible, however, that the glial cells play an important role as metabolic intermediaries between the blood capillaries and nerve cells.

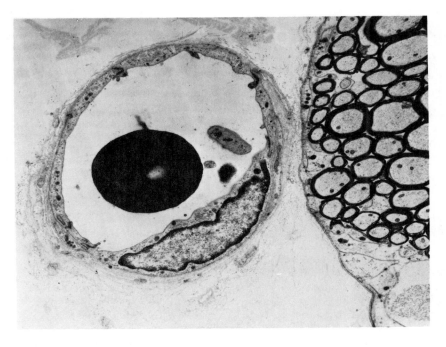

Fig. 6. Section of a rabbit retinal vessel. The direct contact of the vitreous humor with the vessel walls should be noted. Osmium tetroxide fixed tissue embedded in araldite. Sections stained with uranyl acetate and lead citrate.

The BRB is, therefore, located at two levels, forming what may be called an outer BRB and an inner BRB. The main structures involved appear to be, for the outer BRB, the retinal pigment epithelium, and for the inner BRB, the endothelial membrane of the retinal vessels. Both these membranes have tight junctions of the "non-leaky" type. To traverse the BRB a molecule must pass directly either through the retinal endothelial cell or the retinal pigment epithelial cell. It must escape from plasma proteins and water, enter the cell membrane, escape into and traverse the cytoplasm, and similarly penetrate the outer membrane. This transcellular passage probably occurs in general capillaries, but is overshadowed by the efficient nonspecific exchange routes.

III. PERMEABILITY CHARACTERISTICS OF THE BLOOD-RETINAL BARRIERS

The study of the permeability characteristics of a membrane involves an analysis of the different types of molecular movement which take place across its surface. There are two main types of transfer across cell membranes - active and passive. Active transfer is defined as a transfer or movement against an electrochemical concentration gradient. Passive transfer is said to occur when molecules or ions are transferred according to the prevailing electrochemical concentration gradients.

Present knowledge on diffusion and transport mechanisms of the BRB refers generally to both the outer and inner barriers, because there is yet no clear information on differences in permeability rates between the outer and inner parts of the BRB.

1. Passive diffusion. In general, after intravenous injection, test substances penetrate into the vitreous in minimal amounts, always reaching higher values in the anterior vitreous entering from the posterior chamber or ciliary circulation rather than through the BRB (32). This has been observed with proteins, urea (33), sodium (34, 35), potassium chloride (36), phosphate, inulin, sucrose and antibiotics (37).

Personal studies in collaboration with David Maurice produced the first approximate value for the permeability coefficient of a substance at the level of the BRB (17) when the permeability of the BRB for fluorescein was examined by slit-lamp fluorophotometry under conditions of passive diffusion. The results obtained showed that fluorescein, which has a molecular radius of approximately 5.5 Å, has a permeability coefficient at the BRB in the outer of 0.14×10^{-5} cm sec^{-1}. This value is very different from the values obtained for the capillary permeability in other vessels of the body for molecules of similar size (38), but comparable to the value obtained by Crone (39) for the permeability of the BBB. It is especially interesting to compare the value obtained for the permeability of the BRB to fluorescein in a situation of simple diffusion with the value found by Davson and Danielli (40) for the cellular permeability to sucrose. They are exactly similar. It can be concluded, therefore, that the passive transfer at the level of the BRB is extremely restricted, nonselective exchange being prevented by the presence of tight junctions of the "non-leaky" type between adjacent cells.

The ability of a solute in free solution in plasma to penetrate the BBB has been shown to depend upon the relative affinity for plasma water and the endothelial cell plasma membrane. Sufficiently lipid-soluble materials penetrate BBB and these presumably can enter the membrane at a nearly infinite number of sites. Also, certain lipid insoluble substances, such as glucose, penetrate the BBB, and it is presumed that these enter because of the presence in the membrane of specialized proteins having high-affinity sites specific for the transport substances.

Similarly, the BRB penetration can be considered to be lipid-mediated or carrier-mediated.

2. Lipid-mediated penetration. Studies on the BRB have shown that lipid substances penetrate freely into the vitreous after intravenous injection (34) and that their rate of penetration is directly related to their oil/water partition coefficient (35).

The plasma-cell membrane interface can be simulated in vitro by an oil-water (nonpolar versus polar) two-phase system. If a radio-labeled substance is placed in a bottle, some buffered water and oil (such as olive oil) is added, shaken violently, and allowed to separate to oil and water, the concentration in the oil divided by the concentration in the water is the oil/water partition coefficient. This relative affinity appears to be cru ial, rather than the absolute solubility of the labeled molecule in either lipid or water.

3. Carrier-mediated penetration. In the cerebral capillaries seven independent carrier transport systems mediating exchange of essential substances have been described. They are for glucose (and certain other hexoses) short-chain monocarboxylic acids, certain neutral aminoacids, basic aminoacids, certain purines, and certain nucleosides (41).

In vitro studies, using the isolated retinal pigment epithelium of the frog, found evidence for a net flux choroid to retina of labelled glucose (42, 43). With an "in vivo" method, Dollery et al. (44) found evidence for a preferential uptake of D-glucose in the retinal tissue in rats, rabbits and guinea pigs. Intravenously injected labelled D-glucose and L-glucose were followed by determinations of radioactivities in the tissue at different intervals after the injection.

More recently, Tornquist (45) reported on a carrier-mediated net influx of glucose in the retina across the retinal pigment epithelium and the retinal capillary wall. The glucose transport system in the retinal pigment epithelium showed a stereospecific preference for D-glucose. A carrier-mediated net outflux or lactate at both sites of the BRB has been also demonstrated by Tornquist and Alm (45).

Similar results have been obtained with aminoacids. The total aminoacid concentration gradient that exists between the posterior aqueous and the vitreous, and between the posterior and anterior segments of the vitreous, clearly indicates that aminoacids are lost from the vitreous to the retina. Experiments using a non-metabolized aminoacid demonstrated that this is due to an outward oriented aminoacid transport system across the BRB.

4. Active transport by the BRB. Carrier-mediated BRB permeability to glucose and other metabolic substrates are not necessarily energy-dependent, because if the retina is utilizing them, a concentration gradient will be maintained between plasma and retina and no pump mechanism is needed.

There are, however, substantial ionic gradients across the BRB, which cannot be accounted by retinal utilization. Magnesium and potassium, for example, show such gradients. The Mg++ concentration is highest in the posterior vitreous, and naturally in the extracellular fluid of the retina, a situation which is similar to that in the cerebrospinal fluid system. Both in the case of the dog and the rabbit, influx of Mg++ across the BRB must take place against a concentration gradient, i.e., it must represent an active transport process (46). With potassium, the reverse occurs. The highest K+ concentration in the intraocular fluids is found in the posterior chamber and anterior segment of the vitreous. In the absence of lens, the K+ concentration in the vitreous was found to be significantly lower than the plasma dialysate value, suggesting that K+ is actively transported out of the vitreous across the BRB.

Certain of the acidic end products of brain monoamines may also be transported out of brain since probenecid (which competes with organic anion transport) results in an elevation of their concentration in cerebrospinal fluid and brain. This mechanism has been studied at some length in the BRB. The availability of slit-lamp fluorophotometry made possible the study of movements of fluorescein, an organic anion, into and out of the eye, through the BRB (17). The results were of peculiar interest since they provided evidence for an active transport for fluorescein across the entire retina and walls of the retinal vessels. It was found that when fluorescein is injected into the blood, no measurable amount enters the vitreous body of the normal eye. When fluorescein was injected into the vitreous body of the normal eye, its concentration dropped from behind the lens to the retinal surface where it fell to a very low value (fig. 7). This distribution was not affected even if a very high

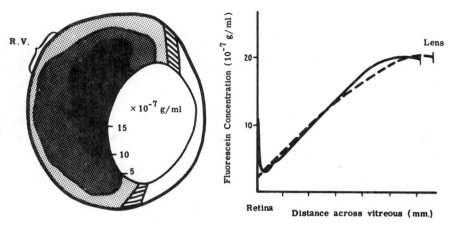

Fig. 7. Intravitreal injection of 15 μl of 0.06% fluorescein in saline. (a) In vivo recordings taken 6 hr after the injection. (b)
Contours from eye frozen 7 hr after the injection. (From ref. 13).

concentration of fluorescein was maintained in the blood. When the
eye is treated with metabolic inhibitors or with competitive inhibitors of the type that influence organic anion transport in other
regions of the body (e.g., probenecid, iodopyracet, penicillins),
the entire pattern of the fluorescein movement in the vitreous alters in the direction of free exchange across the retinal surface.
The transport of fluorescein across the BRB thus appears to be similar to organic anion transport in kidney and liver, and it may be
involved in the protection of neural elements of the retina from toxic action of some waste products of metabolism.

IV. TELEOLOGY OF THE BRB

There undoubtedly are many reasons for the BBB and BRB, but the
most widely held belief is that they protect the brain and retina
from potentially neurotoxic substances in blood. It is a fact that
they perform this function, but their function is better defined by
stating that the BBB and BRB facilitate the optimization of the fluid
environment of the brain and retinal cells, respectively.

Many drugs (such as most antibiotics) are kept out of the retina
by the BRB, and this is an important protective effect, particularly
when it is recalled that when there is retinal disease a barrier alteration is usually present, thus making the retina accessible to
the therapeutic effect of the drug.

It is noteworthy, that once a lipid-soluble molecule is intro-

duced into the body, the usual effect of metabolism is to render the
molecule more polar. This increasing polarity can be thought of as
a protective mechansm on the part of the body since the organism
has no ability to confine or otherwise transport lipid-soluble substances that readily diffuse through all cell membranes and tissue
compartments. Only when rendered polar can biological membranes ef-
ficiently transport these substances.

The ability of the BBB and BRB to obstruct the passage of some
substances is enhanced by enzymatic mechanisms in the cytoplasm of
the capillary endothelial cells. These cells contain monoaminoxidase
(MAO) which probably serves to restrict the passage of biogenic amines in or out of the brain (23). One could readily imagine a burst
of systemic norepinephrine upon jumping into cold water (41). En-
trance of this norepinephrine into the retina could substantially
alter its function and isolation of the retina from such systemic
perturbations probably is a significant effect of the BRB. This enzymatic barrier probably completes simple physical exclusion by the
barrier.

The barrier system behaves as though all substances in plasma
are prevented from entering the brain and retina, but specific classes of molecules are, in effect, issued "passes" to allow entry (41).
Such an arrangement could provide considerable stabilization of the
flux into brain of metabolic substrates such as glucose.To be most
effective as a control mechanism, such a carrier transport system
should be about half-saturated in the presence of the usual concentration of substrate to which the carrier protein is exposed. This
is the case with several of the BBB carriers, including the glucose
carrier. The flux of glucose into brain is, therefore, rendered relatively constant in the event of hyper or hypoglycemia.

Finally, a particularly interesting situation occurs with the
neurotransmitters which play a prominent role in neural function
either by exciting or inhibiting postsynaptic neurons by opening
ion channels so as to change membrane potentials. The percursors of
the recognized neural transmitters (glucose, DOPA, histidine, tryptophan) readily penetrate the BBB and BRB by virtue of various carrier systems. The transmitters themselves, however, are polar substances without affinity for any of the carriers. As a result they
are trapped in the neural tissue by the barriers. The brain and
retina presumably need to keep their transmitters to some degree
localized to the region in which they are released.

V. POSSIBLE ROLE OF BRB IN RETINAL DISEASE

The role of BBB in human disease is still unclear because so
little is known about it. The development of two diagnostic methods
- fundus fluorescein angiography and vitreous fluorophotometry, has,

however, contributed significantly to our understanding of the alteration of the BRB in retinal disease. It appears that there is an intimate relationship between breakdown of the BRB and almost every retinal disease, particularly the vascular retinopathies and the pigment epitheliopathies(6, 10). Whereas, fluorescein angiography shows BRB loss in virtually all lesions in which normal histology is altered, vitreous fluorophotometry, a quantitative method of fluorescein analysis of the vitreous, can detect functional alterations of the BRB (8, 9).

Vitreous fluorophotometry appears to be particularly suitable for early diagnosis and for much needed pharmacological research on the barrier.

Along this line, the preservation of an intact BRB, the diminution of a barrier breakdown, or even a controlled breakdown of the barrier to help drug delivery have obvious clinical significance.

The role of the BRB in retinal disease is now only starting to be envisaged. The retina appears to be, like the brain, dependent on the BRB carrier systems to exchange its metabolites with plasma. If the BRB glucose carrier is somehow inactivated, glucose deprivation would ensue and the retina become irreversibly damaged. In some pathological lesions it is conceivable that the glucose carrier is regionally inactivated, thereby creating what would be, in effect, a regional hypoglycemia (41). This could be quite localized because the diffusion from the surrounding tissue is restricted by the limited diffusional flux of the small retinal extracellular space.

There is also an independent carrier transport for short-chain monocarboxylic acids which increases BRB permeability to lactate and several related acids as pyruvate and B-hydroxybutyrate. This carrier appears to facilitate loss of lactate from the retina where its production exceeds the existing enzymatic mechanisms for metabolizing it. It is known that when the brain becomes acutely hypoperfused, the brain lactate rises within 3 to 5 minutes from its normal 2mM to about 15 mM. This parallels an accumulation of CO_2, and these two factors are largely responsible for the drop in brain pH in hypoperfusion. The cardinal importance of a stable pH to retina and brain is suggested by the observation that it is apparently the regional extracellular pH that is the major parameter used to adjust regional blood flow.

Another important aspect is the possible role played by the BRB in ischemia and other disorders of glucose metabolism. The BRB lactate carrier, probably becomes oversaturated on the presence of high lactate levels and can no longer effectively transport this lactate out of brain and retina (46). The exceptional vulnerability of the nervous tissue to ischemia may be consequence of the barrier system.

It is also interesting to speculate on how much of a limitation on retinal development is imposed by heavily saturated BRB aminoacid carriers in the normal infant and what interactions take place in disease, between various aminoacids using the same carrier system.

REFERENCES

1. Schnaudigel, O. (1913) Albrecht von Graefes Arch. Ophthalmol., 86:93-97.
2. Palm, E. (1947) Acta Ophthalmol., 25:29-33.
3. Goldmann, E.E. (1913) Abhandl Konigl Preuss Akad Wiss, 1:1-60.
4. Ashton, N. and Cunha-Vaz, J.G. (1965) Arch. Ophthalmol., 73:211--223.
5. Majno, G. and Palade, G.E. (1961) J. Biophys. Biochem. Cytol., 11:571-605.
6. Cunha-Vaz, J.G. (1976) Doc. Ophthalmol., 41:287-327.
7. Archer, D.B. (1976) Doc. Ophthalmol. Proceedings Series, New Developments in Ophthalmology, The Hague W Junk, pp 155-167.
8. Cunha-Vaz, J.G., Abreu, J.R.F., Campos, A.J.,et al. (1975) British J. Ophthalmol., 59:649-656.
9. Cunha-Vaz, J.G., Goldberg, M.F., Vygantas, C. and Noth, J. (1979) Ophthalmology, 86:264-275.
10. Cunha-Vaz, J.G. (1979) Survey Ophthalmol., 23:279-296.
11. Adler, F.H. (1962) Textbook of Physiology of the Eye. St. Louis, CV Mosby.
12. Bito, L.Z. (1977) Exp. Eye Res. 25 (Suppl.):273-290.
13. Cunha-Vaz, J.G. and Maurice, D. (1967) J. Physiol., 191:467-486.
14. McMahon, R.T., Tso, M.O.M. and McLean, I.W. (1975) Amer. J. Ophthalmol., 80:1058-1065.
15. Shakib, M. and Cunha-Vaz, J.G. (1966) Exp. Eye Res., 5:229-234.
16. Staehelin, L.A., Mukherjee, T.M. and Williams, A.W. (1969) Protoplasma, 67:165-184.
17. Cunha-Vaz, J.G., Shakib, M. and Ashton, N. (1966) Brit. J. Ophthalmol., 50:441-453.
18. Reese, T.S., Karnovski, M.J. (1967) J. Cell Biol., 34:207-217.
19. Shiose, Y. (1970) Jap. J. Ophthalmol., 14:73-79.
20. Smith, R.S. and Ruth, L.A. (1975) Invest. Ophthalmol., 14:556-560.
21. Nilausen, K. (1958) Acta Ophthalmol., 36:65-69.
22. Wislocki, G.B. and Dempsey, E.W. (1948) J. Comp. Neurol., 88:319--326.
23. Butler, A., Falck, B., Owman, C.H. and Rosengren, E. (1966) Pharmacol. Rev., 18:369-385.
24. Hazlett, L.D. and Meyer, D.B. (1974) Exp. Eye Res., 19:303-308.
25. Cunha-Vaz, J.G. (1966) Permeability of the retinal vessels in health and disease. PhD thesis, University of London.
26. Peyman, G.A., Spitznas, M. and Straatsma, B.R. (1971) Invest. Ophthalmol., 10:181-187.
27. Shakib, M., Rutkowski, P. and Wise, G.E. (1972) Amer. J. Ophthalmol., 74:206-218.
28. Steinberg, R.H. and Miller, S. (1973) Exp. Eye Res., 16:365-372.

29. Gerschenfeld, H.M., Wald, F. and Zadunaisky, T.A. et al. (1959) Neurology, 9:412–425.
30. Brightman, M.W. (1965) Am. J. Anat., 117:193–220.
31. Smelser, G.K., Ishikawa, T. and Pei, Y.F. (1965) Structure of the Eye, vol. 2 Stuttgart, Verlag, p. 109.
32. Davson, H. (1969) The Eye, vol. 1, New York. Academic Press, ed. 2, pp. 67–186.
33. Bleeker, G.M. and Maas, E.H. (1958) Arch. Ophthalmol., 60.1013––1020.
34. Davson, H., Duke-Elder, W.S., Maurice, D.M. et al. (1949) J. Physiol., 108:203–217.
35. Sallman, L. von, Evans, T.C. and Dillon, B. (1949) Arch. Ophthalmol., 41:611–626.
36. Kinsey, K.E. (1960) Circulation, 21:968–975.
37. Havener, W.H. (1974) Ocular Pharmacology. St. Louis, C.V. Mosby.
38. Vargas, F. and Johnson, J.A. (1967) Am. J. Physiol., 213:87–93.
39. Crone, C. (1965) Acta Physiol. Scand., 64:407–412.
40. Davson, H. and Danielli, J.F. (1952) The Permeability of Natural Membranes. London, Cambridge University Press.
41. Oldendorf, W.H. (1975) Permeability of the Blood-Brain Barrier. In "The Nervous System", Donald B. Tower, ed., vol. 1: The Basic Neurosciences, pp. 279–289, Raven Press, New York.
42. Zadunaisky, J.A. and Degnan, K.Y. (1976) Exp. Eye Res., 23:191––196.
43. Miller, S. and Steinberg, R.H. (1976) J. Membrane Biol., 36:337––372.
44. Dollery, C.T., Henkind, P. and D'Orme, M.L'E. (1971) Diabetes, 20:519–524.
45. Tornquist, P. (1979) Acta Univ. Upsaliensis, 326.
46. Bito, L.Z. (1970) Exp. Eye Res., 10:102–116.
47. Cunha-Vaz, J.G. (1972) Trans. Ophthalmol. Soc. UK, 92:111–121.

ALTERATIONS OF AMINO ACID TRANSPORT IN THE CENTRAL NERVOUS SYSTEM

Abel Lajtha and Henry Sershen

Center for Neurochemistry, Rockland Research Institute

Ward's Island, New York   10035

INTRODUCTION

Alterations in the transport and in the levels and regional distribution of amino acids occur under a variety of conditions, including normal development. Since the levels, distribution, and movement of amino acids have important effects on brain metabolism, their changes would be reflected in altered metabolism. An understanding of control of amino acid transport is a goal toward which we have directed much of our research interest. The results obtained suggest that there is no single mechanism that regulates acid transport, but that there are many transport systems with different properties influenced by a number of factors.

The transport system measured in the brain includes low-affinity and high-affinity carrier sites; low-affinity systems have been best measured in brain slice preparations, and high-affinity uptake is most often measured in synaptosomes. Regional differences have been observed for both systems. Properties of transport in brain capillaries are different from those measured in brain slices. Parallel developmental changes in level and transport capacity have been observed, indicating a relationship. Specific differences also exist, however, indicating that specific metabolic changes also occur during development that result in alteration of metabolic distribution.

Possible regulating mechanisms include ions (distribution, fluxes, specific ionic influences), specific energy sources for specific transport systems, hormonal effects (regional effects, specific cellular permeability changes), and nutritional influences.

A survey based to a large extent on data in this area obtained in our laboratory is presented to illustrate a type of approach to an understanding of the complex mechanisms involved in central nervous system regulation of distribution and metabolism of amino acids, peptides, and proteins.

Regional Heterogeneity

The biochemical heterogeneity of brain is parallel to its structural and functional heterogeneity. For the amino acids in brain, such heterogeneity was shown in their distribution, metabolism, and transport. The levels of amino acids and their metabolic products, and their rates of metabolism, are different in the various structural compartments. The distribution pattern is rather specific for each amino acid, with distribution even for some and heterogeneous for others, and an area with the lowest concentration for one amino acid may contain the highest level of another. Several regional studies, including ours, on various species (Table 1) showed the heterogeneity and specificity of this distribution (1,2,3).

When we studied regional differences in cellular amino acid transport by measuring amino acid uptake in slices, considerable heterogeneity was found. The nonessential amino acids were accumulated to a high degree in all areas studied, but there was still considerable variation, sometimes several fold, in the uptake in the various brain areas. The picture was similar with the essential amino acids: they were accumulated to a lower degree, but heterogeneity could be found. We compared tissue levels with cellular uptake, and changes in tissue levels with changes in cellular uptake, in order to study the role of cellular transport in the regulation and determination of intracellular concentration of metabolites in the brain. There was some correlation between levels and uptake in that the uptake of amino acids that are at high levels in the brain, such as glutamate, asparate, taurine, and GABA, was much higher than the uptake of compounds present in the brain at low levels. Regional distribution and regional uptake were also often parallel (Table 2). The closer comparison of level with uptake, and of regional changes in level with such changes in uptake, showed a number of differences. Exit of amino acids from preloaded slices obtained from various areas also showed regional heterogeneity. A similar comparison of developmental changes in levels and changes in uptake also showed some similarities and some differences. We concluded that cellular transport is an important factor in determining tissue levels, but that in addition several other factors are operative in the control of cerebral metabolite distribution.

When the regional uptake _in vivo_, under conditions where brain levels of the amino acid were significantly elevated, was compared

with tissue levels under physiological conditions, a similar correlation was found (4).

Table 1.   Amino Acid Levels in Regions of Cat Brain

Amino Acid	Cortex	Corpus Callosum	Thalamus	Mesencepha- lic Tectum	Cere- bellum
Taurine	1.9	3.0	1.1	1.6	3.1
Aspartic acid	3.1	1.4	2.7	4.1	2.9
Glutamic acid	13	11	12	9.7	13
Glycine	1.3	0.61	1.7	2.8	1.5
Alanine	0.85	0.70	0.59	1.1	0.89
Phenylalanine	0.05	0.06	0.08	0.09	0.08
GABA	1.4	0.96	3.7	5.8	1.5
Lysine	0.19	0.27	0.28	0.38	0.22

Amino acids in regions of cat brain determined with an amino acid
analyzer (3) are shown.   Values given are μmol amino acid per g
fresh brain.

Table 2.   Distribution In Vivo and Cellular Uptake in
            Vitro of Amino Acids in Rat Brain

Brain Area		Relative distribution: whole brain=100				
		Glycine	Leucine	Lysine	GABA	Glutamate
Hemisphere	Level	55	99	75	101	112
	Uptake	90	108	110	100	111
Midbrain	Level	137	110	133	164	73
	Uptake	155	87	107	148	92
Pons-Medulla	Level	317	99	160	76	67
	Uptake	115	76	65	90	65
Cerebellum	Level	55	101	135	66	100
	Uptake	91	96	82	71	89

Regional levels of amino acids (expressed as μmol/g fresh tissue)
are compared with uptake by slices (concentrative uptake μmol/ml
intracellular water per 5 min) from similar regions.   The level in
whole brain or the uptake by slices of whole brain is taken as
100 (4).

Regional variations in uptake in vitro, as in slices, were often
but not in all cases similar to regional variations in tissue concentrations. The fact that uptake capacity and levels are not
always parallel indicates that transport is not the only determinant
and that additional factors are important in determining changes
in levels.

An important difference in transport relates to specificity
of capillary transport. Although ten or more specific amino acid
transport systems can be identified in brain cells, only 4 or 5
of these can be detected in capillaries (5,6). Therefore some
amino acids that are actively taken up by brain tissue are not
transported through the capillaries. Since the properties of the
various transport systems differ, the fact that only a few are
present in capillaries results in differences in the properties of
capillary versus cellular transport. In cells the large neutral
amino acid transport that is Na+, temperature, and energy dependent
predominates; in the capillaries, it is the form that is not very
dependent on these factors (6,7,8).

Changes During Development

The composition of free amino acids in the brain changes during
development. The greatest change in absolute amount is the increase
in glutamate and the decrease in taurine. With the exception of
glutamate and aspartate, the levels of most amino acids are higher
in immature brain than in adult brain. However, changes in uptake
capacity are not strictly parallel with changes in levels (Table 3).
Plasma amino acid level changes occur; however, they are unlikely
to be responsible for changes in brain level and transport of amino
acids. The changes in amino acid levels are the greatest around
birth, and they show a rather complex pattern (10). It is tempting
to think that the non-essential amino acids increase with increasingly complex metabolism, including neurotransmitter production, and
that the essential amino acids decrease with the decreasing rate of
protein metabolism during development.

Uptake of amino acids also changes during development. It has
been established in several studies that the blood brain barrier
is less restrictive in the immature brain. In our studies of 10
amino acids under similar conditions, maintaining increased plasma
levels fairly constant for 90 min (11), each amino acid was taken
up to a greater extent in the immature than in the mature brain.
In spite of greater permeability, in most cases brain levels
remained below plasma levels, indicating that the restrictions to
uptake are less but are not absent. The changes in brain levels
when plasma concentration of an amino acid is increased is influenced by several factors; these include capillary permeability,
capillary and cellular transport, and metabolism. Capillary permeability is greater in newborn mice, and the portion of the passage

through the capillary that is no inhibited by analogs (diffusion ?) is greater in the immature brain (8). When capillary transport of amino acids was compared in vivo in young and adult rats, transport activity was measured by analog inhibition of uptake, that is, brain uptake index in 15-sec perfusion experiments (Oldendorf), was as great or greater in young brain in comparison to adult. This indicated that capillary transport of amino acids is developed early and is highly active during the active growth phase of the brain (8).

The development of cellular activity of the various transport systems was measured by measuring amino acid uptake in slices of brain at different ages (12). In mouse brain, by the 15th day of fetal life the transport systems for essential amino acids were well developed, and the transport systems for neurotransmitter amino acids (taurine, glycine, GABA, proline, glutamic acid) were less developed, but rapidly increased in the 15-19 day of fetal life. These results would indicate that transport systems for these essential amino acids (needed for protein synthesis) develop earlier than those for the amino acids needed for neurotransmitter function.

Table 3. Comparison of Changes of Amino Acid Levels and Transport During Development

Amino Acid	Adult, percent of newborn	
	tissue level	slice uptake
Alanine	72	83
Leucine	44	78
Phenylalanine	48	69
GABA	140	180
Glutamate	230	140
Lysine	84	87
Arginine	130	130
Glycine	40	150
Valine	71	110
Histidine	59	230
Taurine	45	260

Tissue level is μmol/g fresh tissue uptake, intracellular accumulation is μmol/ml intracellular water from 1 mM ^{14}C-amino acid in medium (9). The amino acids in the upper part of the table show parallel developmental changes of level and uptake; the four bottom examples show changes in the opposite direction.

When followed during further development (13) cellular transport activity showed a fairly heterogeneous pattern in that some amino acids reached adult activity levels early, others later, and in some cases activity showed a maximal peak at 2-3 weeks of postnatal age. It seems that amino acid transport is an essential element of nervous tissue, being present at early developmental stages and rapidly reaching mature values.

Ion Dependence

Ion gradients have been studied in a number of systems; they were suggested to be the source of energy for amino acid uptake against a concentration gradient (14). Lowering of Na^+ in brain slice studies decreased amino acid uptake (15), and absence of Na^+ almost completely inhibited uptake (16). In Ehrlich cells Na^+-dependent and -independent uptake of neutral amino acids was measured; the A system was Na^+-dependent and the L system was Na^+-independent (18). In brain slices, accumulative uptake for neutral amino acids occurred primarily via the A system (glycine, proline) and therefore the uptake was Na^+-dependent (6). In contrast, capillary transport of neutral amino acids is via the L not the A system (6,19). Capillary uptake measured in vivo or in isolated capillaries was not Na^+-dependent (8) (Table 4). Evidence was reported that the A system is operative on the outer surface (brain side) of the capillary or near it (20). Thus, heterogeneous distribution of the two (A and L) systems on the outer and inner (plasma side) surface of a membrane would give different properties of transport inward in comparison to that outward (through the membrane). In the case of brain, it may act as "exchange in pumping out" mechanism.

Our studies of ion fluxes indicated an influence of Na^+ movement on amino acid transport. Inward fluxes increased amino acid uptake in adult and newborn brain; the changes were lower in immature brain (21). Outward Na^+ movement slightly inhibited uptake; however, amino acid inflow still occurred under conditions of net Na exit, indicating that amino acid uptake is not exclusively dependent on Na^+ movement in the same direction (Table 5). Movement of K^+ (influx or efflux) did not affect uptake (22). Ion replacement studies depend on depletion methods (22). Incubation in K^+-free medium does not completely remove tissue K^+; initial wash in glucose minus Na^+ medium removes most of the K^+ from the brain slices. Incubation in K^+-free media reduced acidic amino acid transport slightly; L system neutrals were decreased, and lysine and ornithine were increased. High K^+ in the media inhibited lysine and ornithine uptake, and low and high K^+ both decreased GABA uptake (Table 6) (22).

Table 4.   Effect of Na^+ on Amino Acid Uptake in Vivo and in Vitro

| | | Uptake as per cent of control (+Na^+) | | |
		Lysine -Na^+	Leucine -Na^+	Glutamate -Na^+
In Vitro	Brain Slices	63	48	2
	Isolated Capillaries		94	
In Vivo	Capillaries	109	82	

Results are expressed as per cent of uptake of control (Na^+ containing medium)

Table 5.   The Effect of Na^+ Fluxes on Amino Acid Transport

Amino Acid	μmol/ml intracellular water			
	74	74/164 Influx	164/74 Efflux	164 Na^+ concn.
Aspartic Acid	3.9	5.2	2.0	4.5
GABA	2.9	5.2	1.7	3.6
Glycine	2.6	4.2	1.4	2.6
Leucine	1.7	2.2	1.0	1.9
Na^+ Tissue	51.7	95.7	76.5	119
K^+	117	130	125	132

Brain slices were incubated for 30 min in medium containing 74 (or 164) mM Na^+, then transferred and incubated in 164 (or 74) mM Na^+. Results are expressed as μmol amino acid per ml intracellular water.

The accumulation of amino acids especially of the nonessential such as glutamate, aspartate, GABA, and glycine - in brain slices is high, although these amino acids penetrate the brain in vivo very poorly. The high degree of amino acid uptake by slices in comparison to the low degree in vivo is not due to tissue damage (23). An ion gradient does exist between cut and inner area of a single slice, with uptake higher at the cut surface for some amino acids; however, the portion of cut surface constitutes only a small portion of the total slice (23). Swelling of tissue preparations does not account for high amino acid uptake capacity in slices (24). We feel that the major difference is not changes in ion gradients, energy content, or swelling, but that in slices the cellular uptake mechanism is rate-limiting, whereas in the living brain capillary permeability is the limiting factor.

It is likely that the heterogeneous distribution of transport systems results in variations in transport properties not only between capillary and cellular transport but also between various other structural elements - ganglia, peripheral nerves, and glia versus neurons - and in subcellular elements. This may extend to differences in ion dependence. Synaptosomal uptake of amino acids, related to high-affinity uptake, demonstrates strict Na^+ dependence (25). It is not known whether ion gradients are the primary source of energy changes in high-affinity transport, and a Na^+-independent high-affinity uptake for serine and threonine in newborn rat synaptosomes (26).

Some differences in ion dependence was observed in the transport of amino acids, such as glutamate and aspartate, belonging to the same (acidic) transport system (15). Although much of cerebral amino acid transport is abolished in the absence of Na^+, this situation is not likely to occur under physiological conditions. Minor changes in ion distribution, however, are likely to occur, and they would influence different amino acids to varying degree.

Energy Dependence

Energy related changes in ATP levels alter amino acid transport in brain slices (26). Depending on the metabolic inhibitors employed, ATP levels could be altered; however, no direct relationship was found between uptake of amino acids and ATP concentration (27, 28). It was possible to have high amino acid uptake in the presence of low ATP and low amino acid uptake with high tissue ATP levels. Glucose is a primary source of energy, yet mitochondrial enzyme inhibitors (rotenone, antimycin-A, oligomycin) were more potent inhibitors of amino acid uptake than glycolytic enzyme inhibitors (NaF, phlorizin) (Table 7) (29). Glucose can be substituted in the incubation medium by addition of succinate, malate, and pyruvate (SMP) with subsequent restoration of D-glutamate, AIB,

glycine, valine, histidine, GABA, or lysine uptake. The inhibitory
effects of NaF were decreased when the affected glycolytic steps
were bypassed by addition of SMP. These results indicate specific
energy sources, probably mitochondrial at the level of ubiquinone
reduction, and coupling to cytochrome b, which are involved in brain
amino acid transport (29).

Uphill transport (against a concentration gradient) is a process
that consumes energy; therefore it is not surprising that metabolic
inhibitors decreasing available energy have an inhibitory effect
on amino acid transport. The heterogeneity of the properties and
of the distribution of transport systems results in heterogeneous
alterations in amino acid transport as a result of changes in energy
metabolism, similar to the effects of changes in ion levels. Some
of the effects on rapidly metabolized amino acids are not through
transport, since changes in energy, ion levels could affect their
metabolism as well. Changes in tricarboxylic acid cycle activity
often result in changes in alanine and aspartate metabolism,
followed by effects on glutamate and GABA metabolism.

Table 6.   Amino Acid Uptake in High K^+ and K^+-Free Media

Amino Acid	Control C.U. (μmol/ml)	Amino acid uptake Per cent of control No K^+	50mM-K^+
Glu	31	87	94
Asp	31	76*	86
Val	10	73*	83*
Phe	2.2	68*	115
GABA	29	79*	50*
His	17	62*	67*
Orn	5.0	122*	64*
Lys	2.2	112	56*

C.U.=concentrative uptake=μmol/ml intracellular water above
medium level at the end of the uptake incubation. Slices were
incubated in the particular medium for 30 min; then the amino
acid was added, and incubation was continued 30 min. All amino
acids were L isomers. K^+ contents of the tissue at the end of
the incubation were 45, 70 and 115 μeq/ml in media without K^+,
in control medium (5mM-K^+), and in high K^+ (50 mM-K^+) medium
respectively.

    * Significantly different from control P < 0.01
    Averages of 5 experiments are shown (22).

Table 7.   Effects of Inhibition of Glycolytic and Mitochondrial
           Metabolism on Amino Acid Uptake

Inhibitor		Glucose Medium		SMP Medium	
		Glu	AIB	Glu	AIB
None		86	86	106	99
NaF	10mM	25	12	103	75
Iodoacetate	0.3mM	22	56	99	46
Rotenone	0.1µM	50	35	3	15
Antimycin A	0.5µM	40	40	15	28
Oligomycin	11µM	68	60	4	15

Uptake of glutamate and AIB in either normal glucose or SMP medium
in presence of different inhibitors is given as per cent of control
slices (29).

Hormone Effects

       Although endocrine effects on amino acid transport were studied
in a number of tissues and cells in some detail, only a few studies
have investigated transport in brain. This is perhaps due to the
fact that insulin, which affects transport in muscle, does not
influence cerebral amino acid transport. This is not surprising:
tissue specific effects of glucagon on amino acid transport have
been reported (30, 31, 32). In brain the effect of steroid
hormones was studied; in the young, but not in the adult, cerebral
amino acid uptake was increased (33, 34). Synaptosomal uptake was
decreased by thyroid hormone (35). Some endocrine effects may be
indirect, for example, by influencing ATP levels (36). Amino
acid metabolism may also be affected; steroids were found to affect
brain amino acid metabolism, especially of nonessential amino
acids (37).

       To study effects on cellular transport, we studied amino acid
uptake by brain slices in the presence of several hormones (38).
Some hormones that are active in other tissues, such as insulin and
glucagon, had no effect in brain slices. Only a few of those tried
had effects, and these were primarily when the amino acid concentration in the medium was kept low. Hydrocortisone, estradiol,
and progesterone stimulated uptake, and estradiol at higher concentrations caused a net release of tissue amino acid into the medium
(Table 8). The effects were specific in that uptake of only a
few amino acids was altered. The changes in tissue GABA were
especially large. In this case inhibition of metabolism more than
stimulation of uptake resulted in increased retention of the amino
acid. The results show that hormones affect membrane properties,
amino acid metabolism, and energy metabolism, and thereby may

affect amino acid transport indirectly as well as directly.

Table 8.   The Effect of Hormones on Amino Acid Uptake in Brain
           Slices

| Amino Acids | Uptake as per cent of control | | | |
| | Estradiol | | Progesterone | |
	0.05M	0.25M	0.05M	0.25M
Phenylalanine	141	56	103	111
GABA	126	67	180	290
Valine	142	51	112	127
Glutamate	144	27	118	126
Glycine	107	32	127	111

Mouse brain slices were incubated in HEPES medium for 30 min at 37°C, in the absence or presence of hormones; then respective ^{14}C-amino acid was added for an additional 60 min (38).

Nutritional Influence

        It is known that alteration of the levels of plasma acids
can result in changes in brain levels.   Increase of many different
acids in plasma, such as after a protein-rich meal, may not cause
an equivalent increase in brain, because of competitive inhibition
within the same transport class.   Dietary increase of a specific
amino acid such as the neurotransmitter precursor tryptophan can
result in a change in the brain content of the amino acid and its
neurotransmitter product can be of physiological and therapeutic
significance (39).   Changes during malnutrition or specific nutritional deficiencies have not been studied in detail.

        Mild nutritional deficiency has no significant effect on the
composition of the cerebral free amino acid pool (40), but prolonged
severe undernutrition results in changes.   Many amino acids,
especially the essential amino acids, decrease quantitatively; the
greatest change is a very large increase in histidine and homo-
carnosine.   Most but not all of the changes in mice were similar
to that observed in monkeys (41, 42).   In one experiment we compared
changes in the uptake of three amino acids with changes in their
level in the brain caused by protein-free diet.   The changes in
level and in uptake were parallel in that both increased with histidine, decreased with lysine, and remained unchanged with leucine
(Table 9).   In these experiments values were probably influenced
by changes not only in uptake but also in exit and in metabolism.

These experiments tested only a few compounds, under a single
condition; therefore general conclusions can not be drawn, but it
appears that severe undernutrition alters brain uptake of amino
acids in a specific way, which in turn results in changes in cerebral levels.

Table 9.   Effect of Protein-Free Diet on the Uptake of Amino Acids
           in Adult Mouse Brain

	Time Min	Uptake in experiment as per cent of control	Level as per cent of control
Histidine	20	140	340
	60	160	
Leucine	5	100	100
	20	110	
Lysine	5	82	74
	20	54	
Amino Isobutyric Acid	5	94	
	20	100	

Uptake is measured as brain to plasma concentration ratio.   The
amino acids were injected intraperitoneally in a dose sufficient
to increase brain levels 3-4 fold (42).

CONCLUSION

     Amino acid transport into and out of the brain under physio-
logical conditions seems to proceed at fairly constant rates and
is undoubtedly part of the homeostatic mechanisms maintaining the
metabolic environment.   Transport rates and transport systems,
however, are altered under a variety of conditions.   In general,
nutritional variations in plasma amino acid levels would not be
reflected in the brain;   affinity constant (K_m) of transport of
many amino acids is close to the value of plasma concentration,
that is, transport is near saturation levels not too dependent
on plasma concentration.   The fact that nutritional change similarly affects competing members of a transport class also results
in the competitive interactions minimzing changes in transport.
Undernutrition has significant effects; they seem to be variable,
decreasing the uptake of some and increasing that of other amino
acids.

The transport systems are not homogeneously distributed: regional heterogeneity in uptake and in the level of cerebral amino acids has been observed. Not all structures contain all transport systems. Less than half identified in brain could be detected in capillaries - therefore the properties of capillary transport are quite different - not only is the transport for some, e.g., GABA and proline, minimal, but in neutral transport a relatively Na^+ and energy-independent system predominates.

There are important changes during development: the systems for essential amino acids seem to develop earlier than the ones for neurotransmitter amino acids; some systems present early are diluted out or their properties change; most increase in activity.

The mechanisms that control transport activity are not known; changes in available energy, ions, ion gradient (primarily Na^+), and endocrine changes were observed to influence cerebral amino acid transport, but whether some are used for functional needs has not yet been established.

It is clear that transport plays a major role in determining, and at times altering, the level of the amino acid. The metabolic consequences of this are not well established: transmitter synthesis and amino acid metabolism are sensitive to concentration changes; protein synthesis seems less so.

REFERENCES

1.   Shaw, R.K. and Heine, J.D. (1965) J. Neurochem. 12:151-155.
2.   Himwich, W.A. and Agrawal, H.C. (1969) In: Handbook of Neurochemistry, Vol. I, Chapter 3, A. Lajtha, ed., pp. 33-52.
3.   Battistin L. and Lajtha, A. (1970) J. Neurol. Sci. 10:313-322.
4.   Kandera, J., Levi, G., and Levi, A. (1968) Arch. Biochem. Biophys. 126:249-260.
5.   Oldendorf, W.H. and Szabo, J. (1976) Am. J. Physiol. 230:94-98.
6.   Sershen, H. and Lajtha, A. (1979) J. Neurochem. 32:719-726.
7.   Emirbekov, E.Z., Sershen, H., and Lajtha A. (1977) Br. Res. 125:187-191.
8.   Sershen, H. and Lajtha, A. (1976) Exp. Neurology 53:465-474.
9.   Levi, G., Kandera, J, and Lajtha, A. (1967) Arch. Biochem. Biophys. 119:303-311.
10. Lajtha, A. and Toth, J. (1973) Brain Research 55:238-251.
11. Seta, K., Sershen, H. and Lajtha, A. (1972) Brain Research 47:415-425.
12. Sershen, H. and Lajtha, A. (1976) Neurochem. Res. 1:417-428.
13. Piccoli, F., Grynbaum, A., and Lajtha, A. (1971) J. Neurochem. 18:1135-1148.
14. Schultz, S.G. and Curran, P.F. (1970) Physiol. Rev. 50:637-718.

15. Margolis, R.K. and Lajtha, A. (1968) Biochim. Biophys. Acta
     163:374-385.
16. Lahiri, S. and Lajtha, A. (1964) J. Neurochem. 11:77-86.
17. Lajtha, A. and Sershen H. (1975) J. Neurochem. 24:667-672.
18. Christensen, H.N. (1975) In: Current Topics in Membranes and
     Transport, F. Bronner and A. Kleinzeller, eds., Academic Press,
     N.Y., pp. 227-258.
19. Wade, L.A. and Kutzman, R. (1975) J. Neurochem. 25:837-842.
20. Betz, A.L. and Goldstein, G.W. (1978) Science 202:225-227.
21. Lajtha, A. and Sershen, H. (1975) Brain Research 84:429-441.
22. Banay-Schwartz, M., Teller, D.N., Horn, B., and Lajtha, A.
     (1977) J. Neurochem. 29:403-410.
23. Sershen, H. and Lajtha, A. (1974) J. Neurochem. 22:977-985.
24. Banay-Schwartz, M., Gergely, A., and Lajtha, A. (1974) Brain
     Research 65:265-276.
25. Logan, W.J. and Snyder, S.H. (1972) Brain Res. 42:413-431.
26. Petersen, N.A. and Raghupathy, E. (1978) J. Neurochem. 31:989-
     996.
27. Banay-Schwartz, M., Piro, L., and Lajtha, A. (1971) Arch. Bio-
     chem. 145:199-210.
28. Banay-Schwartz, M., Teller, D.N., Gergely, and Lajtha, A. (1974)
     Br. Res. 71:117-131.
29. Teller, D.N., Banay-Schwartz, M., DeGuzman, T., and Lajtha, A.
     (1977) Brain Res. 131:321-334.
30. Wexler, B. and Katzman, R. (1975) Exp. Cell Res. 92:291-298.
31. Sparziani, E. (1975) Pharmac. Res. 27, 207-286.
32. Honoune, J., Chambaut, A.-M., Josipowicz, A. (1972) Arch.
     Biochem. Biophys. 148:180-184.
33. Litteria, M. (1977) Exp. Neurol. 57:817-827.
34. Litteria, M. (1977) Brain Res. 132:287-289
35. Verity, M.A., Brown, Cheung, M.K., and Czer, G.T. (1977) J.
     Neurochem. 29:853-858.
36. Young, D.A. (1969) J. Biol. Chem. 244:2210-2217.
37. Sadasivada, B., Rao, I.T., and Krishna Murthy, R.C. (1977)
     Neurochem. Res. 3:521-532.
38. Banay-Schwartz, M., Zanchin, G., DeGuzman, T, and Lajtha, A.
     (in press) Psychoneuroendocrinology
39. Wurtman, R.J. and Fernstrom, J.D. (1976) Biochem. Pharmacol.
     25:1691-1696.
40. Banay-Schwartz, M., Giuffrida, A.M., DeGuzman, T., Sershen,
     H., and Lajtha, A. (1979) Exp. Neurology 65:157-168.
41. Enwonwu, C.O. and Worthington, B.S. (1974) J. Neurochem. 22:
     1045-1052.
42. Toth, J. and Lajtha, A. (in preparation) The effect of protein-
     free diet on the uptake of amino acids by the brain in vivo.

TRANSPORT FUNCTIONS OF THE BLOOD-RETINAL BARRIER SYSTEM

AND THE MICRO-ENVIRONMENT OF THE RETINA

Laszlo Z. Bito and C. Jean DeRousseau

Laboratory of Ocular Physiology
Research Division, Department of Ophthalmology
College of Physicians and Surgeons
Columbia University, New York, N.Y. 10032 USA

1. Introduction

As we shall see, the blood-retinal barrier system consists of at least three topographically, morphologically and functionally distinct components. Experimental approaches to the demonstration and definition of ocular transport processes across various regions of this barrier system are manifold, and in most cases no single approach can prove the existence of transport. Yet, it appears that with the exception of dissolved gases, virtually all normal solutes and drugs enter into or are removed from the intraocular fluids (IOFs), including the extracellular fluids (ECFs) of the retina, by facilitated or active transport processes across the blood-aqueous and blood-retinal barriers. A complete review of this field is clearly beyond the scope of this article. We shall, therefore, focus on principles rather than details, and will present data and references which are illustrative rather than inclusive.

2. Sites of Passive Exchanges and Transport Processes

The blood-retinal barrier (BRB) is generally regarded as consisting of two components, the endothelium of retinal blood vessels ("inner barrier") and the retinal pigment(ed) epithelium ("outer barrier"). This is, however, an oversimplification. There are no diffusional barriers between the extracellular fluid (ECF) of the retina and the adjacent vitreous (89), nor does the vitreous body itself significantly hinder the diffusion of most solutes (77). Hence, there are free diffusional exchanges between the posterior chamber and retinal ECF, and the epithelia of the ciliary processes (see Section 2a), which serve as the barrier between the posterior chamber and blood, must also be regarded as part of the BRB system.

    2a. Ciliary processes.   Before the advent of electron microscopy and modern techniques of analytical chemistry, the ciliary processes and their secretion, the aqueous humor, were assumed to be very similar to the choroid plexus and its secretion, the cerebrospinal fluid (CSF; 44). Sometimes even a direct analogy between these two systems was advocated (104). However, information developed over the past decades indicates that these systems are not analogous on either physiological or morphological grounds.

    The chemical composition of aqueous is, in fact, grossly different from that of CSF (16, 22). This is not surprising if we consider that aqueous humor has a dual function; it not only provides a suitable chemical environment for the avascular ectodermal tissues, the lens, cornea and trabecular meshwork (16), but also contributes to the chemical composition of retinal ECF.

    Modern techniques capable of distinguishing cellular orientation and revealing different types of intercellular junctions also show that the ciliary processes are morphologically unique among secretory tissues, and are clearly different from the choroid plexus. While the choroid plexus is covered with a single layer of epithelium, the ciliary processes have two distinct epithelial cell layers in a unique apex-to-apex orientation. This orientation need not be regarded as a morphological oddity if these cell layers are considered to be two separate simple cuboidal epithelia. The deep layer should clearly be called the ciliary epithelium. However, the surface ("non-pigmented") layer whose basement lamina covers a connective tissue compartment, the posterior chamber, is more accurately regarded as the epithelium of the posterior chamber. The two cell layers, which appear to form a secretory unit, will be referred to here as the ciliary epithelia rather than epithelium. The "non-pigmented epithelial layer" by itself will be referred to as the epithelium of the posterior chamber and the pigmented layer as the epithelium of the ciliary stroma.

    The transport functions of the ciliary processes, which were originally deduced from observed differences between the chemical composition of aqueous humor and plasma dialysate (44), were demonstrated by in vitro "Ussing chamber" (33, 65) and accumulation studies (5, 55). A better understanding of the scope of these transport functions was achieved by analysis of aqueous humor collected from the posterior chamber, which more closely approxi-mates the composition of freshly secreted fluid (67), and by more detailed studies on the concentration gradients of solutes in the whole IOF system (20, 16). Literature on the transport functions of the ciliary processes (66), the mechanism of fluid production (36), and the chemical composition of the freshly secreted fluid (67, 16) has been reviewed extensively and will be dealt with here only in regard to the influence of these transport functions on the composition of retinal ECF.

2b. Retinal choroid. The choroid consists of a vascular network separated from a simple cuboidal epithelium (the "retinal pigment(ed) epithelium") by a thin layer of connective tissue, and as such, it is morphologically more analogous to the choroid plexus than are the ciliary processes. Indeed, the original description of this structure regarded the posterior uvea, Bruch's membrane and its epithelial covering as a unit, called the "tunica Ruyschiana" (52). Apparently, we can credit Kolliker in the late 19th century with confusing the nomenclature when he demonstrated that the pigmented epithelium is derived from the outer layer of the secondary optic vesicle. This finding led somehow to the conclusion that this epithelium belongs to the retina. However, an epithelium is not necessarily part of the structure whence it was derived; rather, it represents an integral part of the structure to which it is attached through its basal lamina.

In the case of the "retinal pigment(ed) epithelium", there is no morphological, physiological, physical, clinical or semantic basis for considering it to be separate from the choroid. Hogan, Alvarado, and Weddell (63) describe this epithelium as part of the retina, yet regard the "basement membrane of the retinal pigment epithelium" as part of the choroid. Even though Bloom and Fawcett (31) consider it "illogical to assign the pigment epithelium to the retina and its basal lamina to the choroid," they also continue to discuss this epithelium as a part of the retina. This terminology is not only illogical and morphologically untenable, but also mis-leading, and must have contributed to the reluctance of physiologists to study this "retinal" epithelium, which cannot be isolated with the retina from the underlying choroid.

In fact, this epithelium is clearly adherent to the choroid and, together with it, forms a structure which separates with ease from the "neuro-retina". Clinically, it is also the neuro-retina that separates in retinal detachment from the underlying epithelium, which remains firmly attached to the choroid (63). Finally, from a semantic point of view, the term choroid means 'resembling the chorion' (Oxford English Dictionary, 1971), i.e., the outermost, nutritive coat of the embryo which includes a vascular bed, con-nective tissue and a layer of epithelial cells (84). Thus, by any criteria, the epithelium that covers the choroid is correctly called the choroidal or chorioretinal rather than the retinal epithelium, and we will refer to it henceforth by one of these names. It should also be noted that since pigment granules are not a universal feature of these cells, e.g., regions of epithelium that lie in front of a tapetum lucidum are devoid of pigmentation (87, 69), the modifiers "pigment" or "pigmented" are also misleading.

Though these problems appear to be semantic, they are relevant to the understanding of the BRB system. By regarding this epithelium and the underlying connective tissue and vascular network as a unit, it immediately becomes apparent that the "choroid of the retina" refers to a secretory organ which is remarkably similar both morphologically and functionally to the choroid plexus of the brain: both consist of a single tight-junctional epithelial layer, characteristic apical microvilli projecting into an ECF space, and a basal lamina which is attached to connective tissue containing an extensive vascular bed (22). Regarding the choroid plexus of the brain and the choroid of the retina as analogous organs will greatly increase our understanding of the control of the chemical composition of retinal ECF by the choroidal BRB, since much is known about the diversity and orientation of the transport processes of the choroid plexus (22, 32, 88). Furthermore, this perspective orients the researcher to accept more readily the results of in vitro studies on the isolated retinal choroid, which heretofore has been referred to as a "retinal pigment epithelium-choroid preparation."

2c. Retinal vasculature. The tight-junctional endothelium of the euangiotic retina must be analogous to the capillaries of the brain and unquestionably represents a critically important and well-documented permeability barrier (43, 83). Any significant leakage at this site would clearly circumvent the whole BRB system. Morphological (EM, freeze fracture) and physiological (horseradish peroxidase and other molecular markers) studies (40, 41, 89), together with observations that the vitreous of all species studied has a very low concentration of plasma proteins and a solute composition greatly different from plasma ultrafiltrate (see Table 1), clearly demonstrate that the retinal vasculature is indeed an effective permeability barrier.

By analogy with the capillaries of the brain, whose transport functions are much better documented than those of the retina (11, 10), the endothelium of retinal capillaries undoubtedly transports a variety of solutes. Transport functions at this site are further suggested by the observation of Cunha-Vaz and Maurice (42) that fluorescein is removed from the vitreous across "retinal capillaries" of the rabbit eye as well as by experiments on the isolated vascular network of the bovine retina (9) in which transport machinery similar to that found in preparations of brain capillaries was demonstrated. However, in the retina, the proximity of the capillary bed to the choroid makes it nearly impossible to determine the site of transport in most in vivo studies, while the so-called "retinal capillaries" of rabbits which were examined by Cunha-Vaz and Maurice (42) cannot be taken as a typical example of euangiotic retinal capillaries (105). Furthermore, in vitro accumulation of substrates by isolated vascular tissues cannot be regarded as proof of transmembrane transport (see Section 3).

Table 1. Steady-state concentration (mM/kg H_2O) gradients within IOF compartments and between vitreous and blood plasma or plasma dialysate. (Based on values from references 12, 29 and 35).

	Plasma	Q_{dial}*	Aqueous (Aqu)	Vitreous (Vit)	Vit/Aqu	Vit/Plasma*
Chloride						
Human	109		134	114	0.85[+]	1.05[+]
Rabbit	108		100**	104	0.96[+]	0.97[+]
Sodium						
Human	176		163	144	0.88[+]	0.82[+]
Rabbit	143		159**	134	0.84[+]	0.94[+]
Calcium						
Rhesus	2.43	0.58	1.27**	1.31	1.03	0.93*
Cat	2.40	0.63	1.39**	1.61**	1.16	1.07*
Rabbit	3.11	0.67	1.74**	1.61**	0.93	0.78*
Magnesium						
Rhesus	0.62	0.75	0.65**	0.63	0.97	1.37*
Cat	0.98	0.71	0.45**	0.54**	1.20	0.86*
Rabbit	0.94	0.75	0.75**	1.08**	1.44	1.44*
Chicken	0.52	0.77	0.71	1.01**	1.42	2.53*
Potassium						
Rhesus	4.23	0.92	4.12**	3.55	0.86	0.91*
Cat	4.08	1.10	4.70**	4.99**	1.06	1.10*
Rabbit	4.57	0.95	4.69**	4.62**	0.99	1.06*
(aphakic)	4.21	0.95	3.75	3.30	0.88	0.83*
Bicarbonate						
Rabbit	24.9		34.1**	26.2	0.77[+]	1.05
Ascorbate						
Human	0.04		1.06	2.21	2.08[+]	52.6[+]
Cat			0.10	0.12	1.20[+]	
Rabbit	0.04		1.30**	0.46	0.35[+]	11.5
Glucose						
Human	6.33		3.00	3.44	1.15[+]	0.54[+]
Cat	5.96		4.55	3.17	0.70	0.56
Rabbit	8.14		5.60**	4.06	0.73[+]	0.50
Chicken	14.9		12.2	9.70**	0.80	0.65
Lactate						
Rabbit	10.3		9.30	7.22	0.77[+]	0.70[+]
Chicken	3.65		7.40	13.1**	1.77	3.59

*The dialysis quotient was calculated as plasma value divided by in vivo or in vitro plasma dialysate value. In all cases, when the dialysis quotient was available, vitreous/plasma-dialysate ratio rather than vitreous/plasma ratio is given.

**Fluid obtained from the posterior chamber, or from the posterior vitreous segment of enucleated, bisected mammalian globes, or, in the case of chickens, from liquid vitreous adjacent to the retina.

[+]Ratio calculated from values derived from two different sources.

    2d. Relative importance of the three transport sites.   Most
vertebrates do not have an intraretinal circulation, and even among
mammals an euangiotic retina is not a universal feature (105). Some
species possess an extensive preretinal vascular bed lying on the
vitreous or a small highly vascularized organ, a conus papillaris,
pecten or falciform process, protruding into the vitreous. Clearly,
in terms of the potential of retinal vasculature to influence the
chemical environment of a true euangiotic retina, as, for example,
in the human eye, transport activities of the capillary endothelium
could theoretically be more important than either of the other two
regions of the BRB system. On the other hand, a circulatory bed
which is limited to a few percent of the retinal surface, as is the
case in rabbit eyes (76), is unlikely to play an important role in
controlling the chemical environment of the entire retina.

    In contrast to retinal vasculature, which varies greatly among
species in extent, location, distribution and presumably in
function, all vertebrates have well-developed ciliary processes and,
with very few exceptions, retinal choroids. In all species studied,
cells covering these two vascular structures show the typical
morphological characteristics of secretory epithelia. Thus, it is
reasonable to generalize from the few species on which physiological
properties of these tissues have been well established and to regard
the retinal choroid and the ciliary processes as the two universal
components of the mammalian BRB transport system. Although evidence
on transluminal transport function by retinal capillaries is very
limited, so that transport at this site remains almost entirely
presumptive and dependent on analogies to the brain, apparent
transport across this barrier will also be discussed.

    2e. Vitreous.   To understand the relationship between the
retina and vitreous, the vitreous may be regarded as one of the
great cisterns of the brain. In the case of the brain, cisternal
volumes are generally small relative to the depth of adjacent tissues. This suggests that the retina has a privileged position in
that it is a thin brain tissue adjacent to a large cistern. The
vitreous provides the retina with a very large "emergency reservoir"
which contains sufficient nutrients to supply its short-term
metabolic needs and acts as a sink for potentially harmful metabolic
end-products during acute ischemia (16, 29). The vitreous may also
be regarded as a lymphatic drainage route for the retina (16).

    2f. Nomenclature and Summary. Diffusion is a physico-chemical
term directly applicable to dilute solutions or gels. Thus, we can,
in general, refer to diffusion of substances through the vitreous;
this subject is dealt with in detail in another chapter (77).
However, in all other parts of the eye, the movement of solutes can
be expected to be affected by bulk fluid flow (see section 4h),
fixed charges and/or specific transport processes across permeability barriers. The observation that a solute or a marker has moved

in a tissue or fluid compartment from point A to point B must not be interpreted as evidence of diffusion unless it can be specifically shown that this movement is not accounted for by a bulk displacement of the solvent, is non-saturable and, in general, obeys the laws of diffusion.

By transport we shall here refer to saturable (facilitated, carrier-mediated or active) processes that require some intervention as opposed to diffusion and flow which are unaided, unsaturable processes. For example, water in the Tejo River flows downstream to Lisbon, while drinking water may be transported upstream in barges. Shipping water up-river would be an energy-requiring process; in biological terminology, we would refer to it as active transport. Movement of barges down the river would not require energy; thus, it is not an active process. Nevertheless, it is certainly transport, and carrier-mediated transport at that. Thus, we will use the term transport any time there is substantial evidence that movement of a solute is mediated by a specific, saturable mechanism. If there is evidence that this transport is taking place against a chemical concentration gradient and/or it is energy-dependent, we shall refer to it as active transport.

We shall refer here to net transport of any given solute across a blood-tissue barrier from blood to an extracellular fluid compartment as secretory transport, and to a net flux from extra-cellular fluid to blood as absorptive transport. Such transport processes occur across all regions of the blood-retinal barrier system, namely, the tight-junctional retinal capillaries, i.e., the endothelial BRB (inner barrier); the choroidal or chorioretinal epithelium, i.e., the choroidal BRB (outer barrier); and the ciliary processes, i.e., the ciliary BRB. We shall refer to the first two of these together as the blood-retinal barriers (BRBs) and to all three collectively as the blood-retinal barrier system (BRB system).

The choroidal and ciliary BRBs are proven and universal sites of secretory and absorptive transport processes both facilitated and active. The endothelial BRB is, for the most part, a presumptive site of transport functions. In addition, net solute fluxes between retinal ECF and glial elements, and diffusional exchanges between the vitreous and the retinal ECF must play an important role in retinal homeostasis. This latter mechanism may be of primary importance under conditions such as ischemia, when transport processes to and from the circulation are not functional.

3. Methods for Studying the Transport Functions of the BRB System

3a. In vivo evidence for transport. The presence of concen-tration gradients within the IOFs and between IOFs and blood

represents the best physiological criteria for the existence and
direction of transport processes across the BRBs (16).   This
approach is particularly applicable to inert solutes, i.e. substances which are not formed in, or chemically altered by,
surrounding tissues.

It should not be assumed, however, that transport takes place
across the particular region of the barrier system where a concentration gradient is measured. For example, it may be found that the
concentration of K^+ is higher in vitreous adjacent to the retina
than in plasma. This would imply secretory transport across the
BRBs only if it were found that the K^+ concentration is lower in the
posterior chamber than in the vitreous near the retina. In fact, as
we shall see (see section 4b), the opposite is true in most species
implying that K^+ transport across the BRBs is absorptive, not
secretory. Thus, elucidation of the sites of transport processes
from in vivo distribution gradients requires detailed information on
the concentrations of the substance in question within all regions
of the IOF system.

In vivo studies of the steady-state distribution of isotopically labeled solutes and/or measurement of non-steady-state
isotope fluxes can also provide important and sometimes definitive
information on the sites and direction of transport across the
blood-ocular barriers, particularly when a non-metabolized,
biologically inert analogue of the natural substrate (e.g., cycloleucine or 3-0-methyl glucose) is used. These and other non-steady-
state experiments, such as the incubation of enucleated globes in
moist chambers in which the possibility of transport to or from the
blood is eliminated (26), are also useful for clarifying the
contribution of metabolism to the distribution of non-inert
substances. These techniques permit study of the effects of
substrate concentration (saturation), the inhibition of transport by
chemically related compounds (competition), the effects of metabolic
inhibitors (energy dependency) and the transport of structurally
related tracers (selectivity).

Conversely, the rate of loss of intravitreally injected tracers
from the eye can also be used as an indication of facilitated
transport processes across the BRB system. This approach is most
effective when the loss of a putative transport substrate is
directly compared to the rate of loss of a simultaneously injected
tracer of similar molecular weight which is known not to be a
substrate for transport processes (27).

These approaches have been used extensively to elucidate the
permeability and transport properties of the anterior uvea (44, 67),
but only very recently have they been directed primarily toward
clarifying the properties of the BRBs (91, 16).

3b. In vitro evidence for transport. It has been well established that tissues that have secretory or absorptive transport
functions, such as the kidney cortex (37), choroid plexus (39, 88),
or anterior uvea (4), tend to accumulate certain substances in vitro
against an apparent concentration gradient, i.e., yielding tissue-
to-medium (T/M) accumulation ratios greater than unity. Incubation
of tissues with isotopically labeled substrates thus provides a
means to survey large numbers of tissues for transport activity, to
screen for inhibitors, or to study the specificity and kinetics of a
transport system. Such in vitro accumulation techniques have been
used successfully in studies on the anterior uvea for two decades
(5), but have only recently been applied to isolated preparations of
the retinal vasculature (9, 62) and choroid (17).

Interpretation of the concentrative accumulation of some substances, such as those which are normally present in high concentrations in all cells (e.g. potassium and amino acids) or solutes
which can be incorporated into macromolecules or chemically altered,
may be ambiguous or require chemical identification of the accumulated tracer. In general, in vitro concentrative accumulation
should be regarded as only an initial indication of transmembrane
transport, which must then be supported by other in vivo or in vitro
evidence.

Accurate in vitro transmembrane tracer-flux measurements under
short-circuited conditions represent the ultimate proof of, and the
best means for quantifying any transmembrane transport system and
its energy dependence. Modifications of the classical Ussing
chamber, first developed to study electrolyte transport across the
frog skin (102), have been used to measure the electrolyte transport
functions of the anterior uvea (33, 64, 65) and, more recently, the
retinal choroid (71, 79, 96, 106). It must be borne in mind,
however, that the trauma of the isolation procedure and the altered
electrochemical environment may well alter permeability and
transport processes. Thus, even the most rigorous in vitro study
must be supported by in vivo observations before its physiological
significance can be considered.

4.   Active and Facilitated Transport of Solutes
Across the BRB System

The steady-state distribution of the major solutes in the
aqueous, vitreous and blood plasma of a variety of species is
presented in Table 1. As can be seen, many solutes show significant
concentration differences between IOF compartments and/or between
these compartments and blood plasma or blood plasma dialysate.
Although there is considerable variation among species, some typical
patterns are readily apparent.

4a. Sodium, chloride and bicarbonate. These are the major electrolytes in all ECFs, and one or more of these ions is clearly involved with aqueous production in any given species (36). These are also among the best studied ions with respect to the transport function of the ciliary processes (36, 66, 74) and the retinal choroid (96). There is, however, no indication that retinal ECF is uniquely different from the ECFs of other tissues with respect to the concentration of these ions.

Since sodium makes such a large contribution to the total osmolality of ECFs, its concentration in a typical ECF is unlikely to differ by more than a few percent from that of plasma and, since the concentration of sodium is well controlled in the blood, a need for further control at the BRB level is not evident. Furthermore, a rapid osmotic flux of water was found to occur across the blood-brain barrier (54) and can be expected to occur across the BRB system. Thus, a net sodium flux across the BRBs sufficient to cause an osmotic gradient would result in a net water flux (see section 4h) rather than in a significant steady-state ionic gradient across these barriers.

The highest osmolality within the IOFs is found in the posterior chamber, where freshly secreted fluid is clearly hyper-osmotic to plasma (Fig. 1). The osmolality of the vitreous is lowest near the retina, suggesting that the ECF of the retina is iso-osmotic with, or may even be hypo-osmotic to plasma. These osmotic gradients mitigate against net secretion of major electrolytes or net osmotic fluid flow into the retinal ECFs through the BRBs, but are consistent with an absorptive transport of some major solutes at these sites associated with limited osmotic water flow from retinal ECF to blood.

Since chloride and bicarbonate are the two major anions, their total concentration in any ECF must match the total cation concentration, and hence must essentially be fixed. However, the chloride-to-bicarbonate ratios in the aqueous, for example, do show significant species variations (47). Limited data on the vitreous indicates that both pH (95) and bicarbonate ion concentrations (45), especially near the retina, are generally lower than those of aqueous. This may be due to acid production by the retina (44), although in vitro studies indicate the existence of net, possibly seasonally variable, bicarbonate and/or chloride fluxes across the amphibian choroidal epithelium (96).

4b. Potassium. Potassium is one of the most precisely controlled electrolytes in the ECF of the brain (22, 32), and its concentration in CSF, especially in the sub-arachnoid space and, hence, presumably in the ECF of the cortex, is much lower than the simultaneously measured plasma K^+ concentration (21). One would expect, therefore, that the retina also requires a low and well-

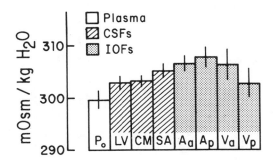

Fig. 1. Steady-state gradient of osmolality in the IOFs of dogs. Osmolalities of blood plasma and CSFs are also given for comparison. The freezing point depression of all samples was measured with an Advanced Osmometer (Advanced Instruments, Inc.). Abbreviations: LV, CM and SA represent CSF taken from the lateral ventricle, cisterna magna and the cortical subarachnoid space, respectively; P=plasma, A=aqueous, V=vitreous. Subscript o refers to the beginning of sample collection; a and p indicate anterior and posterior, respectively. Anterior and posterior segments of vitreous were obtained by rapid bisection of the freshly enucleated globe. Limits are S.E. of the mean; $n \geq 6$. (Modified from Bito, 1977; see reference 16).

controlled K^+ milieu.

Unfortunately, based on K^+ flux measurements on in situ "open eye" preparations, Noell (81) suggested the existence of an active K^+ transport from blood through the retina into the vitreous, a concept which was supported by the high vitreal K^+ value (9.5 mmoles/kg H_2O) reported by Reddy and Kinsey (92). This model, which Noell himself regarded as tentative, implied that K^+ concentration in the ECF of the retina was much higher than that in any other region of the brain. More recent studies on several mammals, including rabbits (12, 20), show that the K^+ concentration in the vitreous is much lower than that reported by Reddy and Kinsey, and, in fact, that the K^+ concentration in the posterior segment of the vitreous adjacent to the retina is typically lower than that in the anterior region of the vitreous (Fig. 2B).

To investigate the steady-state distribution of K^+ without the complicating factor of translenticular K^+ fluxes, which may modify

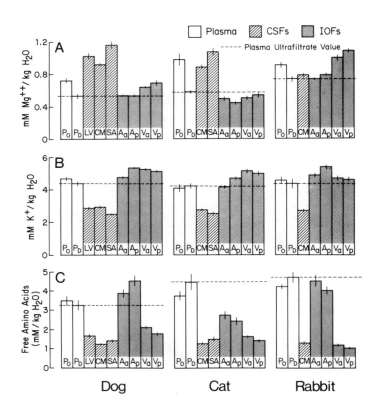

Fig. 2. Steady-state concentration gradients of magnesium, potassium and free amino acids within the IOFs of three mammalian species in relation to their concentration in blood plasma or plasma ultrafiltrate. Concentrations in CSFs are also given for comparison. Subscript D refers to measured or estimated dialysis value. For explanations of other abbreviations, see legend to Fig. 1. (Modified from Bito, 1977; see reference 16).

K^+ distribution within the IOFs (20), similar studies were done on rabbit eyes several weeks after the surgical removal of the lens (29). The concentration of K^+ in the vitreous of these long-term aphakic eyes was found to be 22% lower than that of the contralateral phakic eyes, well below that of aqueous and plasma dialysate K^+ concentrations and, in fact, very similar to that of CSF. These findings can only be accounted for by a net K^+ flux from the ECF of the retina to the blood across the BRBs. Since this flux is against a concentration gradient, the endothelial and/or the choroidal BRBs must have an active, absorptive K^+ transport function (16). Absorptive transport of K^+ across the chorioretinal epithelium is supported by in vitro experiments on the frog choroid (96), and there is reason to believe that the mammalian choroid is functionally similar to that of the frog (97). It should be noted that the rate of K^+ transport across the choroidal epithelium may vary with the physiological state of the retina (82).

Recent experiments on preparations of isolated bovine retinal vessels indicate that the endothelial BRB may also have a transmural K^+ transport function (9). As was pointed out in section 3, such in vitro studies cannot by themselves be regarded as proof of in vivo transport. However, in vivo evidence strongly suggests that cerebral capillaries have a transmural absorptive K^+ transport activity (21, 22), so that similar transport across retinal capillaries might be expected to occur.

4c. Calcium and Magnesium. Ca^{++} concentration in the IOFs is close to the measured or calculated plasma dialysate Ca^{++} concentration, and concentration gradients of this cation within the IOFs are, in general, small. This suggests that freshly-secreted aqueous has a Ca^{++} concentration similar to that of plasma ultrafiltrate and that there is little or no further net Ca^{++} flux across other regions of the BRB system. However, in Ussing chamber experiments on frog choroid, Miller and Steinberg (80) found a net Ca^{++} flux of 5.9 nM/cm^2 per hr oriented toward the retina. At present, the significance of this observation is not clear.

In dog and rabbit IOFs, Mg^{++} concentrations show the following relationships: posterior vitreous > anterior vitreous > plasma dialysate > posterior aqueous ≈ anterior aqueous. All cat IOFs have a curiously low Mg^{++} concentration, lower than plasma dialysate. Still, even in this species, the Mg^{++} concentration in the vitreous near the retina is significantly higher than that of the posterior aqueous (Fig. 2A; 16). The IOFs of chickens show even more pronounced Mg^{++} concentration gradients and higher Mg^{++} concentrations near the retina (98). Mg^{++} is present in similarly high concentrations in the CSF of all mammals studied and may be involved with the moderation of central excitability (11, 32).

Since there are no _in vitro_ studies on Mg^{++} fluxes across any region of the BRB system, the site of Mg^{++} transport processes can only be postulated on the basis of _in vivo_ steady-state Mg^{++} concentration gradients. The following is a working hypothesis of Mg^{++} transport systems in the eye: In most vertebrates, but certainly in all mammals, active secretory transport of Mg^{++} across the choroidal epithelium, and perhaps across the retinal vessels, maintains a Mg^{++} concentration in the ECF of the retina that is significantly greater than that of plasma dialysate or freshly secreted aqueous. In species that do not have an euangiotic retina, the Mg^{++} level in the whole vitreous tends to be elevated in order to maintain a high Mg^{++} concentration in the ECF of inner retinal layers. This may be accomplished by the active secretion of Mg^{++} into the vitreous by the choroid, by preretinal blood vessels, or by a pecten or similar vascular structure which projects into the vitreous of some birds, reptiles and fishes.

Alternatively, in euangiotic retinas, active secretory transport by the choroid could be combined with some reabsorption of Mg^{++} by retinal capillaries located near the inner retinal surface, so that a high intraretinal Mg^{++} concentration would be maintained with little or no elevation in the Mg^{++} concentration of the vitreous. Such mechanisms could account for the low vitreal Mg^{++} concentration observed in the cat eye without necessarily implying that the ECF of the feline retina has a uniquely low Mg concentration. However, the possibility that the ECF of the retina of cats and other nocturnal animals is deficient in Mg^{++} may also be considered since low retinal Mg^{++} levels may maintain the retina in a more readily excitable state.

4d. Ascorbic acid. Because ascorbic acid is actively transported by the ciliary processes into the posterior chamber (7), its concentration in the aqueous humor of most species, including man, is very high (10-25 mg/100 ml), as much as 30 times that of blood plasma (45). Although its concentration in the vitreous was stated to be lower than that of aqueous (44), in guinea pigs (59) and in both hibernating and normothermic woodchucks (25), the concentration of ascorbic acid has been found to be somewhat higher in the vitreous than in the aqueous.

In some other species, the aqueous ascorbate concentration is relatively low, and in rats it was reported to be non-detectable (45). Yet, the vitreous of even this species has a measurable amount of ascorbic acid (35); its retina contains a very high concentration of ascorbate (61), comparable to that of other mammals (59), and accumulates ascorbic acid against a concentration gradient _in vitro_ (60).

Thus, active ascorbic acid transport into the IOFs may be related primarily to some requirement of the retina. Some species may achieve a high retinal ascorbic acid concentration by elevating the ascorbic acid level in all IOFs, while other species, especially those that have an euangiotic retina, may do so by local transport across the BRBs and/or into cellular compartments. Studies on ascorbic acid transport across the endothelial or choroidal BRBs and more detailed studies on steady-state ascorbic acid concentration gradients within the IOF of mammals other than the rabbit will be required before the site(s) and physiological significance of ocular transport of this vitamin can be established.

4e. Glucose. We tend to assume that glucose must be transported from blood into the ECFs of both the brain and retina in order to serve the nutritional needs of these metabolically active organs. While there is clearly a facilitated transport of glucose from capillaries into the brain (73), glucose in the CSF is maintained at a value approximately 40% below that of blood plasma (72). This may be accounted for in part by active absorptive glucose transport from CSF into the circulation (38, 86). Such complex transport systems may be required in order to supply the metabolic needs of neural tissue while preventing build-up of high levels of glucose in the surrounding ECF during episodes of hyperglycemia.

A similar situation may also exist in the eye. Under normal steady-state conditions, the glucose concentrations of the aqueous and vitreous are approximately 20% and 50% below that of blood plasma, respectively (45). Because these low values cannot be wholly accounted for by the metabolic activities of the lens (29), it is reasonable to postulate that retinal metabolism may also be responsible for the normally low vitreal glucose concentration. That the retina can use glucose derived from the vitreous is clearly indicated by the rapid decrease in vitreal glucose concentration in both aphakic and phakic globes during ischemia (29).

These findings imply that under steady-state conditions, there must be a rapid flux of glucose into the posterior chamber. However, since glucose concentration in the posterior chamber is slightly below or equal to the plasma value (46, 92), there is no evidence that this secretory transport normally occurs against a concentration gradient. Based on these considerations and on _in vivo_ isotope flux studies (50, 51), we can only conclude that glucose transport into the IOFs is a saturable, facilitated process.

In _vitro_ studies on isolated bull frog retinal choroid have so far yielded conflicting results. Zadunaisky and Degnan (106) found a net, phloridzin-sensitive flux of 3-0-methyl-D-glucose and D-glucose from the blood side to the retinal side through the frog choroid. Since Miller and Steinberg (78) were unable to confirm these findings, more work on choroidal glucose transport is clearly indicated. Special attention should be paid to the possibility that at least under certain conditions, such as during hyperglycemia, transport of glucose at this site may be absorptive (from retina to choroid) rather than secretory.

Experiments on isolated brain capillaries show a mediated glucose accumulation (10); isolated blood vessels of bovine retina show a similar capacity to accumulate hexoses (9). Whether this accumulation reflects an absorptive or secretory transport across the endothelial BRB remains to be established (see section 3).

4f. Amino Acids. The pioneering work of Lajtha and his co-workers (70) on amino acid fluxes across the blood-brain barrier and between various compartments of the brain itself has revealed a complex system of transport processes. A similar, if not more complex situation exists in the eye.

As is the case with CSF (72), most amino acids are present in the vitreous, especially in the posterior segment, at a concentration much below that of blood plasma or plasma dialysate (16). In fact, the total amino acid concentration (non-protein alpha-amino nitrogen) of the posterior segment of the vitreous is only a fraction of that of blood plasma and is very similar to that of CSF (Fig. 2C; 16). The implied fact that the ECF of both the retina and brain have similar and very low amino acid levels is not surprising if we consider that many amino acids are neurotransmitters or "false transmitters," so that their concentration in the ECF of neuronal tissue must be limited in order to prevent interference with normal neuronal function.

Reddy and co-workers (93, 94) have clearly shown that there is secretory transport of amino acids into the posterior chamber of the eye and absorptive amino acid transport from the vitreous to blood across the BRBs. In some species, secretory transport of some amino acids across the ciliary epithelium appears to be an active process; in other species, some, and possibly all amino acids may enter the posterior aqueous by facilitated transport (23, 90).

Other in vivo experiments (91) on accumulation of amino acids in the vitreous of normal and sodium iodate-treated rabbits indicate that there is absorptive transport of amino acids across the BRBs located primarily at the choroidal epithelium. Measured fluxes of L-methionine and especially of taurine across the frog choroid, which were greater from the apical to basal than from the basal to apical side (78), support this conclusion. Ouabain-sensitive amino acid uptake into isolated blood vessels of the bovine retina has also been observed (9), suggesting that the endothelial cells of retinal vessels, like cells in general, transport amino acids. To what extent this transport contributes to the net flux of amino acids into or out of the retinal ECF (see section 3) is yet to be determined.

It is safe to conclude that amino acids are transported into the IOFs by the ciliary processes and are continually removed from the IOFs by an active transport process across the choroidal regions of the BRB and perhaps across the endothelial regions as well. The possibility that some amino acids enter the retina through facilitated transport across one or both of these BRBs, as well as through diffusion from the vitreous, must also be considered.

4g. The removal of potentially harmful substances from ocular ECFs. Since the first demonstration that some organic acids are removed from the eye by the ciliary processes (5, 55), the so-called organic acid transport system of the anterior uvea has been shown to consist of several separate but overlapping subsystems (1, 2, 4), and a very large number of other substances have been implicated as substrates for such transport processes (Table 2A). Since most of these putative substrates are not produced in the body, and since some of them have, in fact, only recently been synthesized, the physiological role of these absorptive transport processes has been repeatedly questioned (Kinsey, in discussion of paper by Forbes and Becker, 55; 34).

More recently, it has been found that a class of biologically active substances, the prostaglandins (PGs), which are produced but not inactivated or destroyed by intraocular tissues, and which have an adverse affect on the eye when allowed to accumulate in the IOFs, are substrates for the absorptive transport functions of the blood-ocular barriers (13, 14, 17). Concentrative PG accumulation by in vitro anterior uvea obeys Michaelis-Menten kinetics (48) and is not dependent on chemical alteration or incorporation of the PG molecule (18). Furthermore, PG accumulation is inhibited by probenecid and a variety of other organic acids and by conditions that limit the availability of metabolic energy (17). It should be noted that thromboxane (TXB_2) and prostacyclin (PGI_2) are also accumulated by most PG transporting tissues, including the anterior uvea (49).

Intravitreally injected ^{3}H-$PGF_{2\alpha}$ and ^{14}C-sucrose are lost from the in vivo eye with half-times of 3 and 15 hr, respectively, and essentially none of the ^{3}H, but all of the ^{14}C activity passes through the anterior chamber (27). Because the basic cell membrane, such as that of the rabbit erythrocyte, is completely impermeable to E and F PGs (19), and because the existence of transmembrane PG transport has been demonstrated in other in vitro and in vivo systems (17), it is safe to conclude that PGs are removed from the eye by facilitated or active transport processes.

Yet, such a short half-time of elimination of intravitreally injected PGs cannot be accounted for by diffusion into the posterior chamber and removal by the ciliary processes. Instead, these results suggest the existence of facilitated or active absorptive transport across the BRBs (27). Preliminary experiments in our

Table 2. Demonstrated, putative or predicted substrates of the
absorptive, detoxifying transport system of the anterior uvea
and/or retinal choroid.

A. A partial list of substances which are actively accumulated by
the anterior uvea or which inhibit the concentrative accumulation
of another substrate by this tissue.

Substance	References	Substance	References
Acetazolamide	5	Iopanoic acid	3
Benzmalacene	5	Nalidixic acid	3
Bromcresol green	3,28	Naproxen	28
Bromthymol blue	3,5	Norobiocin	3
Chenodeoxycholate	4	Oxybenbutazone	28
Cephalothin acid	3	PAH (p-aminohippurate)	99,5,6,3
Chlorothiazide	5	Penicillin	5
Cholic acid	3,100	Perchlorate	6
Deoxycholate	4	Phenolsulfonphthalin	5
Fluoroborate	6	Phenylbutazone	28
Fursemide	28	Pirprofen	28
Glychocholate	4	Probenecid	3,5,99,24,28
Glycodeoxycholic	3	Prostaglandins	13,18,27
Ibuprofen	28	Prostacyclin	17,49
Indomethacin	24,28	Pyrazinoic acid	3
Iodide	6	Thiocyanate	6
Iodipamide	4,24	Thromboxane-B_2	17,49
Iodohippurate	4	Sulfobromophthalin	3
Iodopyracet	5	Urate	5

B. Some other substrates which are actively accumulated by the
choroid plexus, and thus, by analogy can be assumed to be
substrates for the detoxifying transport processes of the anterior
uvea and/or retinal choroid.

Atropine	88	Lysergic acid	
c-AMP	58	diethylamide	88
Choline	39,72	Methotrexate	39,72
Decamethonium	39	Methylatropine*	88
Dextrophan	39,88	Morphine*	39,88
Dihydromorphine	39,88	Nalorphine	39,88
Folate	72	Nicotinamide	39
Hexamethonium	39	Norepinephrine	39
Homovanillic acid	32,72	Phenol red	32
5-Hydroxyindole-		Serotonin	39
acetic acid	39,72	Thiosulfate	39,88
Levorphan	39,88	Xanthine	39

*In vitro accumulation of these substances may not reflect their
in vivo absorptive transport (72).

laboratory (DiBenedetto and Bito, unpublished results; 17) indicate that the isolated rabbit choroid or choroid attached to the sclera, indeed accumulates ^{3}H-PG against a concentration gradient.   This accumulation, like accumulation by the choroid plexus, is inhibited by probenecid or bromcresol green, suggesting that the retinal choroid does indeed have a PG transport function similar to that of the choroid plexus or anterior uvea.

Although there is no direct evidence of active or facilitated PG transport across the endothelial BRB, recent results of Betz and Goldstein (9) on isolated bovine retinal blood vessel preparations suggest that this vascular endothelium also possesses an organic acid transport system. Furthermore, Cunha-Vaz and Maurice (42) have observed that intravitreally injected fluorescein is removed by the "retinal capillaries" of the rabbit eye.   Since there is reason to believe that PAH, fluorescein and PGs are all substrates for the same organic acid transport complex (17), it is reasonable to conclude that PGs and related compounds such as TxB_2 and prostacyclin are transported across the endothelial BRB as well as across the choroidal BRB and the ciliary epithelia.

The physiological significance of ocular PG transport has been demonstrated by experiments which show that the adverse effects of intravitreally injected PGE_1 on retinal function, as measured by ERG and VER, are greatly enhanced by the systemic pre-treatment of rabbits with PG transport inhibitors (103).   Since accumulation of PGs in the aqueous humor is associated with anterior uveitis and probably contributes to its onset (53), rapid and efficient removal of PGs across the BRB system can also be expected to have significance with regard to the anterior segment of the eye.

Under normal conditions, PGs produced by the retina as a consequence of normal neuronal activity would be rapidly removed across the BRBs.   Any PGs that elude this transport and hence diffuse into the vitreous would be prevented from entering the anterior chamber by the absorptive transport activity of the ciliary processes (27).   It has been found, however, that following one episode of severe uveitis, there can be a long-term and possibly permanent blockade of anterior uveal PG transport capacity (15).   In a like manner, local inflammation and/or other pathologies may block other sites of PG transport, including the endothelial or choroidal BRBs. Such blockade of local PG transport can be expected to render ocular tissues more vulnerable to local PG accumulations and hence may account for the progressive or recurrent nature of some ocular disorders.

There are several other substances of biological importance which are actively accumulated by the anterior uvea in vitro and/or were found to be effective inhibitors of the accumulation of other compounds.   These substances can be expected to be transport substrates themselves (Table 2B).   Two of them, penicillin and indomethacin, are worthy of special note, since absorptive transport of these substances may hinder their therapeutic delivery into the eye.

Penicillin was found to inhibit the concentrative accumulation of iodopyracet by the rabbit anterior uvea (5) and thus it is likely to be a substrate for the organic acid transport system of this tissue.   However, direct experimental evidence seems to be lacking. Rapoport (88) quotes a paper by Goldman, McLain and Smith (57) as having shown that accumulation of penicillin in the aqueous is enhanced by probenecid.   However, that paper only contains results on the effect of probenecid on aqueous humor ampicillin titers, and does not provide data on the effects of probenecid on blood levels of either of these drugs.   Therefore, we cannot draw any conclusions from this paper concerning ocular transport of these antibiotics.

Indomethacin was found to inhibit anterior uveal PG accumulation, and ^{14}C-indomethacin itself is concentratively accumulated by the rabbit anterior uvea in vitro (28).   However, actual transmembrane transport of indomethacin has not been demonstrated in any organ system.   Indeed, even in vivo evidence of rapid indomethacin removal from the eye would not be convincing since cell membranes appear to be highly permeable to this drug (19).

More recently, it has been shown that tetrahydrocannabinol is also accumulated by the isolated rabbit anterior uvea and rapidly lost from IOFs (68).   The significance of this finding is questionable since it was not considered that cellular barriers may be sufficiently permeable to this drug to allow its rapid loss from the IOFs by passive diffusion.

In summary, there is substantial evidence that the ciliary processes and the choroidal BRB, and circumstantial evidence that the endothelial BRB have absorptive transport processes which are capable of removing potentially harmful substances from the ECFs of the eye.   While a large number of substances are potential substrates for these transport system(s), most substances tested thus far are not produced within the eye and are not normally present in the circulation.   With the exception of studies on the PG transport system, there have been no attempts to demonstrate that these transport processes have a physiological function.   Further in vivo and in vitro studies on these absorptive transport processes will be required in order to better understand ocular pharmacokinetics and the detoxification mechanisms responsible for maintaining a normal chemical environment within the retina.

4h. Water flow and solute movements within the retina.   In mammalian eyes, the ciliary processes are primarily responsible for net fluid production, and there is a bulk outflow through the anterior chamber. In other vertebrate eyes, specializations of the retinal and/or optic nerve circulation, such as the pecten, conus capillaris or falciform process, which are very different from retinal capillaries in their fine structure and in permeability properties (8), may also play an important role in total IOF production. In the avian eye, for example, there is a continuous layer of liquid vitreous around much of the pecten and in front of the retina. The possibility that this liquid vitreous is produced by the pecten and flows over the retinal surface must be considered, especially since there is some evidence that the pecten has transport functions (30, 98).

The existence of fluid flow from the posterior chamber through the vitreous and retina has been considered by several authors. Such meridional flow was described in the rabbit eye by Fowlks, Havener and Good (56), but was never confirmed or quantified. This flow, as well as fluid absorption in repair processes following retinal detachment or following experimental introduction of fluid into the subretinal "space" is assumed to result from the transport activities of the "retinal pigment epithelium" (107, 75). However, this cell layer should not be regarded as the only possible source of fluid transport in the retina. In fact, significant fluid movements could occur within the retina even without a net fluid flux between the vitreous and choroidal circulation.

Since the net amount of uptake or loss of H_2O across plasma membranes must differ in different regions of polarized cells, the Muller cells, which span most of the depth of the retina, could by themselves cause a continuous fluid flow through the retinal ECF. For example, a net flux of H_2O from the subretinal space into the distal processes of the Muller cells would, under steady-state conditions, result in an equal volume of H_2O loss across some other region of the Muller cells. A net H_2O flux into the vitreous across these cell processes and the consequent net intracellular H_2O flow could be equalized by a net flow in the opposite direction through extracellular pathways (Fig. 3A). Water movements within and across the retina must be further complicated by metabolic processes which can use or produce H_2O, and by movement of free or bound H_2O from or toward the perikaryon due to axoplasmic flow.

Local bidirectional fluid movements both within the cells and in the ECF compartments must also occur as a result of the ocular pulse transmitted primarily from the choroid, and/or as a result of cellular motility. Thus, the ECF compartment of the retina should not be regarded as narrow tortuous channels through which solutes pass by diffusion alone, but rather as a rapidly moving and highly dynamic system of continuously changing dimensions. The pattern of fluid flow depicted in Fig. 3A is only an example, and in fact, the direction and/or rate of H_2O fluxes across any given region of the retina can be expected to be affected by metabolic activity, state

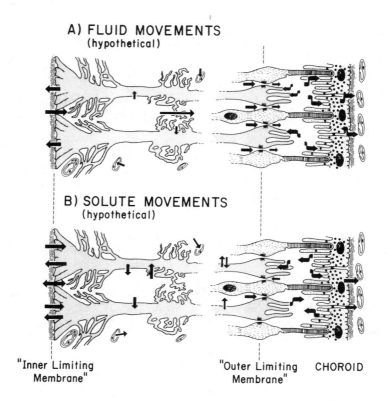

Fig. 3. Fluid (A) and solute (B) movements through the retina.
For simplicity, only the choroidal epithelium, some capillaries
and portions of Muller cells and photoreceptors are shown. Arrows
indicate some hypothetical sites where net fluxes may occur. See
text for details.

of stimulation, hormonal influences, pathological state, etc.

Intraretinal fluid flow in regions of restricted ECF passage, such as the "external limiting membrane" (which should really be called the external band of junctional complexes), must produce region(s) of negative tissue pressure relative to the surrounding areas. Under the hypothetical conditions described above (Fig. 3A), a region of low tissue pressure would occur in the subretinal space. Such low tissue pressure may contribute to and, in fact, could account for the maintenance of an apparent adherence between the retina and choroid. Reversal of the flow patterns through the Muller cells and/or through the choroidal epithelium could result in the accumulation of fluid in the subretinal space and thus cause separation of the retina from the choroid.

Patterns of fluid flow are important with respect to the transport functions of the BRB system in that flow through the ECF space and through the Muller cells may play an important role in the distribution of nutrients and in the removal of potentially harmful metabolic products from avascular regions of the retina. In addition to bulk fluid flow, distribution of solutes within the retina can be expected to be aided by facilitated or active transport of solutes through cells which span considerable distances, such as the Muller cells, which span the whole depth of the retina (Fig. 3B). Although the need for mechanisms, in addition to diffusion, that will distribute nutrients and remove potentially toxic metabolic waste products is especially apparent in the case of the very highly developed, much thicker, but avascular avian retina, the same mechanisms could play a role in the euangiotic retinas of mammals, including man.

In summary, one may assume that there are fluid movements within the extracellular channels of the retina. In fact, it is almost inconceivable that this ECF compartment could be stagnant, or that the distribution of solutes within the retina, especially the avascular retina, could be dependent on diffusion alone. Pulsatile and unidirectional fluid movements, as well as active and facilitated solute transport processes across the plasma membranes of supporting cells, especially the Muller cells, must play an important role in the distribution of nutrients and in the removal of waste products from avascular regions of the retina. Although there is no available technology to test this hypothesis, observations that intravitreally injected horseradish peroxidase (HRP) passes through the ECFs of the retina all the way to the choroidal epithelium (85), while its passage in the opposite direction, i.e. from the subretinal space toward the vitreous seems to be hindered at the "external limiting membrane" (101), support the concept of ECF flow as depicted in Fig. 3A. A better knowledge of intraretinal fluid dynamics will clearly be required in order to understand the mechanisms underlying the development of retinal edema and the accumulation and resorption of subretinal fluid, as well as retinal nutrition, detoxification and pharmacodynamics.

5. Summary and Conclusions

The micro-environment of the retina, which differs from plasma ultrafiltrate but closely resembles the ECF of other regions of the brain, is maintained by facilitated and active transport processes across one or more regions of the blood-retinal barrier system. This system includes the following barriers or transport sites: the capillaries of the retina, which are referred to as the endothelial barrier; the choroidal or chorioretinal epithelium (generally, but incorrectly referred to as the retinal pigment epithelium) called the choroidal barrier; and the epithelia of the ciliary processes, which are referred to as the ciliary barrier. The proven, apparent or predicted sites and directions of transport of some biologically important solutes across these regions of the BRB system were discussed in section 4, and are briefly summarized here (Fig. 4).

The active secretory transport of sodium, chloride and/or bicarbonate by ciliary epithelia represents the main osmotic driving force for the production of aqueous humor. While there is some evidence that these major electrolytes are also transported across the choroidal epithelium, their predicted concentration in the ECF of the retina is similar to that of ectodermal tissues.

A net K^+ flux from retina to blood and a net Mg^{++} flux in the opposite direction across the choroidal, and most likely, also across the endothelial BRB, provides a low K^+ and high Mg^{++} extra-cellular environment in the retina, which presumably resembles the K^+ and Mg^{++} environment of other brain regions. Active secretory transport of Ca^{++} across the choroidal epithelium is indicated by in vitro experiments, but a general pattern of in vivo IOF Ca^{++} concentration gradients indicative of such a transport system has not emerged.

Ascorbic acid is maintained in the IOFs of most, but not all vertebrates at a concentration several-fold higher than that of blood plasma by its active transport across the ciliary epithelia and, at least in some species, possibly also across the BRBs. Much of the total concentration of free amino acids present in the IOFs and at least some of the amino acids present in the retina are derived from the secretory transport activity of the ciliary processes. This transport (facilitated or active), together with absorptive transport of amino acids across the choroidal and possibly also across the endothelial BRBs creates a continuous "flow" of these important precursors through the retina. Thus, the retina is amply supplied with amino acids even though their concentration in the retinal ECF is maintained at a very low level,

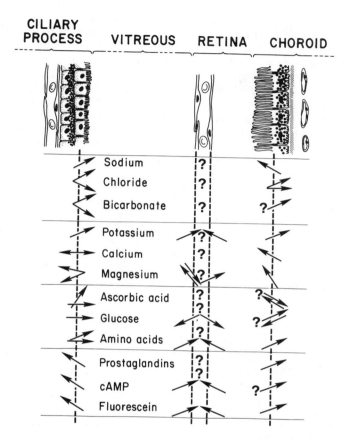

Fig. 4. A schematic summary of the transport processes across the ciliary processes, retinal capillaries, and choroidal epithelium which contribute to the maintenance of a normal retinal micro-environment. Arrows pointing upward indicate proven or presumed active transport against a concentration gradient; horizontal or downward oriented arrows indicate facilitated transport. Arrows directed from blood (ciliary or choroidal stroma, capillary lumen) toward the vitreous or retina represent secretory transport; those pointing in the opposite direction indicate absorptive transport processes. See text for details.

presumably similar to its level in the brain.

Several other classes of substances, most notably organic acids, are removed from the ECFs of the retina by active absorptive transport across the BRB system. Most of the known substrates for these transport functions, such as fluorescein, para-aminohippuric acid and iodopyracet, are not present in blood and/or are not produced within the eye and therefore cannot be regarded as natural substrates for this presumed "kidney-like" detoxification system. In contrast, prostaglandins and some related compounds, which are produced but not metabolized within the eye and which cannot be expected to penetrate blood-ocular barriers passively, represent a major class of natural substrates for absorptive transport by the anterior uvea, retinal choroid and choroid plexus. Furthermore, inhibition of the PG transport process has been shown to enhance the adverse effects of PGE on retinal function. By comparison with the choroid plexus, we can expect that some other autacoids and neurotransmitters and/or their initial metabolites are also removed from retinal ECF by facilitated or active transport processes across the BRBs. Preliminary experiments indicate, for example, that both the anterior uvea and the retinal choroid have saturable concentrative transport mechanisms for cyclic AMP (F.E. DiBenedetto and L.Z. Bito, unpublished observations) similar to those described for the choroid plexus (58).

This review clearly illustrates the complexity of the transport processes which are responsible for the maintenance of a normal retinal micro-environment. While each solute or class of solutes is handled by separate transport system(s), the following generalizations or predictions can be made: The choroid is a site of secretory and absorptive transport in virtually all vertebrates but, by itself, cannot control the environment of the entire retina. The normal composition of the ECF of the inner layers of the retina must be maintained by transport across retinal capillaries and/or by modifying the chemical composition of the adjacent vitreous. This latter mechanism plays a primary role in species that do not have euangiotic retinas or that have avascular retinal regions. In such species, as a result of transport processes across the ciliary processes, preretinal capillaries, and/or special secretory organs which project into the vitreous, the composition of much of the vitreous differs greatly from that of plasma dialysate. Some metabolic precursors are clearly derived from the vitreous, even in species that have highly vascularized retinas, and in all species, solute exchanges between the retina and its adjacent vitreous can be expected to be of primary importance during episodes of acute ischemia. The distribution of solutes within, and their removal from, the retina is undoubtedly aided by bulk fluid movements within retinal ECF channels and by facilitated or active transport of solutes across the membranes of supporting elements such as the Muller cells.

References

1 Barany, E.H., Acta Physiol. Scand., 86 (1972) 12–27.
2 Barany, E.H., Acta Physiol. Scand., 88 (1973) 412–429.
3 Barany, E.H., Acta Physiol. Scand., 88 (1973) 491–504.
4 Barany, E.H., Acta Physiol. Scand., 93 (1975) 250–268.
5 Becker, B., Am. J. Ophthalmol., 50 (1960) 862–867.
6 Becker, B., Am. J. Physiol., 200 (1961) 804–806.
7 Becker, B., Invest. Ophthalmol., 6 (1967) 410–415.
8 Bellhorn, M.B., R.W. Bellhorn and D.S. Poll, Exp. Eye Res., 24 (1977) 595–605.
9 Betz, A.L. and G.W. Goldstein, Exp. Eye Res., in press (1980).
10 Betz, A.L., J. Csejtey, and G.W. Goldstein, Am. J. Physiol., 236 (1979) C96–C102.
11 Bito, L.Z., Science, 165 (1969) 81–83.
12 Bito, L.Z., Exp. Eye Res., 10 (1970) 102–116.
13 Bito, L.Z., Comp. Biochem. Physiol., 43A (1972) 65–82.
14 Bito, L.Z., J. Physiol., 221 (1972) 371–387.
15 Bito, L.Z., Invest. Ophthalmol., 13 (1974) 959–966.
16 Bito, L.Z., The physiology and pathophysiology of intraocular fluids, In The Ocular and Cerebrospinal Fluids. Fogarty International Center Symposium, eds. L.Z. Bito, H. Davson, and J.D. Fenstermacher, Academic Press, London (1977) pp. 273–289.
17 Bito, L.Z., The role of transport processes in the pharmacokinetics of prostaglandins and related cyclooxygenase products, In Prostaglandins and Microcirculatory Function, eds. G. Kaley and E.J. Messina, University Park Press, Baltimore (1980).
18 Bito, L.Z. and R. Baroody, Prostaglandins, 7 (1974) 131–140.
19 Bito, L.Z. and R.A. Baroody, J. Physiol., 229 (1975) 1580–1584.
20 Bito, L.Z. and H. Davson, Exp. Eye Res., 3 (1964) 283–297.
21 Bito, L.Z. and H. Davson, Exp. Neurol., 14 (1966) 264–280.
22 Bito, L.Z., H. Davson, and J.D. Fenstermacher, eds., The Ocular and Cerebrospinal Fluids, Fogarty International Center Symposium, Academic Press, London (1977).
23 Bito, L.Z., H. Davson, E. Levin, M. Murray, and N. Snider, Exp. Eye Res., 4 (1965) 374–380.
24 Bito, L.Z., H. Davson, and E.V. Salvador, J. Physiol., 256 (1976) 257–271.
25 Bito, L.Z. and J.C. Roberts, Comp. Biochem. Physiol., 47A (1974) 173–193.
26 Bito, L.Z. and E.V. Salvador, Exp. Eye Res., 10 (1970) 273–287.
27 Bito, L.Z. and E.V. Salvador, Exp. Eye Res., 14 (1972) 233–241.
28 Bito, L.Z. and E.V. Salvador, J. Pharmacol. Exp. Therapeutics, 198 (1976) 481–488.
29 Bito, L.Z., E.V. Salvador, and L. Petrinovic, Exp. Eye Res., 26 (1978) 47–55.
30 Bito, L.Z. and M.C. Wallenstein, Exp. Eye Res. Suppl. 25 (1977) 229–243.

31 Bloom, W. and D.W. Fawcett, A Textbook of Histology, W.B. Saunders Co., Philadelphia (1975).
32 Bradbury, M., The Concept of a Blood-Brain Barrier, John Wiley & Sons, New York (1979).
33 Cole, D.F., Brit. J. Ophthalmol., 45 (1961) 641-653.
34 Cole, D.F., Aqueous and ciliary body, In Biochemistry of the Eye, ed. C. N. Graymore, Academic Press, London (1970) pp. 105-181.
35 Cole, D.F., Comparative aspects of the intraocular fluids, In The Eye, Vol. 5, Academic Press, New York (1974) pp. 71-161.
36 Cole, D.F., Secretion of the aqueous humour, In The Ocular and Cerebrospinal Fluids, Fogarty International Center Symposium, eds. L.Z. Bito, H. Davson, and J.D. Fenstermacher, Academic Press, London (1977) pp. 161-176.
37 Cross, R.J. and J.V. Taggart, Am. J. Physiol., 161 (1950) 181-190.
38 Csaky, T.Z. and B.M. Rigor, The choroid plexus as a glucose barrier, In Progr. Brain Res. Brain Barrier Systems, Vol. 29, ed. A. Lajtha and D.H. Ford, Elsevier, Amsterdam (1968) pp. 147-158.
39 Cserr, H.F., Physiol. Rev., 51 (1971) 273-311.
40 Cunha-Vaz, J.G., Doc. Ophthal., 41 (1976) 287-325.
41 Cunha-Vaz, J.G., Sites and functions of the blood-retinal barriers, In The Blood-Retinal Barriers, ed. J.G. Cunha-Vaz, Plenum Publishing Co., New York (1980) pp. 101-117.
42 Cunha-Vaz, J.G. and D.M. Maurice, J. Physiol., 191 (1967) 467-486.
43 Cunha-Vaz, J.G., M. Shakib and N. Ashton, Brit. J. Ophthal., 50 (1966) 441-453.
44 Davson, H., Physiology of the ocular and cerebrospinal fluids, J.& A. Churchill Ltd., London (1956).
45 Davson, H., The intraocular fluids, In The Eye, Vol. 1, ed. Davson, H., Academic Press, New York (1969) pp. 67-186.
46 Davson, H. and W.S. Duke-Elder, J. Physiol., 107 (1948) 141-152.
47 Davson, H. and C.P. Luck, J. Physiol., 132 (1956) 454-464.
48 DiBenedetto, F.E. and L.Z. Bito, Exp. Eye Res., in press (1980).
49 DiBenedetto, F.E. and L.Z. Bito, Submitted for publication (1980).
50 DiMattio, J. and J.A. Zadunaisky, Invest. Ophthalmol. Visual Sci. Suppl. (1979) 160.
51 DiMattio, J. and J.A. Zadunaisky, Exp. Eye Res., in press (1980).
52 Duke-Elder, S., System of Ophthalmology, Vol. II. The Anatomy of the Visual System, The C. V. Mosby Co., St. Louis (1961).
53 Eakins, K.E., Prostaglandin and non-prostaglandin mediated breakdown of the blood-aqueous barrier. In The Ocular and Cerebrospinal Fluids, Fogarty International Center Symposium, eds. L.Z. Bito, H. Davson and J.D. Fenstermacher, Academic Press, London (1977) pp. 483-498.

54 Fenstermacher, J.D. and J.A. Johnson, Am. J. Physiol., 211 (1966) 341-346.

55 Forbes, M. and B. Becker, Am. J. Ophth., 50 (1960) 867-873.

56 Fowlks, W.L., V.R. Havener, and J.S. Good, Invest. Ophthalmol., 2 (1963) 63-71.

57 Goldman, E.E., J.H. McLain, and J.L. Smith, Amer. J. Ophth., 65 (1968) 717-721.

58 Hammers, R., P. Clarenbach, T. Lindle, and H. Cramer, Neuropharm., 16 (1977) 135-141.

59 Heath, H., T.C. Beck, and A.C. Rutter, Vision Res., 1 (1961) 274-286.

60 Heath, H. and R. Fiddick, Exp. Eye Res., 5 (1966) 156-163.

61 Heath, H., A.C. Rutter, and T.C. Beck, Vision Res., 2 (1962) 431-437.

62 Hjelle, J.T., J. Baird-Lambert, G. Cardinale, S. Spector, and S. Udenfriend, Proc. Natl. Acad. Sci. USA, 75 (1978) 4544-4548.

63 Hogan, M.J., J.A. Alvarado, and J.E. Weddell, Histology of the Human Eye, W.B. Saunders Co., Philadelphia (1971).

64 Holland, M.G., D. Mallerich, J. Bellestri, and B. Tischler, Arch. Ophth., 64 (1960) 693-696.

65 Holland, M.G., D. Mallerich, B. Tischler, and J. Bellestri, Am. J. Ophth., 51 (1961) 1027-1032.

66 Kinsey, V.E., Ion movement in ciliary processes, In Membranes and Ion Transport, Vol. 3, ed. E.E. Bittar, Wiley, New York (1971) pp. 185-209.

67 Kinsey, V.E. and D.V.N. Reddy, Chemistry and dynamics of aqueous humor, In The Rabbit in Eye Research, ed. J.H. Prince, Charles C. Thomas, Springfield, Ill. (1964) pp. 218-319.

68 Krupin, T., C. Fritz, J. J. Dutton, and B. Becker, Exp. Eye Res., in press (1980).

69 Kuwabara, T., Species differences in the retinal pigment epithelium, In The Retinal Pigment Epithelium, ed. K.M. Zinn and M.F. Marmor, Harvard University Press, Cambridge, Massachusetts (1979) pp. 58-82.

70 Lajtha, A. and H. Sershen, Alterations of amino acid transport in the central nervous system, In The Blood-Retinal Barriers, ed. J.G. Cunha-Vaz, Plenum Publishing Co., New York (1980) pp. 119-132.

71 Lasansky, A. and F.W. de Fisch, J. Gen. Physiol., 49 (1966) 913-924.

72 Lorenzo, A.V., Factors governing the composition of the cerebrospinal fluid, In The Ocular and Cerebrospinal Fluids, Fogarty International Center Symposium, eds. L.Z. Bito, H. Davson and J.D. Fenstermacher, Academic Press, London (1977) pp. 205-228.

73 Lund-Andersen, H., Physiol. Rev., 59 (1979) 305-352.

74 Maren, T.H., Ion secretion into the posterior aqueous humor of dogs and monkeys, In The Ocular and Cerebrospinal Fluids, Fogarty International Center Symposium, eds. L.Z. Bito, H. Davson and J.D. Fenstermacher, Academic Press, London (1977) pp. 245-247.

75 Marmor, M.F., A.S. Abdul-Rahim and D.S. Cohen, Invest. Ophthalmol. Visual Sci., in press (1980).
76 Maurice, D.M., J. Physiol., 137 (1957) 110-125.
77 Maurice, D., Drug exchanges between the blood and vitreous, In The Blood-Retinal Barriers, ed. J.G. Cunha-Vaz, Plenum Publishing Co., New York (1980) pp. 165-178.
78 Miller, S. and R.H. Steinberg, Exp. Eye Res., 23 (1976) 177-189.
79 Miller, S.S. and R.H. Steinberg, J. Membrane Biol., 36 (1977) 337-372.
80 Miller, S.S. and R.H. Steinberg, Exp. Eye Res., 25 (1977) 235-248.
81 Noell, W.K., J. Optical Soc. Amer., 53 (1963) 36-48.
82 Oakley, B., S.S. Miller and R.H. Steinberg, J. Membrane Biol., 44 (1978) 281-307.
83 Palm, E., Acta Ophthal. 25 (1947) 29-35.
84 Patten, B.M., Human Embryology, McGraw-Hill Book Co., New York (1953).
85 Peyman, G.A., M. Spitznas and B.R. Straatsma, Invest. Ophthalmol. 10 (1971) 181-189.
86 Prather, J.W. and E.M. Wright, J. Membrane Biol., 2 (1970) 150-172.
87 Prince, J.H., Comparative Anatomy of the Eye, Charles C. Thomas, Springfield, Ill. (1956).
88 Rapoport, S.I., Blood-Brain Barrier in Physiology and Medicine, Raven Press, New York (1976).
89 Raviola, G., The structural basis of the blood-ocular barriers, In The Ocular and Cerebrospinal Fluids, eds. L.Z. Bito, H. Davson, and J.D. Fenstermacher, Academic Press, London (1977) pp. 27-63.
90 Reddy, D.V.N., Invest. Ophthalmol., 6 (1967) 478-483.
91 Reddy, D.V.N., B. Chakrapani, and C.P. Lim, Exp. Eye Res., 25 (1977) 543-554.
92 Reddy, D.V.N., and V.E. Kinsey, A.M.A. Arch. Ophthal., 63 (1960) 715-720.
93 Reddy, D.V.N. and V.E. Kinsey, Invest. Ophthalmol., 2 (1963) 237-242.
94 Reddy, D.V.N., M.R. Thompson, and B. Chakrapani, Exp. Eye Res., 25 (1977) 555-562.
95 von Sallmann, L., Arch. Ophthal., N.Y., 33 (1945) 32-39.
96 Steinberg, R.H. and S.S. Miller, Transport and membrane properties of the retinal pigment epithelium, In The Retinal Pigment Epithelium, eds. K.M. Zinn and M.F. Marmor, Harvard University Press, Cambridge, Mass. (1979) pp. 205-225.
97 Steinberg, R.H., S.S. Miller, and W.H. Stern, Invest. Ophthalmol., 17 (1978) 675-678.
98 Stetz, D.E., F.E. DiBenedetto and L.Z. Bito, Invest. Ophthalmol. Suppl. (1979) 281.
99 Stone, R.A., Invest. Ophthalmol., 18 (1979) 807-818.
100 Stone, R.A., Invest. Ophthalmol., 18 (1979) 819-826.
101 Tso, M., Pathology of the blood-retinal barrier, In The Blood-Retinal Barriers, ed. J.G. Cunha-Vaz, Plenum Publishing Co., New York (1980) pp. 235-250.

102 Ussing, H.H., and K. Zerahn, Acta Physiol. Scand., 23 (1951) 110–127.
103 Wallenstein, M.C. and L.Z. Bito, Invest. Ophthalmol., 17 (1978) 795–799.
104 Wegefarth, P. and L.H. Weed, J. Med. Res., 31 (1914) 167–176.
105 Wise, G.N., C.T. Dollery, and P. Henkind, The Retinal Circulation, Harper and Row, New York (1971).
106 Zadunaisky, J.A. and K.J. Degnan, Exp. Eye Res., 23 (1976) 191–196.
107 Zauberman, H., Adhesive forces between the retinal pigment epithelium and sensory retina, In The Retinal Pigment Epithelium, eds. K.M. Zinn and M.F. Marmor, Harvard University Press, Cambridge, Mass. (1979) pp. 192–204.

Acknowledgments

Work originating from the authors' laboratory was supported in part by U.S.P.H.S. Research grants EY 00333 and EY 00402 from the National Eye Institute. The authors wish to thank Ann S. Zaragoza and Adrienne B. Backerman for their assistance in the preparation of this manuscript.

DRUG EXCHANGES BETWEEN THE BLOOD AND VITREOUS

David M. Maurice
Division of Ophthalmology

Stanford University, Stanford, California, U.S.A.

The vitreous body, corresponding in function to the space between the lens and the film of a camera, is very properly ignored by most sensible people. However, as a large unstirred fluid space contiguous with the retina it provides unusual opportunities for characterizing solute exchanges with the central nervous tissue and its vasculature and has attracted some attention from a limited number of investigators (1-10). Unfortunately, it is the nature of such a stagnant pool to provide excellent conditions for the growth of microorganisms whether introduced by trauma or the surgeon's knife. These infections are particularly resistant to chemotherapy, and so the question of drug exchanges between the blood and the vitreous body is of considerable clinical importance.

The treatment of endophthalmitis has brought into being a considerable body of literature concerned with the intraocular kinetics of drugs injected systemically, around the globe, or into the chambers of the eye. These studies have generally been carried out on a pragmatic basis, and the experimental techniques that have been adopted frequently do not allow their results to be interpreted in any theoretical framework. This makes it difficult to compare the findings with different drugs or to relate them to their chemical properties. In particular it is not even possible to take the preliminary step of determining what proportion of the exchange takes place directly across the barrier between the vitreous and the retina and its blood vessels, and what indirectly with the newly formed aqueous humour at the base of the vitreous body.

In order to develop methods to elucidate this question, inert tracers, radioactive or fluorescent, have been used, since the measurement of drugs by bacterial or pharmacological assay is tedious and relatively inaccurate, especially at the low levels encountered. Two experimental situations have been studied: the penetration of solutes into the vitreous after systemic administration and the loss from the vitreous of material injected directly into it. The analysis is simpler in the latter case, and this will be considered first.

LOSS FROM THE VITREOUS BODY

Diffusion and Flow in Vitreous

The vitreous body is a very loose structure containing only about 0.01% of collagen, which implies that the distance between its fibrils is of the order of 1-2 μm (2, 26). These fibrils are braced apart by expanded hyaluronic acid molecules (26) which do not appear to offer a great resistance to the diffusion of small molecules, as indicated by direct measurements of its electrical conductivity (1) or of the diffusion of fluorescein within it (3). The observations on fluorescein show that the fluid is virtually stagnant; the suggestion that has sometimes been advanced of an appreciable backward flow would require the production of a volume of fluid by the ciliary body greater than that passing through the anterior chamber. In man some stirring of the fluid might be expected as a result of eye movements, especially in the elderly where the structure is liquefied.

Diffusional Pathways

As far as the experimental animal is concerned, loss from the vitreous will take place by diffusion, either relatively slowly over to the interface with the posterior chamber (Fig. 1a) or more quickly across the shorter path to the retinal surface (Fig. 1b). The rate of loss to be expected by the operation of the former pathway alone has been solved by means of a thermal analogue and was calculated to be 0.15/day in the case of serum albumin (2). In the case of the latter pathway, recourse has been made to mathematical approximations based on simplified models of the vitreous geometry (9). On the assumption that the resistance offered by the retinal surface is negligible so that the concentration at this surface is zero, the rate of loss can be calculated to be about 10 times greater than that possible through the anterior route.

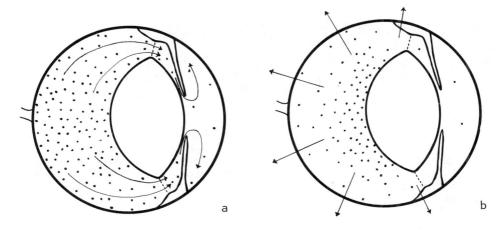

Figure 1.   Illustration of the two principal pathways of loss from the vitreous body: a, anterior route via drainage of the aqueous humor; b, across the retinal surface.

Measurement of Loss

The rate of loss of a tracer injected into the vitreous can be determined experimentally by collecting and analyzing the fluid at various periods thereafter.   It is more economical of animals to follow the drop in concentration in a single eye with an external counter for radioactive tracers (1,2,4,5,6) and with a slit-lamp fluorophotometer for those which are fluorescent (9). This is generally not possible when drugs are used.

For all test substances the fall in concentration has been found to be exponential for as long as it can be followed, up to 20 days in the case of albumin.   The rate of loss for this substance averaged 0.16/day (4 days half-life), similar enough to the value derived from the thermal analogue to encourage the belief that it was leaving the vitreous body entirely by the anterior route.

Aqueous Outflow

There is another, more direct, approach to estimating the amount of tracer diffusion forward into the posterior chamber. In order to leave the eye this material must enter the anterior chamber and be removed by the well established aqueous humor loss mechanisms, principally drainage through the angle of the eye but also diffusion across the iris. Where the coefficient of outflow from the anterior chamber, k_o, is known, the loss of material from the eye is given by $k_o C_a$, where C_a is its concentration in the aqueous humor. The total amount of material dissolved in the vitreous is its average concentration multiplied by the vitreous volume, $C_v V_v$. Then the proportion of the vitreous decay constant represented by anterior diffusion is given by

$$k_v = \frac{k_o C_a}{V_v C_v} \tag{1}$$

The quantities k_v, k_o and V_v might be expected to remain constant with time, and measurements of the ratio C_a/C_v show that it does indeed remain constant for various tracers as they leave the eye (1,2,9).

Using the value of k_o corresponding to bulk outflow, k_v can be plotted against C_a/C_v (Fig. 2). Substances that have experimental values falling on this line must leave the vitreous almost entirely by way of the aqueous humor (15). In the literature, figures are available for sucrose (7) and albumin (2) which place them in this category. Data has also been provided for hyaluronic acid in the owl monkey which also falls on the same base line (11). Although the geometry of the eye differs, some confidence can be placed in this point because the half-life has been reported to have the same value, two weeks, in the rabbit as it does in the monkey (14).

The thermal analogue mentioned before allows the decay constants for vitreous loss to be related to the diffusion constant of the injected material. These diffusion constants can be converted to the approximate molecular weights, assuming free diffusion in the vitreous body, and an excellent correspondence with the experimental data is shown.

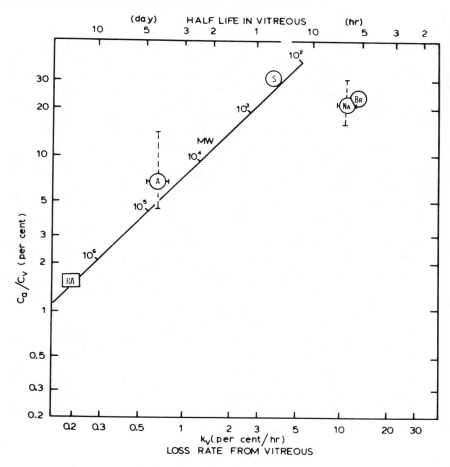

Figure 2. Relationship between the average concentrations in aqueous and vitreous humors, C_a/C_v, of substances leaving the eye principally through the anterior chamber after vitreous injection and their rates of loss from the vitreous, k_v. The straight line represents a theoretical relationship for loss only through the anterior chamber. Experimental values are shown for ^{22}Na, ^{82}Br, $[^{14}C]$sucrose (S), and $[^{131}]$albumin (A) in the rabbit and for hyaluronic acid (HA) in the owl monkey. The data were recalculated and replotted where necessary to find C_v and k_v. Limits indicated for albumin and sodium are extreme values.

Retinal Loss

     A number of tracers give experimental points lying below the
line of simple aqueous outflow, indicating that there is a
component of loss across the retina. The two ions Na and Br fall
a short distance below the line, and for these the retinal loss
is not overwhelming, being 60% of the total for the former (1)
and 50% for Cl (12). Three substances, iodide (5), iodopyracet
(6), and fluorescein (3), fall very much off the line and have a
markedly lowered aqueous-to-vitreous concentration ratio (Fig.
3). For these substances the retinal surface has to be the major
pathway out of the vitreous. The rate of loss, a half-life of
2-3 hr, is considerably faster than that corresponding to
anterior diffusion but is not as rapid as would be expected if
zero concentration were maintained over the entire retinal
surface. Slit-lamp fluorophotometry within the vitreous body
shows that the concentration of fluorescein is not zero at the
retina; however, there is a gradient from the lens to the retina,
confirming the existence of the outflux of the dye across this
surface (3). As a result of saturation or by the use of
competitive or metabolic inhibitors, the rate of loss of these
three substances can be slowed and their aqueous humor
concentrations raised such that the experimental data point
almost falls on the line corresponding to aqueous outflow. Thus
it appears that the low concentration at the retinal surface is
maintained by an active transport mechanism. This has been
confirmed in the case of these substances by showing that they
cannot penetrate the vitreous from the blood and that loss across
the retinal surface takes place against a considerable
concentration gradient (3,5,6).

Drugs

     There are several series of measurements on the decline in
concentration of drugs injected into the vitreous body of the
rabbit's eye (15). In a few of these the aqueous-vitreous
concentration ratio was established also (16-20), and these are
displayed in Fig. 4. It is seen that sulphacetamide and
streptomycin leave only by way of the aqueous humor, whereas
penicillin and novobiocin appear to be lost predominantly across
the retinal surface.

     Rapid passage across the retinal barrier can be mediated by
active transport as already noted, but it could also be a result
of lipid solubility of the drug, which allows it to pass through
cell membranes. In the case of penicillin it is more probable

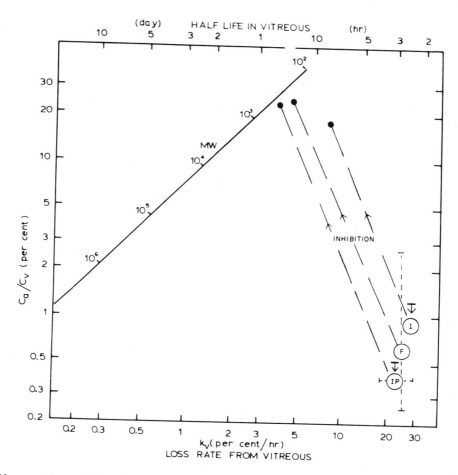

Figure 3. Relationship between the average concentrations in aqueous and vitreous humors, C_a/C_v, of substances actively transported across the retina after vitreous injection and their rates of loss from the vitreous, k_v. The straight line represents a theoretical relationship for loss only through the anterior chamber. Experimental values for fluorescein, [131I] iodopyracet, and 131I in the rabbit are represented by the symbols F, IP, and I. The data were recalculated and replotted where necessary to find C_v and k_v. The limits shown for F and IP correspond to extreme values. The value of C_a was reported to be zero for IP and the arrow symbol corresponds approximately to the lower limit of sensitivity of detection. The points joined to the symbols by lines show the experimental values on inhibition of the transport mechanism.

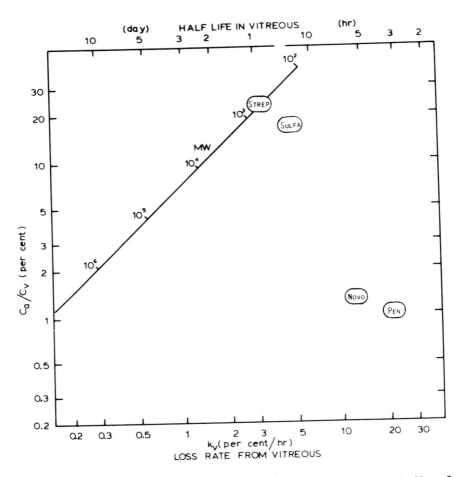

Figure 4. Plot of experimental values of k_v and C_a/C_v for antibiotics injected into the rabbit vitreous body. Data were collated from the following sources: sulfacetamide[16,17]; streptomycin[18]; penicillin[17,20]; and novobiocin[19]. The first two drugs appear to leave the vitreous through the anterior route, and the latter two leave across the retina.

that active transport is involved both because this drug has been found to inhibit the loss of fluorescein and because its partition coefficient does not indicate lipid solubility. There appears to be no such data readily available for novobiocin.

For the majority of intravitreally injected drugs only the half-life in the vitreous was measured. These results are displayed in Table I. The longer-lived ones have decay constants and molecular weights consonant with simple aqueous humor loss. The ones that leave quickly can only do so by taking the short diffusion path across to the retina. Apart from the two extremes, there would seem to be a number of drugs that leave by both pathways to a comparable degree.

TABLE I

RATE OF LOSS OF DRUGS FROM VITREOUS OF RABBIT

Major route of loss (Assumed from half-life)	Drug	Half-life (hr)
	Tobramycin	30
	Gentamycin	20
Anterior Chamber	Streptomycin	20
	Sulfacetamide	11
	Kanamycin	10
	Novobiocin	7
Retina	Methicillin	6
	Pencillin	5
	Carbenicillin	3 1/2
	Clindamycin	3
	Dexamethasone	2 1/2

PENETRATION OF VITREOUS BODY

Penetration Kinetics

Essentially, the kinetics of penetration from the bloodstream are the same as those of loss from the vitreous body. Substances can enter either directly across the retinal surface or indirectly from the posterior aqueous humor. The time constants corresponding to either pathway would be expected to be the same in both directions. From the experimental point of view investigation of penetration is more complex. First, instead of the concentrations in the blood and freshly-formed aqueous humor being zero at all times, they are subject to constant change, even if attempts are made to hold them at a fixed level. This is particularly the case in the initial stages of the introduction of the tracer into the blood stream at which time the penetration is also the fastest. Mathematical (1) and electrical (12) analogues have been used to treat this situation, but they rely on experimental data in the form of analysis of fluid tapped from the posterior chamber. Second, analysis of the data requires a knowledge both of the steady state level of the tracer in the newly-formed posterior aqueous and of the steady state concentration ratio between blood and vitreous across the retina, which can be influenced by protein-binding as well as active transport. Third, whereas in the loss experiments the bulk of the tracer is in the center of the vitreous where it can be easily collected, it tends to be more toward the surfaces during penetration (Fig. 5). This makes for potential problems when only partial sampling of the humor is carried out.

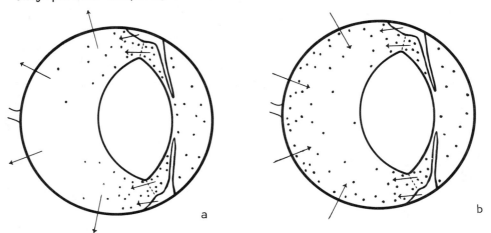

Figure 5. Penetration of drugs into the vitreous (a) when there is an active transport mechanism removing the drug across the retinal surface (b) with entry both from the ciliary body and across the retina.

Tracer Studies

The literature on the penetration of inert tracers into the vitreous of rabbits is sparse. The accumulation of radiosodium has been measured (13), and in spite of the difficulties listed above the time constant of the penetration is almost identical with that found for loss, and the same is true for bromide (4). An interesting result with the very lipid-soluble ethyl-thiourea can be noted (10), which enters with a half-life of about 1 hr. This is about the quickest possible rate of penetration if entry is limited solely by the diffusional resistance in the vitreous body, and it appears that the retina offers no barrier in this case.

At the opposite extreme, fluorescein does not enter across the retina to any measurable extent. The dye that penetrates from the posterior chamber, which can be distinguished by plotting concentration contours (3), is transported out across the retina before it can diffuse a great distance into the vitreous body.

Drug Penetration

In contrast to the few studies on inert tracers there have been many series of experiments on the penetration of systemically administered drugs into the eyeball and into the vitreous body, most of which have been listed by Barza (21). Because of the generally low concentration in the eye, the uncertainties inherent in biological assays, and the rapidly falling blood levels generally encountered in these studies, it is impossible to carry out a kinetic analysis of the data in nearly every case. In some instances one is able to arrive at a rough estimate of the steady state ratio between the vitreous humor and the blood, a figure whose value is enhanced if the degree of plasma protein binding of the drug is also established.

In theory, it should be possible by means of this data to decide whether a drug which is found to be lost across the retina after intravitreal injection is being transferred by active transport or as a result of its lipid solubility. In the case of active transport the penetration from the blood should be small, as with fluorescein; in the case of lipid solubility the penetration should be rapid and a high level in the vitreous body should be found. In fact, the yield of useful results is small. Of the drugs listed in Table I, the penetration of only five seems to have been investigated. Because the plasma levels have not been always determined, the peak vitreous concentrations are compared to the total dose in Table II. No correlation between penetration and loss rates is evident. The entry of about one-half the drugs tested is below the level of sensitivity of the assay that is used. Since this usually involves the inhibition of growth of a similar microorganism, the results have some practical value in determining which drugs are likely to be of therapeutic interest in man. Those drugs that do enter generally show a short-lived peak in the vitreous fluid during the first and second hours. This peak probably results from a combination of the pulse-delivery effect of the rapidly dropping plasma concentration and the inadequacy of a control tap as a sample of the entire volume, alluded to earlier.

TABLE II

COMPARISON OF RATE OF LOSS OF DRUGS FROM VITREOUS OF RABBIT
AND RATE OF PENETRATION FROM SYSTEMIC DOSE

Drug	Loss	Penetration	
	Half-life (hr)	$\dfrac{\text{Max. Conc.}}{\text{Total Dose}}$	x 100,000
Gentamicin	20	<4 [34]	
Streptomycin	20	2 [33]	
Methicillin	6	<0.4 [29-32]	
Penicillin	4	0.6 [22-25]	
Carbenicillin	3.5	<0.6 [27,32]	
Clindamycin	3	2 [28]	

Penicillin

In the case of this substance a number of workers have measured the changes with time of the concentration in the vitreous, as well as that in the aqueous humor and plasma. Studies after both intravenous and intramuscular or subcutaneous injection have been published (22,23,24,25). There is little concordance between their results, even in the changes in blood concentration, but as a very rough consensus it would appear that the plasma-to-vitreous concentration ratio, when the latter peaks, is of the order of 10:1. This steady state figure is supported by studies with a depot penicillin, which gave a very slow decline in concentration and a plasma:aqueous:vitreous ratio of 10:3:1 (23). The proportion of free penicillin in the plasma is close to 40%, and this would make the steady state level in the vitreous 25% of the free drug in the plasma.

If penicillin crossed the blood-vitreous barrier by virtue of its lipid solubility, the level should approach 100%. There is some support from the penetration data, then, for the conclusion that a unidirectional transfer is taking place at the retinal boundary.

CONCLUSIONS

It would be useful to know about the mechanisms by which drugs pass across the retinal barrier in order that the chemical properties or molecular structures which lead to rapid penetration could be identified and incorporated in new antibiotics. It is possible, also, that these findings could be applied to drug penetration into the brain.

From a study of the literature I have concluded that, for technical reasons, observations on the loss of a drug injected into the vitreous body give more useful information than those in which penetration from the blood is observed. It would be valuable to have the penetration data in addition, but workers in the field could make their results more interpretable by the design of their experiments. In particular, it would be an advantage if, instead of following a clinical modality of treatment, an attempt was made to maintain a steady level of the drug in the blood and the rise in concentration in the humors toward steady state was followed.

ACKNOWLEDGMENTS

This preparation of this paper was supported by National Institutes of Health Grant EY 00431.

1. Maurice, D.M., J. Physiol. 137:110, 1957.
2. Maurice, D.M., Amer. J. Ophthalmol. 47:461, 1959.
3. Cunha-Vaz, J.G. and Maurice, D.M., J. Physiol. 191:467, 1967.
4. Becker, B., Arch. Ophthalmol. 65:97, 1961a.
5. Becker, B., Amer. J. Ophthalmol. 200:804, 1961b.
6. Forbes, M. and Becker, B., Amer. J. Ophthalmol. 50:867, 1960.
7. Bito, L.Z., and Salvador, E.V., Exp. Eye Res. 14:233, 1972.
8. Palm, E., Acta Ophthal. Suppl. 32, 1948.
9. Cunha-Vaz, J. and Maurice, D., Doc. Ophthalmol. 26:61, 1969.
10. Davson, H., J. Physiol. 129:111, 1955.
11. Hultsch, E. and Balazs, E.A., Arvo Abs. 1975, Personal comm.
12. Kinsey, V.E. and Reddy, D.V.N., Doc. Ophthalmol. 13:7, 1959.
13. Friedenwald, J. and Becker, B., Arch. Ophthalmol. 54:799, 1955.
14. Widder, W., Graefe Arch. Ophthalmol. 164:550, 1960.
15. Maurice, D.M., in Symposium on Ocular Therapy, Vol. 9, Ed.
    Leopold, I.H. and Burns, R.P. John Wiley and Sons, Inc., 1976.
16. vonSallman, L., Trans. Amer. Ophthalmol. Soc. 45:570, 1947.
17. Duguid, J.P., Ginsberg, M., Fraser, I.C., Macaskill, J.,
    Michaelson, I. and Robson, J.M., Brit. J. Ophthalmol. 31:193,
    1947.
18. Gardiner, P.A., Michaelson, I.C., Rees, R.J.W. and Robson, J.M.,
    Brit. J. Ophthalmol. 32:449, 1948a.
19. Sery, T., Paul, S.D., and Leopold, I., Arch. Ophthalmol. 57:100,
    1957.
20. Gardiner, P.A., Michaelson, I.C., Rees, R.J.W., and Robson,
    J.M., Brit. J. Ophthalmol. 32:768, 1948b.
21. Barza, M. Treatment of bacterial infections of the eye. In
    press.
22. Tanaka, M., Acta Soc. Japan 67:252, 1963.
23. Trichtel, F. and Papapanos, G., von Graefes Archiv fur Oph-
    thalmol. 164:42, 1961.
24. Salminen, L., Jarvinen, H., and Toivanen, P., Acta Ophthalmol.
    47:115, 1969.
25. Bloome, M., Golden, B. and McKee, A., Arch. Ophthalmol. 83:78,
    1970.
26. Balazs, E., In The Structure of the Eye, Ed. Smelser, G.
    Academic Press, New York, 1961, p.293.
27. Barza, M., Baum, J., Birkby, B. and Weinstein, L. Amer. J.
    Ophthalmol. 75:307, 1973.
28. Tabbara, K. and O'Connor, G.R. Arch. Ophthalmol. 93:1180, 1975.
29. Faris, B. and Uwaydah, M. Arch. Ophthalmol. 92:501, 1974.
30. Green, W.R. and Leopold, I.H. Amer. J. Ophthalmol. 60:800, 1965.
31. Calmettes, L., Deodati, F., Monnier, J., Bec, P. and Delpech,
    J., Therapie 16:934, 1961.
32. Deur, H.A. and Maas, E.R., Ophthalmologica 144:316, 1962.
33. Leopold, I.H. and Nichols, A., Arch. Ophthalmol. 35:33, 1946.
34. Golden, B. and Coppel, S., Arch. Ophthalmol. 84:792, 1970.

DRAINAGE OF INTRAOCULAR FLUIDS

Anders Bill

Department of Physiology and Medical Biophysics
Uppsala University, Box 572, Uppsala, Sweden

The fluids that will be considered in this communication are the tissue fluids of the uvea and the retina and the vitreous and aqueous humors. Retinal tissue fluid and the vitreous and aqueous humor are very special fluids located outside barriers with a low permeability to most solutes. In the choroid and the ciliary processes on the other hand the capillaries have a high permeability to all low molecular weight substances (Törnquist, Alm and Bill, 1979). As a consequence the tissue fluids in these regions are practically at equilibrium with the plasma with regard to most low molecular weight solutes and contain considerable quantities of plasma proteins (Bill, 1968a, b).

In most tissues where there is leakage of plasma proteins into the tissue fluid there is a drainage of such fluid by the lymph vessels. In the eye there are no lymph vessels and there is thus a need for drainage of tissue fluid in some other way. An essential factor here is the intraocular pressure, which enables a continuous flow of aqueous humor into the extraocular veins and leakage of modified aqueous humor and tissue fluid into the extraocular tissues.

Much of our knowledge about fluid dynamics in the eye comes from experiments in animals. Such studies have demonstrated very clearly that there are important differences between primates and lower animals such as cats and rabbits and there are probably important differences also between sub-human primates and man.

THE CHOROID

In rabbits there is an outflux of IgG from the choroidal vessels that corresponds to about 0.06 ul plasma/min (Bill, 1968a). The con-

centration of IgG in choroidal tissue fluid is about 50 % of that
in plasma (Bill, 1968b). Then if it is assumed that the IgG leaves
the eye by tissue fluids flow – this flow would correspond to about
0.06/0.5=0.12 ul/min. A similar amount may come from the ciliary
body. The routes involved in the drainage of these fluids were investigated both with dyes and radioactively labelled albumin (Bill,
1964). Small amounts of fluid were injected into the suprachoroid
through a needle via the cornea and sclera. Albumin-bound Evans
blue could be seen passing through the sclera at a low rate around
the site of injection. With larger amounts injected there was almost
immediate drainage also around the nearby vortex vein. These results
indicated that even high molecular weight substances can pass out
of the eye by filtration and diffusion through the scleral substance
and also by flow via perivascular spaces. With radioactively labelled
albumin it was possible to demonstrate that after leakage through
the sclera the macromolecules entered the lymph vessels of the conjunctiva and were returned to blood via the lymph vessels.

The relative roles of the perivascular spaces and the scleral
substance in the normal drainage of ocular tissue fluid are not
clear. In vitro experiments have been performed to study diffusion
through the sclera (Maurice and Polgar, 1977). Diffusion seems to
be influenced both by steric hindrance and negative charges in the
sclera.

An attempt to determine the hydrodynamic conductance of the
sclera under in vivo conditions was made by Kleinstein and Fatt
(1977). They applied a suction device over a small part of the
sclera and determined the relationship between flow and suction
pressure. They calculated that under normal conditions there could
be a flow of about 1.1 ul/min through the sclera. This flow most
probably did not include movement through perivascular spaces.

Fig. 1 illustrates one of the problems encountered in in vitro
experiments with the sclera. Scleral pieces were incubated with a
mixture of 125I-myoglobin and 131I-albumin. Both substances entered
the sclera rapidly over the first 30 min and there was then a slow increase in concentration over many hours. There was also an increase
in weight of the scleral pieces. Such swelling of the sclera in vitro complicates interpretation and prevents compartmental analysis.

I have tried to measure the pressure at the tip of a cannula
introduced into the suprachoroid before, during and after infusion
of a small amount of 3 % albumin. The animal was under general anesthesia and treated with i.v. indomethacin (20 mg/kg b.w.) and no-
vesin topically to prevent as much as possible inflammatory changes.
Before the infusion was started the pressure in the suprachoroid was
1-5 cm lower than the intraocular pressure. An infusion of 0.25 ul/
min increased the pressure to a level 4-10 cm higher than the intra-

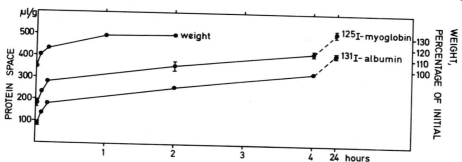

Fig. 1. Accumulation of labelled albumin and myoglobin in rabbit
sclera. Incubation at room temperature in 3 % serum albumin
in saline. The change in weight is also shown.

ocular pressure. After infusion the pressure fell to a level almost
identical with the intraocular pressure and the difference between
the two pressures was less than 1 cm H_2O for more than 10 min. Evans
blue was observed in the whole suprachoroid of the quadrant of infusion and passed through the sclera - near as well as far from the
needle tip.   These admittedly crude experiments confirmed the observation of van Alphen in cats (1961) that the suprachoroidal pressure
is lower than the intraocular pressure and suggest that under conditions of increased leakage from the choroidal vessels the pressure
in the suprachoroid and choroid can build up to levels higher than
the intraocular pressure. Direct measurements of the pressure in the
conjunctiva with a fine needle resulted in values between 0 and 1 cm
H_2O.

We may conclude then that in rabbits there is a need for drainage of tissue fluid from the suprachoroid and that such drainage
seems to occur through the scleral substance as well as through
perivascular spaces.

The pressure difference existing between the suprachoroid and
the extraocular tissue is a prerequisite for the drainage of uveal
tissue fluid. It is not surprising then that in hypotonic eyes there
is strong tendency to fluid accumulation in the suprachoroidal and
supraciliary spaces and choroidal detachment. The elasticity of the
uvea in such a situation may even tend to cause a subatmospheric
pressure in the suprachoroid (Moses, 1965).

In primates and cats the pressure difference between the anterior chamber and the suprachoroidal space results in significant inflow of aqueous humor from the anterior chamber into the suprachoroid as will be discussed later.

THE RETINA

In the retina there are narrow spaces between the cells and
these spaces contain small amounts of tissue fluid. Very little is
known about this fluid but a number of suggestions can be made concerning its origin and fate. Experiments by Smelser, Ishikawa and
Pei (1965) and Peyman and Bok (1972) have demonstrated that ferritin
and horse radish peroxidase injected into the vitreous humor can
pass between the cells of the retina up to the pigment epithelium.
The inner limiting membrane of the retina thus is no efficient barrier between the vitreous and retina.

The density of the retina is slightly higher than that of the
vitreous. Then if there were free communication between the potential space inside the pigment epithelium and the vitreous and no
drainage through the pigment epithelium the force of gravity would
result in retinal detachment – at least under conditions of liqui-
fied vitreous. This problem was considered some years age by Maurice,
Salmon and Sauberman (1971) and Fatt and Shantinath (1971). Maurice
et al. worked with the hypothesis that there might be a flow from
the vitreous into the choroid and that under such conditions the
pressure just inside the pigment epithelium should be somewhat lower
than that in the anterior chamber. They implanted a tubing between
the pigment epithelium and the photoreceptors and measured the two
pressures but found no difference. The approach of Fatt and Shantinath
was indirect. They determined the density of the retina and the vitreous and the hydraulic conductance of· the retina. They could then
calculate the pressure difference across the sensory retina that
would be required to keep the retina in place. It was very low indeed. About $0.1 \cdot 10^{-3}$ mm Hg. The negative result of Maurice et al.
then becomes less surprising – such a small pressure difference could
not be determined experimentally.

According to Fatt´s hypothesis the hydrostatic pressure difference alone could result in sufficient flow from the vitreous
body through the retina into the choroid and out through the sclera.
The presence of colloids in the choroid adds another driving force–
a difference in colloid osmotic pressure across the pigment epithelium which in rabbits is about 10 mm Hg. In addition there will be
small differences in the concentration of glucose across the pigment epithelium which also will have an osmotic effect tending to
cause reabsorption into the choroid. The pigment epithelium has
systems for active transport (see Miller, Steinberg and Oakley,
1978) but it is not clear if these are engaged in transporting fluid
out of the retina. The sodium pump is in fact transporting sodium
from the choroidal side into the retina. All the evidence taken together suggests very strongly that the sensory retina is sucked
against the pigment epithelium by osmotic and colloid osmotic forces.

An interesting observation concerning the movement of water through the retina was reported recently by Marmor (1979); injection of 50 µl 500 mOsm NaCl solution into the vitreous humor resulted in retinal detachment. The injection no doubt made the tissue fluid of the retina hypertonic compared to the tissue fluid in the choroid and probably reversed the normal movement of water through the pigment epithelium.

The quantity of fluid leaving the retina for the choroid per minute is not known. It is probably very small. The fluid most probably comes from the posterior chamber. It is of some interest then that the movement of the aminoacid cycloleucine from the posterior chamber into the vitreous humor is not appreciable affected by a rise in IOP (Bill, 1969). Insensitivity to changes in IOP of course can be expected if the main driving force is a difference in oncotic and osmotic pressure across the pigment epithelium.

With a hole in the sensory retina, part of the resistance to outflow via the retina and the pigment epithelium is abolished. The clinical result is hypotony, most probably due to aqueous outflow through the pigment epithelium. One could expect then that eyes with retinal detachment should have a high facility. But facility determinations in patients, as well as in rabbits with experimental detachment, have failed to indicate increased facility (see Foulds, 1968). This observation adds further to the hypothesis that osmotic and oncotic pressures are the main driving forces for fluid reabsorption through the pigment epithelium.

THE VITREOUS AND OPTIC NERVE

It seems very likely as discussed above that small amounts of fluid pass from the posterior chamber into the vitreous and out through the retina and sclera. In rabbits it is possible to demonstrate another route of drainage: from the vitreous into the perivascular spaces around the vessels of the retina and optic nerve. Dyes injected into the vitreous soon appear around the blood vessels where they leave the optic nerve. In primates such drainage via perivascular spaces seems to be of much smaller magnitude. Hayreh (1966) compared different species and found no significant drainage in primates when colloidal iron was used as a tracer. The difference seems to be quantitative rather than qualitative, however. Peyman and Apple (1972) demonstrated that even in monkeys small amounts of horse radish peroxidase can pass through the inner limiting membrane into the spaces between the astrocytes and nerve fibres of the optic nerve and also along the perivascular spaces.

Oddly, the lens may contribute somewhat to the drainage of fluid from the vitreous. Fowlks has (1973) demonstrated that in the lens the water balance is such that small amounts are pumped out at

the anterior surface. The fluid most probably comes from the vitreous. Such drainage may help to explain a tendency for small particles to accumulate behind the lens. In a recent study on the elimination of microspheres from the vitreous body in rabbits (Algvere
and Bill, 1979) such a tendency was observed.

It should be mentioned also that the retinal capillaries may
be engaged in the drainage of fluid from the retina and vitreous
body; the hydrostatic pressure difference across the capillary wall
may well be lower than the oncotic pressure difference tending to
cause some reabsorption.

THE AQUEOUS HUMOR

It seems clear now that most of the aqueous humor leaves the
eye via the irido-corneal chamber angle. Here part of the fluid
passes through the meshwork into the canal of Schlemm, another part
passes in a more diffuse way through the chamber angle tissue and
the ciliary muscle into the supraciliary and suprachoroidal spaces.
Before embarking on a discussion on the role of the chamber angle
it is of interest to consider some physiological results obtained
with techniques that have been described previously (Bill and Hellsing, 1956; Bill, 1977). Fig. 2 shows the rate of disappearance of
different radioactive substances from the anterior chamber expressed
as percentage of that of albumin.

The values shown are means of at least 5 determinations. It is
clear from the figure that albumin, IgG and myoglobin leave the anterior chamber at almost exactly the same rates indicating that
they move out of the anterior chamber with a bulk flow of aqueous
humor through relatively wide channels. Tritiated water and low
molecular weight solutes leave the chamber at higher rates indicating that for these substances there are additional routes with
a high degree of discrimination. Movement through such routes might
be by diffusion and convection into the cornea and into the iris
vessels.

It was once thought that the cornea played an important role
in the drainage of aqueous humor but studies by Maurice (1972) have
indicated that the role of the cornea in the drainage of aqueous
humor is negligible. Small amounts of fluid enter the tissue from
the anterior chamber but equal amounts seem to be "pumped" back by
the endothelial cells.

With regard to the iris morphological studies have demonstrated very clearly that there is no layer of endothelial or epithelial cells covering the anterior surface. The stroma is in fact
open to the anterior chamber aqueous humor (Inomata, Bill and Smelser, 1972a). One advantage of such an open system is obvious: when

the pupil is dilated fluid can be squeezed out of the iris. Another consequence is that the iris vessels normally are in very close contact with the aqueous humor which might result in drainage of the fluid into the capillaries.

To test if movement of aqueous humor into the iris is of practical significance we have tried to determine the conductance using osmotic methods (Bill, 1974). The reasoning was simple. If there are routes permitting reabsorption into the iris due to the colloid-osmotic pressure of plasma such convection should be reduced, stopped or reversed by perfusion with an albumin solution through the anterior chamber. We found that if one anterior chamber was perfused with 0.1 % albumin and the other with 2.5-6 % albumin there was only a very small extra inflow into the anterior chamber on the side with a high albumin concentration. The results indicated that the filtration coefficient of the iris capillaries was so low that any net movement of fluid into the capillaries was negligible. Calculations of the conductance of the pores in the iris capillaries suggested a value of $0.5 \cdot 10^{-4}$ ul$\cdot$min$^{-1} \cdot$mm Hg^{-1} (Bill, 1977). Experiments with hyper and hypotonic solutions of NaCl were performed in a similar way; moderate changes in osmolarity had no appreciable effects.

The experiments discussed above indicated that the difference in rate of outflux from the anterior chamber between low molecular weight solutes and macromolecules is due essentially to diffusion, one labelled water molecule entering the iris vessels being replaced by one unlabelled from the plasma.

Uveoscleral Drainage

In some early experiments with perfusion of labelled plasma proteins through the anterior chamber in monkeys we found that part of the protein leaving the anterior chamber did not appear in the general circulation. An analysis of the eyes indicated that movement into the ciliary body, the choroid and the sclera and episcleral tissues was an alternative route. Some movement from the anterior chamber into the uvea had been observed long ago but received little recent interest (see Leber, 1903). The questions then become: was the accumulation of radioactive material in the ocular tissues due to diffusion or to convection from the anterior chamber and was the movement into the tissue fast enough to indicate significant flow from the anterior chamber.

By determining the concentration of labelled substance in the anterior chamber fluid and the amounts recovered in the different tissues it was possible to calculate the volume of aqueous humor that apparently had moved into the tissues. Such calculations demonstrated that sometimes more than 50 % of the labelled material

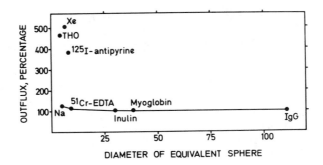

Fig. 2.   Rate of outflux from the anterior chamber of different
          labelled substances, expressed as percentages of the out-
          flux of labelled albumin, was plotted against the dia-
          meter of the equivalent spheres. The solid line connects
          values for solutes, soluble in water but not in lipid.

leaving the anterior chamber had accumulated in the tissues. Thus
in monkeys it was an important question whether the movement into
the uvea and sclera was due to diffusion or to convection.

The observation discussed above that substances with greatly
different molecular weights left the anterior chamber at the same
rate was of great importance in indicating that the accumulation
of labelled material in the uvea and sclera was due mainly to convection. A second important factor was the fact that the tissue
pressure in the suprachoroid is slightly lower than the IOP as
discussed already. It was clear then that there are routes from
the anterior chamber through the uvea and sclera into the episcleral
tissues.

Another question concerned the fate of the fluid passing out
through the uvea and sclera. It was obvious that the fluid moving
through the ciliary muscle mixed with the locally produced tissue
fluid and that there was diffusional exchange with the plasma in
the blood vessels. It was obvious also that while passing through
the suprchoroid there was exchange with the choroidal vessels.

When albumin and IgG were perfused simultaneously through the
anterior chamber the amounts of IgG recovered in the uvea and sclera
were slightly higher than those for albumin (Bill, 1966). This result indicated that small amounts of albumin were passing through
the uvea into the blood vessels. This was not unexpected. Other
experiments in rabbits had demonstrated that in the choroid small
amounts of extravascular plasma albumin tend to return into the
blood vessels (Bill, 1968a). With myoglobin,which is a smaller molecule, the difference was more marked − the amounts recovered in
the tissue were much lower than expected from the contents of al-

bumin (Bill, Hellsing, 1965). Much of the myoglobin moving through the uvea thus entered the capillaries locally.

It was clear from the experiments with myoglobin and albumin that the aqueous humor entering the uvea in the chamber angle did not pass through the tissues into the episclera unaltered. Since myoglobin was lost to a large extent smaller molecules could be expected to pass rather freely between the tissue fluid and the blood vessels. Such a movement by diffusion and convection might result in almost complete absorption of the fluid entering the uvea or the net effect might be a drainage through the sclera and perivascular spaces corresponding to the inflow via the chamber angle plus some locally produced fluid. One possibility to detect marked reabsorption was obvious. If there was a continuous inflow of aqueous humor into the uvea of fluid containing labelled albumin and reabsorption left most of the albumin outside the vessels the concentration of labelled albumin would increase with time. If the amounts of aqueous humor present in the tissue was calculated one might find "impossible values" such as 1 000 ul/g tissue or more. We found no such values in any of the tissues investigated and concluded that the inflow into the uvea from the anterior chamber probably was similar to the drainage via the sclera and perivascular spaces (Bill, 1971). Experiments in dead animals (Bill, 1966) were there could be no reabsorption of fluid into the uveal vessels indicated that under such conditions uveoscleral flow was increased. Reabsorption of fluid into the uveal vessels thus is not a prerequisite for uveoscleral flow.

Morphological studies (Inomata, Bill and Smelser, 1972b; and Inomata and Bill, 1977) indicated that even 0.1 um particles, which are too large to pass through the sclera, can pass out of the eye via spaces around the blood vessels and nerves. It was reasonable then to call the unconventional outflow "uveoscleral flow" since both the uvea and sclera were engaged.

The magnitude of the uveoscleral flow in monkeys under general anesthesia has been reported for cynomolgus and vervet monkeys (Bill, 1971) and corresponds to about 50 % of the total outflow with much variation between individuals. In cats uveoscleral flow is about the same as in monkeys but a small fraction of the total outflow. In rabbits very little fluid passes from the anterior chamber through the ciliary body into the suprachoroid, but there is some drainage through the scleral substance and through perivascular spaces in the limbus region (see Bill, 1975). Observations in some other monkey species which have not been reported previously are shown in Table 1.

Uveoscleral flow has been determined in a few experiments in humans. These studies could be performed only in eyes which had to

Aqueous Drainage in Monkeys

	Body weight	Uveoscleral flow	Flow via Schlemm's canal
Squirrel	0.70	0.11	0.73
monkeys	0.53	0.14	0.71
(Saimiri	0.70	0.18	0.80
sciureus)	0.75	0.13	0.60
	0.70	0.20	0.72
Capuchin	4.5	0.59	0.87
(Cebus	4.5	0.66	1.05
capucinus)	2.4	0.43	0.86
	2.4	0.23	0.87
Baboon	9.4	0.70	1.51
	12.3	0.40	1.97
	13.2	0.77	1.18
Mangabey	11.2	0.46	2.14
(Cercocebus	6.6		
albigena)			
Stump-tailed	10.0	0.40	1.94
macaque (Ma-	9.5	1.92	1.34
caca speciosa)			

be removed because of tumors and the values obtained may not be representative for normal eyes. In man uveoscleral flow was lower than in most monkeys accounting for some 10 % of the total outflow (Bill and Phillips, 1971).

Rhesus monkeys have been used in recent studies on the movement of material from the anterior chamber into the uvea and the conclusions have been somewhat in variance with those in other species. Sherman, Green and Laties (1978a) injected fluorescein intracamerally and observed rapid movement of fluorescein into the ciliary body. Small amounts were recovered within the blood vessels, but there was no appreciable penetration into the sclera from the suprachoroid. Experiments with fluorescein-labelled dextran gave essentially the same results. It was concluded that the fluid entering the uvea seemed to enter the blood vessels, scleral outflow being negligible.

Pedersen, Gaasterland and MacLellan (1977) have made similar observations. They perfused the anterior chamber in rhesus monkeys with a mixture of labelled albumin and fluorescein. The blood flow from a vortex vein was collected continuously. It was possible then to determine the rate of movement of labelled albumin and fluorescein from the anterior chamber into the blood drained by the vor-

tex veins. There was little movement of albumin into the vessels
but the addition of fluorescein to the blood corresponded to
0.45-0.86 ul/min. Fluorescein is not an ideal substance in determinations of aqueous flow since it can be expected to leave the
anterior chamber both by bulk flow and diffusion. Recent experiments with ^{51}Cr-EDTA, which has a molecular weight similar to that
of fluorescein indicate, however, that diffusion into the iris
vessels of molecules of this size introduces only a small error in
aqueous flow determinations, - about 0.1-0.2 ul/min (see Fig. 2).
Diffusion out of and into the choroidal vessels of small molecules
is very rapid (Törnquist, 1979). It can be expected then that the
values reported by Pedersen et al. are good measures of uveoscleral
flow. But they give no proof for uveal resorption of all the aqueous
humor entering via the ciliary muscle: it was not possible to distinguish between the fluorescein entering by diffusion as compared
to that entering by convection.

     According to Pedersen at al. resorption into the uveal ves-
sels of aqueous humor was of crucial importance for the flow via
the ciliary muscle; it produced the pressure difference driving the
flow. No experiments were performed, however, to demonstrate that
such flow was stopped by stopping the blood flow through the eyes.
In other monkey species uveoscleral flow tends to be enhanced after
the death of the animal, if the intraocular pressure is maintained
at a normal level.

     In an attempt to estimate the relative importance of uveoscleral
drainage in monkeys Pedersen et al. calculated the normal rate of
aqueous formation from assumed values for episcleral venous pressure,
intraocular pressure and outflow facility. The value obtained,
4-9 ul/min, was such as to indicate that uveoscleral flow is normally less than 10 % of the total outflow. The normal flow rate in
monkeys is not known but 4-9 ul/min is a very high figure when compared to values obtained in anesthetized monkeys, Table 1.

     Studies on the physiology and pharmacology of the uveoscleral
outflow have indicated that the tone of the ciliary muscle is of
great importance. Contraction of the muscle as caused by pilocarpine
almost stopped uveoscleral flow (Bill and Wåhlinder, 1966; Sherman,
Green and Laties, 1978), relaxation causes increased flow. These results indicate that under normal conditions uveoscleral flow varies
with the degree of accommodation and, interestingly, this variation
is accompanied by changes in outflow resistance in the routes via
Schlemm´s canal tending to cause opposite effects on the flow via
that route.

     Increments in the intraocular pressure which markedly increase
the outflow via the canal of Schlemm have only small effects on the
flow via the uveoscleral routes: in a study with labelled proteins
a rise in pressure of 27 mm Hg increased this out − flow by

0.10 ul/min (Bill, 1967). The increase was not statistically significant. In the study of Pedersen et al. uveal facility measured
with fluorescein was 0.034±0.012 ul/min/mm Hg. If these routes have
a facility it is thus very low.

Flow via Schlemm´s Canal

The drainage of aqueous humor from the anterior chamber via
Schlemm´s canal has been reviewed recently (Svedbergh, 1976; Bill,
1977). After considerable debate there now seems to be agreement
that the aqueous first moves through the large openings of the uveal
meshwork and then through the less wide openings in the corneoscleral
meshwork into the peculiar loose connective tissue represented by
the endothelial or juxtacanalicular meshwork. From here the fluid
moves through invaginations in the inner wall endothelium of the
canal of Schlemm and out into the canal through the transcellular
pores (Inomata, Bill and Smelser, 1972b). Around the normal intraocular pressure the flow is almost proportional to the intraocular
pressure. But if a more marked increase in intraocular pressure is
produced by injecting fluid into the anterior chamber the resistance
to outflow may change. The changes observed are due to complex alterations in the outflow routes: deepening of the anterior chamber
tending to increase outflow, compression of the meshwork and canal
of Schlemm probably tending to reduce facility (see Moses, 1977).
In addition increments in eye pressure tend to change the structure
of the inner wall of Schlemm´s canal; there is an increase in the
number of invaginations and also the number of pores increases(Grierson and Lee, 1974, 1975; Svedbergh, 1976, 1977).

At pressures lower than the episcleral venous pressure there
is practically no reversal of the flow through the chamber angle
tissue (Bill, 1977). Such flow is prevented by collapse of the invaginations of the inner wall endothelium and compression of the endothelial and trabecular meshwork (Johnstone and Grant, 1973; Grierson and Lee, 1974).

The rather complex structure of the outflow routes ensures such
a resistance to flow that a small drainage of aqueous humor from the
anterior chamber into the canal of Schlemm is sufficient to create
the moderate intraocular pressure necessary for good optical function of the eye. The narrow paths through the meshwork that are required to give a suitable resistance is a risk since there is a continuous inflow of small amounts of debris from the anterior chamber.
Such debris might clog the meshwork, if there was no mechanism for
"cleaning". Experiments by Rohen and van der Zypen (1968) indicate
that this problem is handled by the endothelial cells of the trabecular and endothelial meshwork. These cells are phagocytotic; they
engulf and degrade debris, thereby enabling an intact drainage of
aqueous humor over a lifetime in most eyes.

Recent studies on the mode of action of different agents influencing the outflow resistance indicate that the effects may be
directly on the outflow routes or secondary to contraction of the
ciliary muscle. Cholinergic agents seem to exert their effects
mainly via the muscle, pilocarpine which normally produces a marked increase in outflow facility having practically no effect after
disinsertion of the muscle from the trabecular meshwork (Kaufman
and Bárány, 1977). Pilocarpine has been reported to affect the inner wall endothelium of Schlemm's canal. Holmberg and Bárány (1966)
found that the number of vacuoles or invaginations in the inner
wall endothelium was reduced by pilocarpine. Griersen, Lee and Abraham (1979) have observed opposite results, but they found also
that the effect seemed to be more related to the outflow rate
through the chamber angle than to the drug. Recent experiments
(Svedbergh and Bill, unpublished) indicate that in eyes treated with
pilocarpine small particles perfused with gelatine through the
meshwork can enter and pass through the endothelial meshwork more
readily than in eyes treated with atropine. Part of the pilocarpine
effect thus seems to be exerted close to the inner wall of Schlemm's
canal, most probably as a result of pulling of the ciliary muscle
on the trabecular meshwork.

Both cytochalacin B (Kaufman and Bárány, 1977; Svedbergh et al.,
1978) and chelating agents, such as EDTA and EGTA (Bill, Svedbergh
and Lutjen-Drecoll, 1979) have very marked-partly reversible effects
on the outflow facility in monkeys. The resistance to outflow is
in fact reduced to a level that has been ascribed to the collector
channels in the sclera. The two agents produce somewhat different
changes in the ultrastructure of the outflow routes but with both
agents there is distention of the endothelial meshwork with wash-
out of material and disruption of the inner wall of Schlemm's canal at places.

The mode of action of adrenergic substances on the outflow
routes remains an enigma but it seems likely that the effect is
exerted in the endothelial meshwork.

In summary: Small amounts of aqueous humor are likely to pass
from the posterior chamber into the vitreous humor and from there into the retina and optic nerve. Retinal fluid is probably sucked
into the choroid, the colloid-osmotic pressure of choroidal tissue
fluid playing a considerable role. In the anterior chamber aqueous
humor can pass into and out of the iris freely but elimination of
the aqueous takes place almost exclusively in the chamber angle,
partly via the canal of Schlemm into the general circulation and
partly into the ciliary muscle, supraciliary and suprachoroidal
spaces. Fluid passing through these spaces mixes with locally produced tissue fluid and is modified by exchange with the capillaries.
As a result there are changes both in composition and volume. Elimination of fluid from the suprachoroid occurs partly through spa-

ces around the blood vessels and nerves and partly through the
scleral substance.

ACKNOWLEDGEMENTS

Supported by grant B79-14X-00147-150 from the Swedish Medical Research Council and Grant 2 R01 EY00475-13 from the National
Eye Institute, US Public Health Service.

REFERENCES

Algvere, P. and Bill, A., Arch. Ophthalmol. In press.
Bill, A., Exp. Eye Res. 3:179, 1964.
Bill, A. and Hellsing, K., Invest. Ophthalmol. 4:920, 1965.
Bill, A., Exp. Eye Res. 5:45, 1966.
Bill, A., Invest. Ophthalmol. 6:364, 1967.
Bill, A., Acta Physiol. Scand. 73:204, 1968a.
Bill, A., Acta Physiol. Scand. 73:511, 1968b.
Bill, A., Exp. Eye Res. 11:195, 1971.
Bill, A., Jap. J. Ophthalmol. 18:30, 1974.
Bill, A., Physiol. Rev. 55:383, 1975.
Bill, A., Exp. Eye Res. 25: (suppl) 291, 1977.
Bill, A. and Phillips, C.I., Exp. Eye Res. 12:275, 1971.
Bill, A., Lutjen-Drecoll, E. and Svedbergh, B., Invest. Ophthalmol.
     Vis. Sci. In press.
Bill. A. and Phillips, S.I., Exp. Eye Res. 12:275, 1971.
Fatt, I. and Shantinath, K., Exp. Eye Res. 12:218, 1971.
Foulds, W.S., Mod. Probl. Ophthalmol. 8:51, 1968.
Fowlks, W.L., Experientia, 29:548, 1973.
Grierson, I. and Lee, W.R., Exp. Eye Res. 19:21, 1974.
Grierson, I. and Lee, W.R., Am. J. Ophthalmol. 80:863, 1975.
Grierson, I., Lee, W.R. and Abraham, S., Invest. Ophthalmol. Vis.
     Sci. 18:346, 1979.
Hayreh, S.S., Exp. Eye Res. 5:123, 1966.
Holmberg, A.S. and Bárány. E.H., Invest. Ophthalmol. 5:53, 1966.
Inomata, H. , Bill, A. and Smelser, G.K., Am. J. Ophthalmol. 73:
     760, 1972a.
Inomata, H., Bill, A. and Smelser, G.K., Am. J. Ophthalmol. 73:893,
     1972b.
Inomata, H. and Bill, A., Exp. Eye Res. 25:113, 1977.
Johnstone, M.A. and Grant, W.M., Am. J. Ophthalmol. 75:365, 1973.
Kaufman, P.L. and Bárány, E.H., Invest. Ophthalmol. 15:793, 1976.
Kaufman, P.L. and Bárány,E.H., Invest. Ophthalmol. Vis. Sci. 16:47,
     1977.
Kleinstein, R.N. and Fatt, I., Exp.Eye Res. 24:335, 1977.
Leber, T., Graefe-Saemisch: Handbuch der gesamten Augenheilkunde
     II Band, 2, Abt. Leipzig, p. 281, 1903.
Marmor, F.M., Stanford University Medical Center, Stanford, Calif.,
     and Veterans Administration Hospital, Palo Alto, Calif.

Maurice, D.M. and Polgar, J., Exp. Eye Res. 25:577, 1977.
Maurice, D.M., J. Physiol. London, 221:43, 1972.
Maurice, D.M., Salmon, J. and Zauberman, H., Exp. Eye Res. 12:212,
    1971.
Moses, R.M., Invest. Ophthalmol. 4:935, 1965.
Moses, R.M., Survey of Ophthalmol. 22:88, 1977.
Miller, S.S., Steinberg, R.H. and Oakley, B., J. Membrane Biol.
    44:259, 1978.
Pederson, J.E., Gaasterland, D.E. and MacLellan, M., Invest.
    Ophthalmol. Vis. Sci. 16:1008, 1977.
Peyman, G.A. and Apple, D., Arch. Ophthalmol. 88:650, 1972.
Peyman, G.A. and Bok, D., Invest. Ophthalmol. 11:35, 1972.
Rohen, J.W. and van der Zypen, E., Graefes Arch. Ophthalmol. 175:
    143, 1968.
Sherman, S.H., Green, K. and Laties, A.M., Exp. Eye Res. 27:159,
    1978a.
Sherman, S., Green, K. and Laties, A., Suppl. to Invest. Ophthal-
    mol. and Vis. Sci. 5:206, 1978b.
Smelser, G.K., Ishikawa, T. and Pey, F., In: The structure of the
    eye, II Symp., edited by J.W. Rohen, Stuttgart: Schattauer-
    Verlag, p. 109, 1965.
Svedbergh, B., Acta Univ. Upsal. 256:1, 1976.
Svedbergh, B., In: Yamada, E., and Mishima, S., editors: The struc-
    ture of the eye III, Tokyo, 1976, Japanese Journal of Ophthal-
    mology, p. 197.
Svedbergh, B., Lutjen-Drecoll, E., Ober, M. and Kaufman,P.L., In-
    vest. Ophthalmol. and Vis. Sci. 17:718, 1978.
Törnquist, P., Acta Univ. Upsal. 326:1, 1979.
Törnquist, P., Alm, A. and Bill, A., Acta Physiol. Scand. In press.
van Alphen, G.W., Ophthalmologica 142, Suppl. 1, 1961.

VITREOUS FLUOROPHOTOMETRY

JOSE CUNHA-VAZ, M.D., Ph.D.
Department of Ophthalmology, University of Coimbra,
Coimbra, Portugal
Department of Ophthalmology, University of Illinois Eye
and Ear Infirmary, Chicago, U.S.A.

There are numerous examples of restricted permeability in the ocular tissues, particularly between the ocular humors and the blood that protect them from multiple variations to which the blood is constantly subjected. Information accumulated in the last decade has shown that two main barrier systems are present in the eye. The first, the blood-retinal barrier (BRB), separates the retinal neural tissue from the blood. The second, the so-called blood-aqueous barrier (BAB), regulates the exchanges between the blood and the intraocular fluids.

Information regarding these barriers is desirable in that the intraocular fluids (aqueous and vitreous) bathe important structures such as the cornea, lens and retina, and equilibrate with the extracellular spaces of these tissues. Furthermore, changes in these tissue often result in altered visual function.

Soon after we initiated our studies on the permeability of the retinal vessels with Ashton (1) and proposed for the first time the existence of a BRB it was considered desirable to extend our investigations with large molecular weight tracers to more diffusible substances.

Maurice, who at the time had developed a new sensitive slit-lamp fluorophotometer (2) suggested fluorescein, a nontoxic molecule of 5.5 Å radius as being particularly suitable to study molecular movements across the BRB.

Initial experimental studies using the slit-lamp fluorophotometer of Maurice allowed us (3) to determine the distribution of fluorescein within the axial regions of the vitreous body of the living rabbit. The measurements of the gradient in the vitreous immediately

in front of the retina should give a value for the flux of dye across
its surface and so lead to a value of the permeability of the surface
at the point of observation. The rabbit is particularly suitable for
these experiments, since its retinal vessels lie in contact with the
vitreous humor virtually free from any surrounding glial tissue;
furthermore, they are restricted to a limited zone of the retinal
surface, and so direct comparisons can be made between vascularized
and non-vascularized areas.

It soon became evident that both these areas showed a unidirectional permeability to fluorescein in the direction from the inside
of the eye to the blood. The _in vivo_ observations on the concentration gradients were then supplemented by measurements taken on frozen
sections of the eye, which showed the direction of movement of fluorescein across the boundaries of the entire vitreous body.

The results obtained showed that when fluorescein is injected
into the blood no measurable amount enters the vitreous body of the
normal eye (fig. 1). Our in vivo measurements showed that the level
in the vitreous body remained well below 10^{-8} gm/ml when the free
fluorescein in the blood was in the region of 10^{-4} gm/ml for many
hours, suggesting an inward retinal permeability no greater than
10^{-5} cm/hr. A small entry in the most anterior portion of the vitreous body, originating from the region of the ciliary body, could
be seen in the frozen sections.

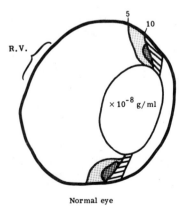

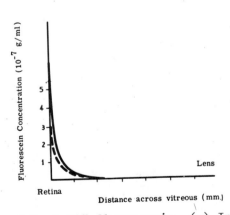

Fig. 1. Intraperitoneal injection of 3 ml 10% fluorescein. (a) In
vivo recordings taken 1 hr and 45 min. after the injection. (b) Contours from eye frozen 2 hr after the injection. (From ref. 3).

Immediately after the fluorescein is injected into the vitreous body, in the normal eye, it may be seen as a discrete mass, but it spreads readily and its outlines become diffuse. After a few hours the fluorescence of the aqueous takes up a constant ratio to that of the vitreous humor, though this is well below 1%. It may be assumed then that the fluorescein has assumed a fixed pattern of distribution within the vitreous body at this time. This distribution correlated well both in frozen sections and in vivo observations. The concentration was greatest immediately behind the lens and it dropped to a low value around the entire retinal surface. Prolongation of the in vivo curves suggested that they would in any case reach zero concentration less than 1 mm behind the retinal surface. This indicates that the minimum value of the outward permeability of this surface is equivalent to that of a layer of vitreous humor 1 mm thick. There is evidence that molecules even as large as serum albumin move relatively unhindered within the vitreous body of the rabbit (4) and so the diffusion rate of fluorescein in this cavity may be taken as its value in free solution, 6×10^{-6} cm^2/sec at 37° C. The outward permeability of the dye must, then, be greater than 0.2 cm/hr.

It is evident from the concentration contours that the principal movement of fluorescein is outward across the entire retinal surface.

This pattern of fluorescein distribution within the frozen vitreous body remained essentially unchanged when very high concentrations of the dye were maintained in the plasma as a result of intravenous or intraperitoneal injection. In several frozen sections, the gradient in the vitreous body showed an outward movement across the retinal surface, including the vascularized region, when the concentration of fluorescein at the surface was apparently 100 times less than that of the unbound dye in the plasma (fig. 2).

However, under conditions designed to inhibit the active transport of anions, the pattern of fluorescein distribution within the vitreous body was modified in a typical manner. With high concentrations of a inhibitor, the fluorescein distribution was as shown in fig. 3. It is evident that the movement of fluoresccin out of the eye has been blocked over the entire retinal surface.

If the retinal circulation is occluded by diathermy, the movement of fluorescein out of the vitreous body ceases in this region, showing that the vessels themselves are participating in active transport.

Similarly, in the inhibited eye, fluorescein was found to enter over all the retinal surface after an intraperitoneal injection of the dye. The entry pattern was similar whether metabolic or competitive inhibitors were injected into the eye or whether Benemid was

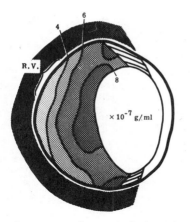
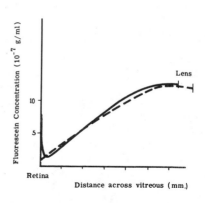

Fig. 2. Intravitreal injection of 20 µl of 0.025% fluorescein. Intraperitoneal injection of 5 ml 10% fluorescein 3 hr later (concentration of free fluorescein in the blood 2 x 10^{-5} g/ml). (a) In vivo
recordings taken 4 hr after the intraperitoneal injection. (b) Contours from eye frozen 5 hr after the intraperitoneal injection. (From
ref. 3).

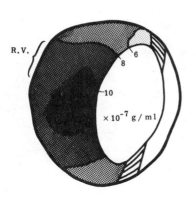
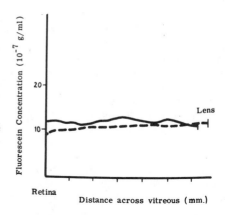

Fig. 3. Intravitreal injection of 15 µl of 1 M benzylpenicillin in
a solution of 0.03% fluorescein. (a) In vivo recordings taken 24 hr
after the injection. (b) Contours from eye frozen 25 hr after the
injection. (From ref. 3).

administered systemically (fig. 4). Very high concentrations of fluorescein in the blood forced an entry by some mechanism of saturation,
which gave a similar distribution.

    The profile of the concentration within the vitreous body con-
formed approximately to that which would be expected if the dye were

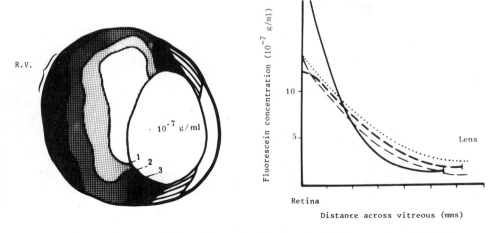

Fig. 4. Intravitreal injection of 15 μl of 1 M benzylpenicillin.
Intraperitoneal injection of 3 ml 10% fluorescein 5 hr later. (a)
In vivo recordings taken 2 hr and 30 min. after the fluorescein
injection. Fine dotted and dashed lines show curves calculated for
spherical and plane models as described in text, with arbitrarily
chosen vertical scale. (b) Contours from eye frozen 3 hr after the
fluorescein injection. (From ref. 3).

liberated at the retinal surface at a constant rate, diffused through
the vitreous humor at the rate of movement found in free solution
and met a barrier to further progress at the lens surface. The geometry of the rabbit's eye, curved lens surface placed 6-7 mm from
the spherical retina of 8 mm radius, leads to a very difficult com-
putation. For the present purpose two simple approximations were
used between which the **true** condition might be expected to fall. In
one, the retina and lens were taken as large plane sheets 6 1/2 mm
apart and, in the other, the retina was assumed to be as complete
sphere 6 1/2 mm in radius. The distributions at any time, corresponding to these approximations, can be interpolated between the
examples plotted by Crank (5). The experimentally determined distribution of the fluorescein concentration was generally similar, sometimes closely so, to one or other of these curves.

These observations showed that in the normal eye, the rapid outflux of fluorescein across the boundary of the vitreous, even against
a high concentration gradient, compared with the great resistance to
its penetration from the blood points to an active transport system
operating over the entire surface of the blood-retinal barrier. These
studies contributed significantly to the understanding of intraocular
dynamics and of the behavior of fluorescein angiography, and slit-
-lamp fluorophotometry of the vitreous immediately appeared as a most
promising field for clinical and experimental research.

VITREOUS FLUOROPHOTOMETRY TECHNIQUE

Principles. Fluorescein, a weak dibasic acid of the xanthene group, has a molecular weight of 330. It is very deeply colored, and the conversion of the absorbed light to fluorescein light is almost 100%. It is this property that is used to detect minimal concentrations of this substance in the eye. Previous studies have shown that there is no problem in detecting values between 10^{-8} and 10^{-9} gm/ml in the anterior chamber or vitreous body. Another important feature is that the weak acidity of fluorescein accounts for its extremely poor staining qualities; it never forms a firm bond to any vital tissues. Finally, when mixed with blood in usual concentrations, a high proportion (about 20%) remains free. Fluorescein, therefore, is particularly appropriate for measurements in the intraocular fluids.

Equipment. Since our initial studies with the slit-lamp fluorophotometer of Maurice, we have been using a different set-up, essentially a modified version of the slit-lamp fluorophotometer presented by Waltman and Kaufman, in 1970, for the examination of the anterior chamber (6). To measure the fluorescein concentration in the vitreous a model 360 Haag-Streit slit lamp and fundus contact lens are used. The instrument is modified by adapting a new source of illumination, appropriate filters, a photometric detection system similar to that described by Waltman and Kaufman, and a device for electrical registration of the movement of the instrument in the antero-posterior (AP) axis (as the retina, vitreous and lens are sequentially brought into focus for fluorescein measurements; fig. 5).

The incandescent bulb normally present in the slit lamp is replaced by a fiberoptic system connected to a 300 W unit with ventilation. A holder containing the removable exciter filter is mounted on the arm in front of the light source. The lamp and microscope arms are locked at an angle of 20° from each other for taking measurements.

The photometric detection system consists of a modified eyepiece containing a fiberoptic probe. It is connected to a photomultiplier tube, an autoranging photometer, and an oscilloscope with storage and Polaroid camera. The sensor tip of the probe is in focus with the optical section, allowing the fluorescein concentration to be measured in all parts of the eye visible in the ocular of the slit-lamp. As the instrument scans through the eye in the A-P axis, it registers electrically through the use of a linear carbon potentiometer clamped to the slit-lamp table and a sliding contact is moved by a rod held against the base of the instrument. All the measurements are made after application of a low-vacuum contact lens to the eye under examination. A Spectrotech pair of appropriate interference filters is used.

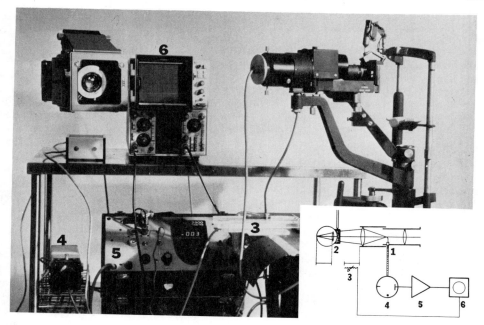

Fig. 5. Vitreous fluorophotometer. Insert, Diagram of photometric system. 1, Eyepiece of slit-lamp microscope with fiberoptic; 2, Eye with contact lens; 3, Linear carbon potentiometer; 4, Photomultiplier; 5, Photometer; 6, Oscilloscope. (From ref. 12).

A standard fluorescein solution in phosphate buffer (pH 7.4) or a standard fluorescence glass are tested before each examination.

A few additional considerations must be kept in mind. It is important to use a thin slit to minimize internal light scatter. If lens opacities are present, the light transmission will be decreased. Also, the pupil must be well dilated to permit adequate focusing and illumination during the entire vitreous scanning.

It is particularly important to note that a good correlation has been demonstrated between measurements performed in the media of the eye in vivo and in fluorescein solutions of known concentrations in vitro. Also, vitreous fluorophotometry is not limited by the phenomenon of absorption of the exciting light beam by the dye, in the range of practical use.

Examination techniques. A simple basic examination serves to detect an alteration of the BRB, if present; however, more sophisticated special examination techniques may be used to obtain additional information about the functional activity of the barrier and the location of the breakdown.

Basic examination. An intravenous (IV) injection of sodium fluorescein in a dose of 14 mg/kg of body weight is given one hour before the vitreous fluorophotometry examination. The pupils are well dilated and a low-vacuum contact lens is applied to the eye under examination.

For the basic vitreous fluorophotometry examination, the light slit and the fiberoptic probe of the eyepiece are initially focused over the macular area immediately superficial to the retina in the vitreous. The linear carbon potentiometer on the table of the slit lamp is then set against the moveable base of the slit-lamp. The window of the photomultiplier is open, and the image of the fiberoptic probe is moved away from the surface of the retina toward the lens along the illumination light path by using the joy stick of the slit-lamp. The final recording is documented with the Polaroid camera of the oscilloscope.

Although the fluorescein is administered according to the weight of the patient, determination of the fluorescein concentration in the blood at the time of the examination is indicated whenever liver or kidney disease may be significant. This can be done by taking samples of blood from a finger prick into a 50 µl Microcap pipette and discharging these samples into a convenient volume of saline; readings are taken in the supernatant fluid when the cells have been centrifuged down. By using the standardized equipment and the technique described, repeatable results can be obtained.

The results, in effect, represent vitreous fluorescein concentration curves. They are semiarbitrarily divided into three approximately equal parts that are ascribed to posterior, middle and anterior vitreous. Information about the concentration of fluorescein in the blood permits the determination of an approximate value for BRB permeability (cm/hr) using a theoretic treatment previously reported. If the value obtained for the mean fluorescein concentration in the posterior vitreous is normal (less than 1.0×10^{-8} gm/ml) the vitreous fluorophotometry findings are considered negative, and the examination is finished (fig. 6). If higher fluorescein concentration are detected in the posterior vitreous, indicating an alteration of the BRB, the basic examination may be followed by additional examination techniques.

Kinetic vitreous fluorophotometry. Kinetic vitreous fluorophotometry is the study of the changes in vitreous fluorescein concentration in relation to time. It consists of a series of vitreous fluorophotometry recordings and anterior chamber measurements that are performed at 3, 4, 4 1/2 and 5 hours after the time of the initial IV fluorescein injection. Average values for the posterior vitreous, aqueous humor and blood from each examination are then plotted against time. The rate of loss of fluorescein from the vitreous and aqueous humor is obtained by determining the half-periods of both

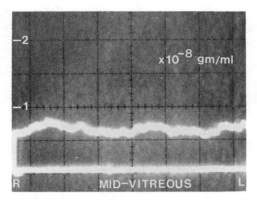

Fig. 6. Vitreous fluorophotometry of eye of normal volunteer.(From ref. 12).

curves (fig. 7). The successive recordings give important information regarding the direction and rate of movement of the fluorescein in the vitreous and aqueous.

Topographic vitreous fluorophotometry. Topographic vitreous fluorophotometry is performed whenever a localized breakdown of the BRB is expected; it is important to differentiate such a situation from a generalized BRB breakdown. To this end, a basic vitreous fluorophotometry examination, using the macula as the starting point is complemented by recordings performed by scanning from other retinal areas to the lens.

VITREOUS FLUOROPHOTOMETRY STUDIES IN DIABETES

The first report on vitreous fluorophotometry, which appeared in 1975 (7) opened a new area of research by showing an early breakdown of the BRB in diabetes mellitus. This finding served subsequently as a basis for a series of clinical and experimental studies investigating the role of the alteration of the BRB in the development of diabetic retinopathy and in other retinal diseases (8-15).

Clinical studies. The application of vitreous fluorophotometry to a series of predominantly adult-onset diabetics with apparently normal fundi revealed the presence of a significant breakdown of the BRB. The disturbance of the BRB, as evidenced by vitreous fluorophotometry, appeared before microaneurysms or capillary closure could be demonstrated by fundus fluorescein angiography. These patients consistently showed fluorescein concentration values in the posterior vitreous greater than 2×10^{-8} gm/ml. These studies have since been extended to a much larger number of patients. Using a dose of IV fluorescein of 14 mg/kg, the average value recorded in the posterior vitreous of diabetic eyes with normal fundi is $4.2 \pm 1.2 \times 10^{-8}$ gm/ml.

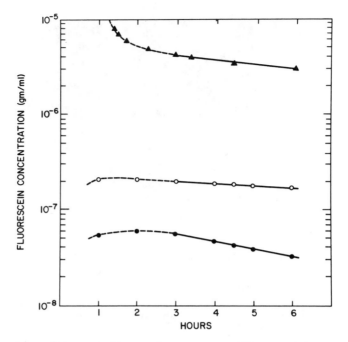

Fig. 7. Kinetic vitreous fluorophotometry. Fluorescein concentrations in blood (▲), aqueous humor (O), and vitreous (●) plotted against time in hours. (From ref. 12).

This contrast with a background value of a $0.7 \pm 0.08 \times 10^{-8}$ gm/ml recorded in the posterior vitreous in a series of normal patients from different age groups who had no personal or family history of diabetes and who had normal findings in ophthalmologic examination. The fluorescein concentration curves in the vitreous in the diabetic patients followed a typical pattern, the gradient indicating penetration of fluorescein across the BRB (fig. 8).

These results were confirmed recently by Waltman and co-workers, who reported on the vitreous fluorophotometry examinations of 99 juvenile-onset, insulin-dependent diabetics and 31 control subjects (8, 9).

Kinetic vitreous fluorophotometry may also prove useful in studying diabetic retinopathy (12). This technique shows that, in the diabetic with an alteration of BRB, the concentration of fluorescein in the vitreous rises and reaches its maximum value between one and three hours after the IV injection. Afterwards, the fall is logarithmic with a half-period of about 4 1/2 hours (kv = 2.3×10^{-3}/min). After the peak concentration in the vitreous is reached the profile of the concentration of the fluorescein in the vitreous inverts. Five hours after the initial IV injection, there is a concentration gradi-

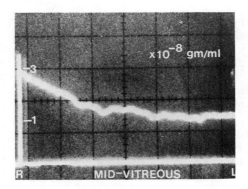

Fig. 8. Basic vitreous fluorophotometry. Examination of eye of diabetic patient that revealed no abnormality with fluorescein angiography.

ent from the anterior vitreous to the retina that is consistent with
an efflux across the entire retinal surface. The concentration profi-
les observed in the diabetic eye without retinopathy confirm that
the active transport for fluorescein, although still operating, appears to be disturbed and operating at a lower rate. The obtained
value for the coefficient of fluorescein loss from the vitreous in
the diabetic eye is lower than the value calculated for the normal
eye ($kv = 3.3 \times 10^{-3}$/min), including both anterior and posterior
routes. Kinetic vitreous fluorophotometry, allowing for the determination of the coefficient of fluorescein loss from the vitreous may
play an important role in the study of the early functional changes
that occur in the BRB in diabetes.

Another aspect of the ocular diabetic disease which has been
studied by vitreous fluorophotometry is the correlation between
breakdown of the BRB and development of retinal lesions (10). Although the reports available have been somewhat contradictory, a correlation between the severity of the vascular lesions and higher vitreous fluorophotometry readings is apparent, suggesting a possible
role for the alteration of the BRB in the progression of diabetic
retinopathy.

Finally, the correlation between early alteration of the BRB
and the degree of systemic metabolic deviation has been also examined by vitreous fluorophotometry.

In a study using a set of criteria to evaluate metabolic control, vitreous fluorophotometry was performed in a series of 100 diabetic eyes, all of which has no visible changes in funduscopy or
fluorescein angiography (11). The eyes were grouped according to
whether the patient was insulin dependent or noninsulin dependent
and whether the duration of the diabetes was less or more than five

years. Insulin-dependent diabetics who had diabetes for less than
five years and relatively good metabolic control had vitreous fluorophotometry values significantly lower than those registered in a
similar group of diabetic patients under poor metabolic control (Table 1). In the same way, noninsulin-dependent patients who had diabetes of less than five years' duration and who were under relatively
good metabolic control had vitreous fluorophotometry values significantly lower than those observed in a similar group of diabetic patients under worse metabolic control (Table 2). A correlation was
also observed between vitreous fluorophotometry values and duration
of the diabetic disease.

Table 1. Vitreous Fluorophotometry Values in Insulin-Dependent
         Diabetics

| | Vitreous Fluorophotometry (Posterior Vitreous $- x\ 10^{-8}$ gm/ml $-$ Mean $\pm$ SD) | | |
| Diabetic Metabolic Control | | Duration of Diabetes | |
	No. Eyes ($<$5 yr)	No. Eyes ($\geqslant$5 yr)	P Values
Relatively good	16 3.1 ± 1.3	3 5.9 ± 0.8	$<$.005
Poor	13 5.0 ± 2.5	3 7.7 ± 1.5	NS
P values	$<$.025	NS	

Table 2. Vitreous Fluorophotometry Values in Noninsulin-Dependent
         Diabetics

| | Vitreous Fluorophotometry (Posterior Vitreous $- x\ 10^{-8}$ gm/ml $-$ Mean $\pm$ SD) | | |
| Diabetic Metabolic Control | | Duration of Diabetes | |
	No. Eyes ($<$5 yr)	No. Eyes ($\geqslant$5 yr)	P Values
Relatively good	25 4.0 ± 1.4	26 6.1 ± 1.8	$<$.001
Poor	10 7.4 ± 2.9	4 8.7 ± 3.4	NS
P values	$<$.005	$<$.0125	

It appears, therefore, that at least in the early stages of the disease, there is a direct correlation between the retinal disturbance that occurs in diabetes, as judged by breakdown of the BRB, and the diabetic metabolic deviation.

Experimental studies. Experimental vitreous fluorophotometry studies performed in rats made diabetic with streptozotocin (STZ) have opened an entirely new avenue of approach to the investigation of diabetic retinopathy. These studies, initiated by Waltman and co-workers, have shown that insulin reverses the breakdown of the BRB that occurs in STZ - diabetic rats (13).

We have been able to confirm those studies and extend them by using kinetic vitreous fluorophotometry. Diabetic rats showed significantly prolonged half-periods of fluorescein loss when compared with controls (2.1 ± 0.12 vs 1.3 ± 0.06 hr; mean $\pm$ SEM), $p < 0.001$. Insulin treatment reduced these values to near normal values (1.6 ± 0.05 hr) without associated normalization of blood glucose. Subsequent discontinuation of insulin resulted in return to diabetic values (2.1 ± 0.12). These studies suggest that insulin availability is more important than normalization of blood glucose in recovery of barrier function (14).

Krupin et al. (15) have also shown that the alteration of the BRB that occurs in STZ-diabetic rats is reversed 13 days following pancreatic islet transplantation.

Noteworthy   is that electron microscopical examination of the retinae of these STZ-diabetic rats has shown that the alteration of the BRB is probably due to lesions located in the retinal pigment epithelium (16).

VITREOUS FLUOROPHOTOMETRY STUDIES ON ARTERIAL HYPERTENSION

Recently vitreous fluorophotometry studies were initiated in experimental systemic hypertension by Waltman and co-workers (17). Arterial hypertension was produced by complete ligation of one kidney combined with daily injection of desoxycorticosterone-acetate (0.2 mg) and saline drinking water. Vitreous fluorophotometry performed before and at various times after the production of hypertension showed an increased accumulation of fluorescein in the vitreous, which correlated well both with the duration and magnitude of the induced systemic hypertension.

VITREOUS FLUOROPHOTOMETRY STUDIES IN HEREDITARY RETINAL DISEASE

Four carriers of X-linked recessive retinitis pigmentosa, one patient with Usher's Syndrome, and another with Best's dystrophy were evaluated by vitreous fluorophotometry, by Gieser et al. (18). All six subjects showed abnormal findings indicative of an alteration of the blood-retinal barrier.

Vitreous fluorophotometry, therefore, appears to be able to detect a subclinical dysfunction of the retinal pigment epithelium not detected by other means like fluorescein angiography or electrophysiological testing.

This new method of clinical investigation appears to have value in the identification of carriers for X-linked recessive retinitis pigmentosa and allows for interesting speculation as to the pathogenetic changes occurring in some hereditary retinal disease.

VITREOUS FLUOROPHOTOMETRY STUDIES ON PHOTOCOAGULATION

A variety of retinal diseases are, at some time of their evolution, treated by photocoagulation. This appears to be somewhat contradictory, in that photocoagulation has been shown by fluorescein angiography and histologic studies using a variety of tracer materials to induce a breakdown of the BRB. Our studies, using vitreous fluorophotometry showed that after localized photocoagulation of the retina there is an abnormal increase in the permeability of the BRB (19). This alteration followed a well-defined pattern. Higher values that were demonstrated during the first 3 days after photocoagulation recovered progressively afterwards. The permeability of the BRB returned to near-normal levels in the period between 10 and 14 days after photocoagulation (fig. 9). A direct correlation between higher initial values and heavier photocoagulation was observed.

In another study, kinetic vitreous fluorophotometry was used to evaluate the effect of pan-retinal argon laser photocoagulation on BRB (20). Similarly, the alteration of the barrier recovered progressively with time, depending on the intensity of the photocoagulation burns. When minimal pan-retinal laser photocoagulation was used, the transport activity was markedly altered at 6 days, but there was almost complete recovery at the end of 30 days. However, when heavier photocoagulation was performed, very little recovery was observed, even 90 days afterwards.

COMMENTS

Vitreous fluorophotometry is mainly a diagnostic technique, the only available method that can quantitate an alteration of the BRB. It appears also to be particularly suited for the early detection of functional changes of the BRB, before lesions are visible in the retina using less refined methods of detection like ophthalmoscopy and

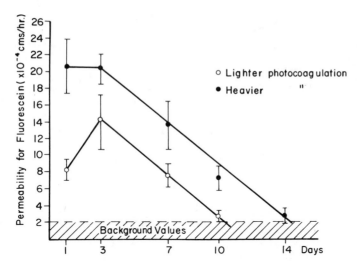

Fig. 9. Permeability of the blood-retinal barrier for fluorescein after xenon photocoagulation.

fluorescein angiography. Kinetic vitreous fluorophotometry is specially promising as a functional test of the BRB and is expected to be of particular prognostic value.

The detection of an alteration of the BRB can also contribute significantly to understand the pathophysiology of a variety of retinal diseases where a breakdown of the BRB is suspected to play a major role. In this way diseases involving the retinal vessels and the retinal pigment epithelium are natural targets for the use of this technique.

Finally, new hope is offered for a variety of retinal diseases associated with early alteration of the BRB, where treatment at a reversible stage may now be an attainable goal.

REFERENCES

1. Ashton, N. and Cunha-Vaz, J.G. (1965) Arch. Ophthalmol., 73:211--223.
2. Maurice, D.M. (1963) Exp. Eye Res., 2:33-38.
3. Cunha-Vaz, J.G. and Maurice, D.M. (1967) J. Physiol., 191:467-486.
4. Maurice, D.M. (1959) Am. J. Ophthal., 47:361-367.
5. Crank, J. (1956) The Mathematics of Diffusion, 1st edn. pp. 59 and 93, Oxford: Clarendon Press.
6. Waltman, S.R. and Kaufman, H.E. (1970) Invest. Ophthalmol., 9:247--249.

7. Cunha-Vaz, J.G., Abreu, J.R.F., Campos, A.J. et al. (1975) Brit.
   J. Ophthalmol., 59:649-656.
8. Waltman, S.R., Oestrich, C., Krupin, T. et al. (1979) Diabetes,
   27:85-87.
9. Krupin, T., Waltman, S.R., Oestrich, C. et al. (1978) Arch. Ophthalmol., 96:812-814.
10. Cunha-Vaz, J.G., Fonseca, J.R. Abreu, J.R.F. et al. (1978) Am.
    J. Ophthalmol., 86:467-473.
11. Cunha-Vaz, J.G., Fonseca, J.R. Abreu, J.R.F. et al. (1978) Diabe
    tes, 28:16-19.
12. Cunha-Vaz, J.G., Goldberg, M.F., Vygantas, C. et al. (1979) Oph-
    thalmology, 86:264.
13. Waltman, S.R., Krupin, T., Hanish, S. et al. (1978) Arch. Ophtha
    mol., 96:878-879.
14. Jones, C., Cunha-Vaz, J.G., Zweig, K. et al. (1979) Arch. Ophtha
    mol., (In press).
15. Krupin, T., Scharp, D., Waltman, S.R. et al. (1978) ARVO 1978:22
16. Tso, M.O.M., Shih, C.Y., Cunha-Vaz, J.G. et al. (1979) Invest.
    Ophthalmol.
17. Waltman, S.R., Oestrich, C., Hanish, S. et al. (1977) ARVO 1977:
    37.
18. Gieser, D., Cunha-Vaz, J.G. and Fishman, G. (1979) Arch. Ophthal-
    mol. (In press).
19. Noth, J., Vygantas, C. and Cunha-Vaz, J.G. (1978) Invest. Ophtha
    mol. Vis. Science, 17:1206.
20. Zweig, K., Cunha-Vaz, J.G., Peyman, G. et al. (1980) Invest. Oph-
    thalmol. Vis. Science.(In press).

FLUORESCEIN ANGIOGRAPHY AND THE BLOOD-RETINAL BARRIER

Gabriel Coscas

Clinique Ophtalmologique de Creteil-Universite Paris XII

40, avenue de Verdun, 94010 Creteil (France)

Fluorescein is a real "providence" for the study of barriers. And reciprocally, the existence of barriers is a real "providence" for the analysis of angiograms.

Retinal vessels normally appear to be impermeable to fluorescein according to the usual photographic techniques. The same can be observed for large choroidal vessels. On the other hand, fluorescein normally escapes easily through the permeable walls of the choriocapillaris into the extravascular tissue, but fluorescein is blocked by the retinal pigment epithelium and the very tight junctions between each of the cells, acting as a screen. Fluorescein angiography, from a morphological point of view, and vitreous fluorometry, from a quantitative point of view, enable us to study the possible clinical changes of these barriers.

The breakdown of outer and inner blood-retinal barriers results in abnormal hyperfluorescence (except for some very particular cases). Hyperfluorescence may be related either to abnormal transmission of fluorescent light (across the altered retinal pigment epithelium) or to leakage of fluorescein molecules themselves when R.P.E. and/or retinal vascular walls are involved.

The transmission of choroidal fluorescence is an optical phenomenon: it is the abnormal visibility of the choroidal background fluorescence by changes of the pigmentary screen without failure of the cellular membrane; this is the classical "window-defect". This hyperfluorescence appears early, increases rapidly but decreases at the same time as choroidal fluorescence.

Real leakage is the abnormal diffusion of fluorescein molecules
through retinal vascular walls or altered retinal pigment epithelium:
this hyperfluorescence begins more or less early but increases
progressively during the angiographic sequence and even at very
late stages.

It is essentially the leakage in fluorescein angiography which
is to be studied during this Symposium on the Blood-Retinal Barrier.
As a matter of fact, an important part of the interpretation of
fluorescein angiography is devoted to the analysis and the location
of breakdown of the blood-ocular barriers in the retina, the optic
disc and even the iris.

FLUORESCEIN AND NORMAL BARRIERS

I.   Fluorescein

Fluorescein is a real biological tracer allowing to test the
value of blood-ocular barriers.

The fluorescein molecule has a diameter of only 5.5 $\overset{o}{A}$: consequently it is very small and its molecular weight is: 376.

After intravenous injection, it binds easily to plasma
proteins and especially to albumin. In the circulating blood, 80%
of fluorescein molecules are bound to albumin molecules, which have
a diameter of approximately 100 $\overset{o}{A}$. This combination is easily
reversible, but only a slight fraction (20%) of fluorescein remains
free in the circulating blood. It is nevertheless this fraction
which is the most fluorescent.

During angiography, one can only analyse transit or fluorescein leakage "photographically detectable", but this is not equivalent to histochemical observation. In fact, angiography consists
in registering on a film the light emitted by fluorescein appropria-
tely excited by blue light. It depends on the concentration of the
dye. Below concentration of 10^{-5} g/l, fluorescence is no longer
detectable.

II.   Angiography and Normal Barriers

A.   The normal fundus. The two barriers which protect the
retina against leakage of large-sized molecules, the retinal
pigment epithelium and the retinal vascular endothelium are also
barriers for fluorescein.

On the contrary, the absence of a barrier in the choriocapillaris determines the aspect of the choroidal background in angiography.

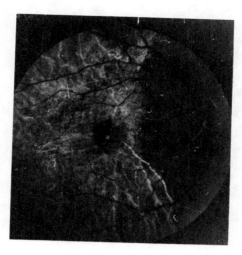

Figure 1

Choroid: The walls of choroidal arteries and veins do not allow any apparent leakage of the dye. Choroidal arteries are clearly visible in patients with weak opacity of the pigment epithelium just before the filling of choriocapillaris. In certain cases, choroidal veins are also clearly visible when filled with the dye (Fig. 1).

On the contrary, choroidal capillaries have a fenestrated endothelium, easily permeable to large molecules and free fluorescein. This leakage is immediate in the choroidal extravascular space. The absence of barrier in this location explains that details of choroidal circulation are difficult to observe because of the rapid hyperfluorescence of the extravascular space.

In late stages of the angiogram, the choroidal background remains fluorescent except the large vessels which appear hypofluorescent. The large choroidal vessels lying in the pool of extravascular dye appear relatively hypofluorescent during the late stages of angiography.

Leakage in the choriocapillaris is easily visible in some clinical cases at the border between healthy and abnormal areas, as for example in this case of fundus flavimaculatis: during early stages, choroidal vessels are abnormally visible through the retinal pigment epithelium "window". They are few in numbers and do not leak. During arterio-venous stages, leakage appears to be escaping from the normal choriocapillaris at the border of the atrophic area (Fig. 2a, b).

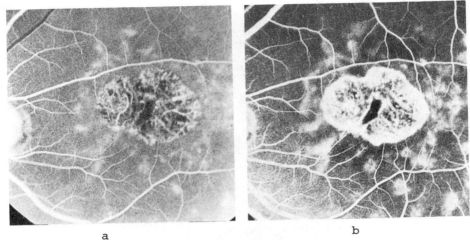

a   b

Figure 2

As far as Bruch's membrane is concerned, it may slow down the leakage of circulating macro-molecules, but is not a real barrier.

In the retina, blood-retinal barriers are located at two levels: retinal pigment epithelium and retinal vascular endothelial cells.

The retinal pigment epithelium has a double function in angiography: Screening function - it partly masks details of the underlying choroid. This is especially true for the melanoderm patients in the macular area. Barrier function between the choroidal extravascular space and the retina. The presence of "zonulae occludentes" between retinal pigment epithelium cell constitutes a complete barrier against fluorescein leakage from the choriocapillaris towards the retina.

Retinal vascular endothelial cells are impermeable to fluorescein: there are "zonulae occludentes" on the whole intercellular surface. These "tight-junctions" restrict molecular movements across the vascular walls and especially for circulating macromolecules.

The passive transfer of free molecules of fluorescein is nonsignificant and photographically not detectable (permeability coefficient 0.14×10^{-5} cm/sec., i.e., 50 times less than other capillaries of the body).

The optic disc. Angiography is very useful for studying flow of interstitial fluid in the anterior part of optic nerve head.

Blood vessels of the optic nerve head exercise a blood-optic nerve barrier. Their filling by the dye contributes to papillary fluorescence during early angiographic stages but there is no fluorescein leakage in the nerve tissue.

On the contrary, a considerable amount of fluid seems to flow from the peripapillary choriocapillaris into the anterior part of the optic nerve. Through large pores in the choriocapillaris, fluorescein leaks out and escapes freely through the border tissue of Elschnig to enter the pre-laminar region of the optic nerve head but not into the superficial layer of the optic fibers (Fig.3a, b).

There is also a free leakage from the cerebro-spinal fluid in the sheaths of the optic nerve towards the optic nerve head. However, there is a blood-brain barrier similar to that of the eye and there is no evidence that the cerebro-spinal fluid becomes sufficiently concentrated in fluorescein. Thus, the interstitial fluid in the anterior part of the optic nerve is probably derived from many sources but there are fluorescein leaking junctions only in choriocapillaris and border tissue of Elschnig.

The later hyperfluorescent ring at the border of the disc seems to be due to the leakage of the dye through Elschnig's border tissue.

The progressive disc staining may be explained as a staining of the collagenous tissue of the cribrosa lamina and the glial tissues in the prelaminar region.

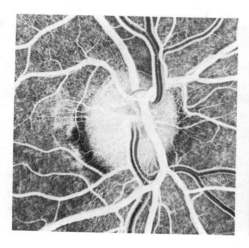
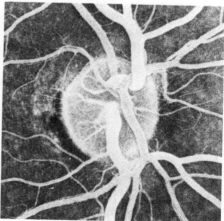

a   b

Figure 3

B. Iris and ciliary body. Endothelial cells of the iris vessels have a structure similar to that of the retinal vessels. Endothelial cells are joined by tight-junctions and "macula occludens" less stable than in retinal vessels. Intercellular impermeability is less complete than in the retina: a slight leakage of free molecules of fluorescein may be observed but it does not produce a photographic effect.

During angiography, normal iris vessels appear impermeable to fluorescein. However, in approximately 20% of cases, a pupillary leakage exists, especially in patients over 50. Certain authors consider that no precise value should be attributed to this leakage because of the frequency of this observation. But this peri-pupillary leakage in the anterior chamber is regarded by others as a change in the blood-anterior chamber barrier, perhaps related to previous diseases like uveitis and glaucoma.

Blood vessel walls of the ciliary body allow free leakage of the dye as in choriocapillaris. The non-pigmented layer of the ciliary epithelium presents tight junctions but spaced out and allows slow leakage of free fluorescein which can be observed in the anterior chamber. In fact, during angiography, ciliary processes become very fluorescent.

III. Fluorescence and Hyperfluorescence

Normal fluorescence. The normal angiogram is essentially a morphological and dynamic record of the two fundus circulations, retinal and choroidal that are separated by pigment epithelium. A retinal vessel becomes visible when it is filling with the dye and if its diameter is not lower than the resolution power. Retinal capillaries are large enough to be photographed by current cameras.

Abnormal fluorescence. Barrier changes resulting in hypofluorescence are poorly known. Breakdown of blood-ocular barriers usually results in hyperfluorescence. When hyperfluorescence appears, there are two major reasons for its presence:

-Hyperfluorescence due to abnormal transmission: Isolated changes in the retinal pigment epithelium result in an increase in the visibility of the normal choroidal fluorescence. There is no extravasation of the dye through the retinal pigment epithelium but only an optical effect of transparency and no rupture of the biological barrier. This is the so-called "window defect".

-Hyperfluorescence due to leakage: Alteration of the normal vascular wall's permeability in the fundus results in leakage. This hyperfluorescence appears early during angiography, as soon as the dye diffuses through altered structures. According to the delay of appearance of the dye, this leakage could be of choroidal or retinal origin and could be of arterial, capillary or venous origin. During the angiography, the surface and the intensity of fluorescence increases more or less rapidly, due to the quantity of extravasated dye.

When leakage occurs into normal or abnormal tissue, it is referred to as staining. When it occurs into an anatomic space it, is called pooling. Leakage Always shows late hyperfluorencence.

BREAKDOWN OF THE OUTER BLOOD-RETINAL BARRIER: ALTER- ATION OF RETINAL PIGMENT EPITHELIUM

Alteration of the retinal pigment epithelium causing break-down of the outer blood-retinal barrier is observed in association with many circumstances like: mechanical damage, inflammation, defective epithelial cells, choroidal ischemia, biochemical and metabolic influences.

I.   RETINAL PIGMENT EPITHELIUM SEROUS DETACHMENT

Definition. R.P.E. serous detachment is not properly due to ruptures of the R.P.E. barrier but rather to a decrease or a local-ized loss in adherence between the R.P.E. and Bruch's membrane, resulting in pooling of fluid, escaping from the choriocapillaris into the usually virtual sub-retinal space.

Usual angiographic aspects. Idiopathic R.P.E. serous detach-ment appears as an area of early hyperfluorescence of deep origin with rounded and distinct contours. There is no evidence of abnormal leakage from retinal vessels. The full extent of the late hyperfluorescence is already evident on the early angiogram; hyperfluorescence increases progressively; it is usually homogeneous and fills the entire R.P.E. detachment with accumulation and abnormal persistance of the dye even in very late stages of angio-graphy. Sometimes, a cruciate pigmented figure results in localized masking of the hyperfluorescence (Fig. 4a, b, c).

Evolution is rather variable: sometimes it does not progress for several years; sometimes the area extends towards the foveola and/or shows subretinal new vessel proliferation.

Morphological aspects. In clinical cases, many morphological aspects may be observed: large R.P.E. serous detachment extending over the entire macular region; R.P.E. serous detachment which may increase in size, change in shape or enlarge; R.P.E. serous

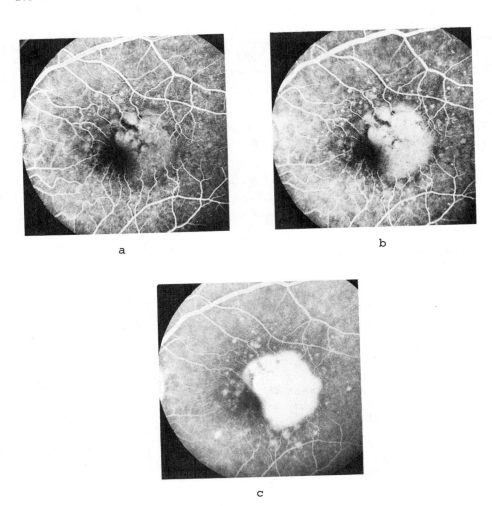

a

b

c

Figure 4

detachment may persist small, silent, or asymptomatical for years
even if multiple; R.P.E. serous detachment may be associated with
central serous chorioretinopathy in the same fundus; but, the
most important association is with subretinal neovascularization
suggested by alterations in the normally sharp margins of the
fluorescence and appearance of a localized area of intense hyperfluorescence or "hot spot".

Physiopathogenesis of the hyperfluorescence of R.P.E. serous
detachment. One more problem remains to be solved: is the hyperfluorescence of R.P.E. detachment only due to the amount of fluid

pooling beneath the R.P.E. and transudating from the choroid?
In this case, the intensity of hyperfluorescence should remain
similar to that of normal choroidal background; it should stop
increasing in the late stages when choroidal fluorescence decreases.
On the contrary, the hyperfluorescence of R.P.E. serous detachment
still increases.

Another hypothesis is therefore necessary. The fluid in
R.P.E. detachment could be particularly rich in proteins and
bound molecules of fluorescein. The transfer of fluorescein molecules is not necessarily similar to that of interstitial fluid.
This should explain why R.P.E. detachment becomes and remains very
intensively hyperfluorescent. The role of an optimal pH or, maybe,
the role of a "release" of fluorescein molecules into the transu-
date could also be considered.

II.   Serous Detachment of Sensory Retina and Idiopathic
Central Serous Chorio-Retinopathy (C.S.C.R.)

Definition. Idiopathic central serous retinopathy is defined
by sensory retinal detachment in macular area. This detachment
is isolated, but fluorescein angiography brings evidence of very
localized changes of the R.P.E.

Typical angiographic aspects. The fluorescein angiogram
typically shows a pin-point leak at the level of the pigment epithelium beneath the bullous sensory retinal detachment, during
the arterio-venous or venous phase of the retinal vascular transit.

The leak is rarely evident in the very early stages of the
angiogram, but gradually increases, as some pooling of the dye
occurs in the subsensory retinal space. In the later stages of
the angiogram, the dye continues to pool in the bullous retinal
detachment, but never completely fills it.

The most frequent hyperfluorescent pin-point is often described as an "ink blot". The hyperfluorescent point enlarges
concentrically and remains localized but with fuzzy margins.

The second variety of leak is referred to as a "jet type" or
"umbrella type" of leak: hyperfluorescence is often very intensive
and begins to ascend rapidly in the subsensory retinal space
towards the superior limits of the sensory retinal detachment
(convectional currents). When it reaches a point close to the
upper limit, it continues to extend nasally and/or temporally
(Fig. 5a, b).

Morphological aspects. In clinical cases, many morphological
aspects may be observed: small detachments with a weak leakage

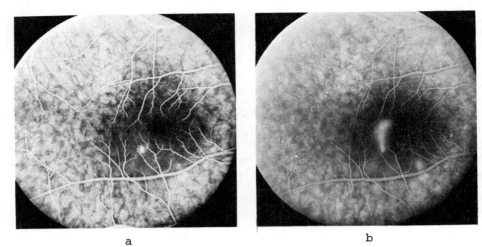

a   b

Figure 5

point, even in late stages; multiple leakage points and multiple
sensory retinal detachments; giant bullous serous detachment;
association with R.P.E. serous detachment

Physiopathogenesis of the hyperfluorescence of C.S.C.R. The
origin of the dye leakage, which is the main aniographic sign, is not
yet fully understood; alterations in the junctional complexes of
the pigment epithelium have been implicated; some have suggested
that the primary event is that of an occlusive change in the choriocapillaris; according to Gass, the anatomical change resulting in
retinal detachment   could be a pigment epithelium detachment,
usually so small that it cannot be seen biomicroscopically and
sometimes not clinically detectable.

Stereoscopic views show that fluorescein is leaking from R.P.E.
level towards the subretinal space. The spontaneous disappearance
of the subretinal fluid is usually accompanied by the healing of
the leakage point. Elective photocoagulation of this point results
in resorption of the subretinal fluid.

The leakage of fluorescein in the "jet-type" form evokes a
rapid and important fluid flow. This would imply the possibility
of equivalent resorption so as to restitute an equilibrium. It
could also be considered that the leakage of the dye is selective
and not proportional to the plasmatic diffusion.

III. Subretinal Neovascularization

Subretinal neovascularization is a histopathologic manifestation
associated with a number of macular diseases. The clinical recog-

nition of subretinal neovascularization is very important in terms
of management and fluorescein angiography allows a major advance
in clinical ophthalmology.   Subretinal vascular membranes are
formed of one or several vascular trunks.   Their ramifications
constitute a peripheral anastomotic arcade.   These new vessels
usually develop beneath the pigment epithelium and may represent
poorly developed junctional complexes.   Their proliferation is also
accompanied by a proliferation of R.P.E. cells (Archer) which
explains that the neovascular membrane appears to be greyish
and surrounded by a pigmented halo.

   During angiography, an early hyperfluorescence (in the choroidal
phase) of the new vessels and the anastomotic capillary arcade
develops.   There is an immediate leakage of the dye into the
subretinal space.   There is no real breakdown of the blood-ocular
barrier as the neocapillaries of choroidal origin have a quite
normal structure but have proliferated in an ectopic position.
Nevertheless this causes a mechanical damage in retinal pigment
epithelium.

   Hyperfluorescence is early and very intense, it increases
progressively in intensity and surface during the course of the
angiography.   There is late hyperfluorescence with staining of
fibrovascular membrane and fuzzy limits indicating leakage into the
sensory retinal detachment.

   In clinical cases many morphological cases may be observed:
small neovascular membrane with a capillary anastomotic arcade; (Fig. 6).

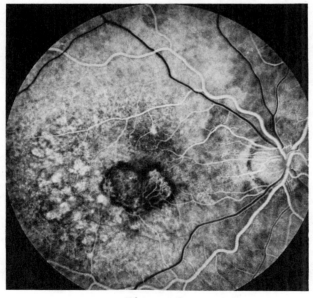

Figure 6

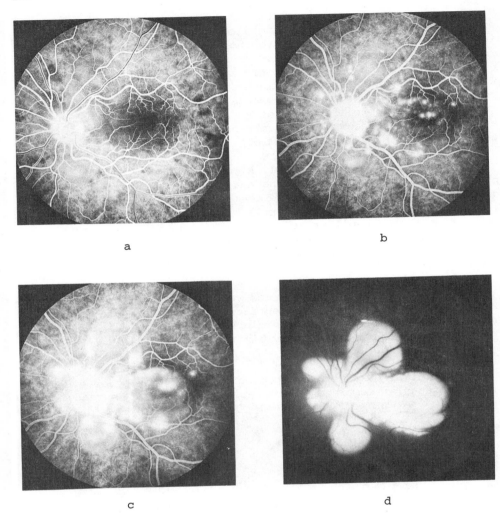

a
b
c
d

Figure 7

more extensive membrane with radial vessels; presumed histoplasmosis;
subretinal neovascular membrane with R.P.E. serous detachment
("hot spot"); subretinal neovascular membrane associated with
retinal bullous detachment simulating idiopathic central serous
chorioretinopathy.

IV.   Particular Cases

Harada's disease.   This disease is rare in Europe, at least
in its typical form. This uveo-meningeal syndrome is characterized
by the presence of multiple detachments of the retinal pigment

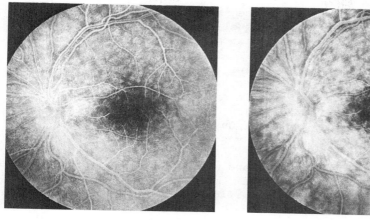

a

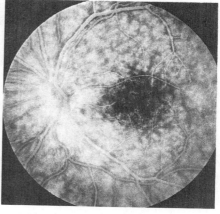

b

c

Figure 8

epithelium associated with a bullous sensory retinal detachment.
This entity produces leaks from the choroid, at the level of the
R.P.E. beneath a sensory retinal detachment.

During angiography, the choroidal vessel filling is irregular.
Many leaking spots appear very soon, showing extensive pooling
into the subsensory retinal space from multiple R.P.E. detachments.
In the late phases of the angiogram, hyperfluorescence is evident
from the filling of the subsensory retinal detachment. Hyperfluorescence of the disc is usually associated, (Fig.7a,b,c and d).

The mechanism of this leakage is still controversial: is it
a primary disease of the R.P.E. or is it an inflammatory disease

of the choriocapillaris with excessive exudation? Usual recovery
leaves very few angiographic sequelae in the R.P.E. and this
suggests that it could be a choriocapillaris inflammatory disease.

Posterior uveitis. Posterior uveitis and pars planitis may
show diffuse retinal edema with cystoid macular edema, moderate
papilledema and slight changes in the retinal venous walls (dilatation and sheathing). Alteration of the blood-retinal barrier
is a common finding in posterior uveitis, especially when
associated with chronic retinal vasculitis (Fig. 8a, b, c).

During angiography, rapid and marked hyperfluorescence of the
choroidal background is observed , associated with dilatation of
the retinal capillaries and significant leakage of the dye.

Retinal edema could also be due to fluid diffusion from the
choriocapillaris through the R.P.E., altered by the inflammation.
The dye is pooling in small juxtaposed "cysts". Should this aspect
be related only to cystoid retinal edema or furthermore be related
also to the disposition of the units of choriocapillaris.

Focal chorioretinitis. Focal or multifocal chorioretinitis
results in an acute but localized breakdown of B.R.B. Fluorescein
angiography has shown first hypofluorescence during the early
choroidal phase due to the filling defect of the choriocapillaris
in the area of the focal choroiditis. During later stages, hyperfluorescence appears progressively, first located at the choroidal
level, with staining of necrotic tissues: choriocapillaris, R.P.E.,
and retina. There is also some leakage towards retina, through
altered R.P.E., resulting in retinal edema.

Retinal vessels crossing the chorioretinitis area may be
altered by the inflammatory process causing more or less marked
changes of the vascular walls and inner blood-retinal barrier,
associated with the alteration of R.P.E. This damage is also
observed in a group of situations which include thermal or cold
injury, photocoagulation and trauma.

Acute multifocal posterior placoid pigment epitheliopathy
(A.M.P.P.P.E.). This disorder is a bilateral acute inflammation of
the R.P.E. and choriocapillaris. The ophthalmoscopic examination
demonstrates yellowish multifocal flat lesions in the posterior
pole.

The characteristic fluorescein angiogram demonstrates, in
the acute stage, hypofluorescence of the yellowish lesions during
the early phase. Later in the angiogram, progressive and moderate
hyperfluorescence can be seen, indicating fluorescein staining of
the lesions which remain well limited. There is no intraretinal
leakage as in acute focal chorioretinitis (Fig. 9 a, b).

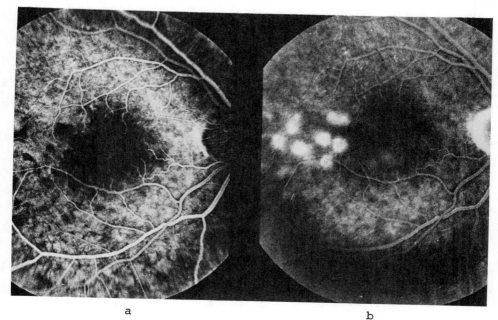

a   b

Figure 9

The interpretation of the angiographic aspect is still controversial: is it only epitheliopathy with thickening or swelling of
the pigment epithelium? In this case, early hypofluorescence
could be blocked fluorescence. The late staining could be explained
by diffusion of fluorescein through altered retinal pigment epithelium. However, this does not result in an extensive sensory
retinal detachment.

Choriocapillaris could be involved with inflammatory cellular
infiltration. Early hypofluorescence could be suggestive of non-
perfusion of the choriocapillaris, caused by acute occlusion of
the precapillary arterioles induced initially by inflammation.
Late hyperfluorescence would be due to the staining of R.P.E. and
the necrotic underlying retina: leakage of the dye would have his
origin from the adjacent units of choriocapillaris.

Serpiginous choroidopathy. Serpiginous choroïdopathy or
geographic helicoid peripapillary choroidopathy is a disorder of
the peripapillary pigment epithelium, choriocapillaris and choroid.
The condition is unilateral in most cases, occurs in older subjects,
and is progressive, extending out from the disc and advancing into
the macula with recurrent attacks. It is more destructive than
acute placoid pigment epitheliopathy (Fig. 10 a, b).

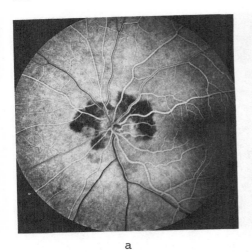 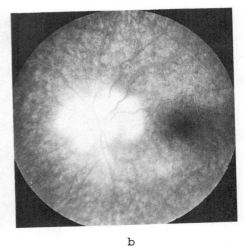

a   b

Figure 10

The fluorescein angiogram of this lesion is very characteristic: in early phases of the angiogram, the main part of the lesion is dark and hypofluorescent; in the late phases appears spotty hyperfluorescence without leakage. The older portion of the lesion shows hyperfluorescent staining caused by subretinal scanning. Sequelae are more severe than in acute placoid epitheliopathy and atrophy of R.P.E. and choriocapillaris is usually marked in the center of the lesion.

<u>Argon laser burns</u>. Argon laser photocoagulation results in local destruction of R.P.E., of the adjacent retina, and of the adjacent choriocapillaris. The immediate whitish appearance taken by each spot is probably due to burning and to intracellular edema of R.P.E.

The angiographic aspect of a recent argon laser burn is similar to that of acute placoid epitheliopathy: early hypofluorescence of the lesion and late staining. The aspect of late lesions is similar to chorioretinal atrophic localized area.

Following argon laser photocoagulation, the R.P.E. barrier appears to be temporarily destructed. Later it recovers partially, showing no permeability to plasma proteins; but it allows diffusion of small-sized molecules, as demonstrated by experimental studies with dextrans of molecular weight ranging between 3.000 to 150.000.

These findings explain the retinal edema which always follows argon laser photocoagulation. This edema is probably related to the massive passage of proteins. It may become very extensive and durable in cases of excessive photocoagulation.

Moreover, photocoagulation could have a beneficial effect on macular edema. The persistence of a certain degree of permeability of the R.P.E., together with the hydrostatic pressure of the vitreous on the retina, could explain the possibility of resorption of intraretinal edema towards the choroid.

Choroidal tumors. Choroidal nevi and melanomas frequently demonstrate degenerative changes of the overlying R.P.E. The area corresponding to a nevus shows hypofluorescence but some nevi have overlying drusen with early focal hyperfluorescent spots. In some cases, when exudative changes develop over a nevus, the fluorescein angiogram will show late hyperfluorescence, small R.P.E. serous detachments and spots of leakage (Figs. 11 a, b).

Choroidal melanoma shows hyperfluorescence during the entire angiogram, but there are usually many complex features. Hyperfluorescence begins in focal areas scattered diffusely throughout the tumor. This results from leakage of dye through Bruch's membrane and areas of R.P.E. degeneration. Later, fluorescein begins to leak into the outer retinal layers. In the later phases, the persistent hyperfluorescence is due to the pooling of dye in small serous detachments of R.P.E. and into subretinal space and in serous detachment of sensory retina. Pin-point hyperfluorescent spots may be observed during angiography. They most likely represent tiny areas of degeneration within the retinal pigment epithelium.

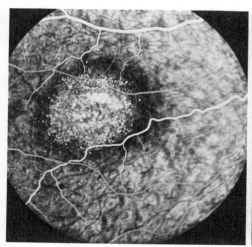 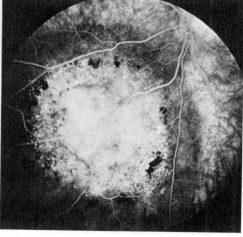

a   b

Figure 11

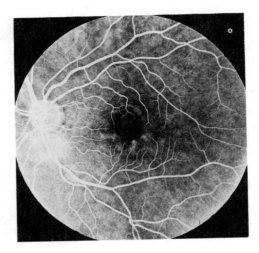

Figure 12

BREAKDOWN OF THE INNER BLOOD-RETINAL BARRIER

Breakdown of the blood-retinal barrier with a significant
degree of alteration of the retinal vessel walls permeability has
been demonstrated in almost every retinal vascular disease:
arteries, capillaries and veins may be involved. Experimental
and clinical observations point to one or more of the following
six causes of breakdown of the barrier: acute distention of the
vessel walls; ischemia-hypoxia; biochemical influences; inflammation; defective endothelial cells; failure of the active transport
processes. However, in most cases, tissular consequences of this
breakdown of the inner blood-retinal barrier are the same: diffuse
edema and/or cystoid edema, retinal serous detachment, retinal
hemorrhages and, later, hard exudates.

A. Arteries. The arterial walls resist well to the agressions.
In some cases transient leakage may be observed, especially in
arteritis or following intensive photocoagulation.

B. Retinal capillaries. Involvement of the endothelium of
retinal capillaries is seen in a great number of retinal vascular
diseases. Three types of elementary lesions can be described:
dilatation, leakage, and exclusion or non-perfusion.

Isolated leakage with or without visible dilatation of the
retinal capillaries is probably the initial sign of the 2 main
types of retinal vasculopathies.

In diabetes and especially juvenile diabetes (Fig. 12),
multiple leakage spots of the dye from retinal capillaries were

seen   in the absence of microaneurysms.   This leakage is probably
the earliest clinical symptom of barrier alteration.   This alteration is reversible after treatment and clinical studies have
shown that there is a correlation between the alteration of B.R.B.
and the diabetic metabolic control.

In severe hypertension, the increase in wall-permeability of
the terminal arterioles or of the capillary bed is an early sign of
hypertensive retinopathy.   This change in the vascular barrier is
due to the elevated blood pressure with acute distension of vessel
walls and/or to the action of excessive secretion of angiotensin.

Microaneurysms often coexist with an alteration of the vascular endothelium (hypertension, diabetes, venous occlusion).   Their
angiographic aspect is variable and is probably related to the
state of the endothelium

   -filling without leakage
   -filling with more or less severe leakage (Fig. 13a, b)
   -absence of filling

The extent of capillary dilatation may be important and permanent like in diabetic retinopathy and edematous central vein
occlusion.   This capillary dilatation may be very easily defined
by fluorescein angiography.

The capillary bed fills more or less rapidly, depending on
arterial flow and venous resistance.   The capillaries are "too
easily" visible because they are dilated and they appear to be
more spaced out from each other than normally.   Leakage of the

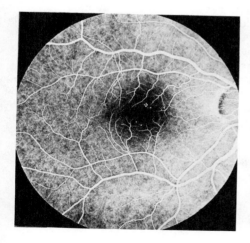 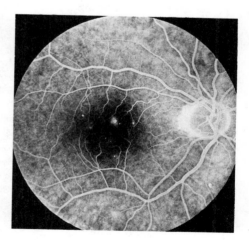

a   b

Figure 13

dye appears progressively in the retinal tissue and rapidly masks
capillary details.

Hyperfluorescence increases at the late stages producing
cloudy diffuse edema. In some cases, the dye collects in intraretinal spaces producing cystoid or microcystic retinal edema.

In diabetic retinopathy, the initial change probably occurs
in the basal membrane of the capillary endothelium. In venous
occlusions, capillary dilatation is directly related to stasis
and venous hyperpressure. In venous stasis retinopathy, dilatation
and dye leakage are the main features and justify the term of
edematous capillaropathy. Obstruction to flow produces both
dilatation of some capillaries and non-filling of others.

Hyperpressure and stasis causes vascular distension and some
degree of breakdown of the barrier at the level of endothelial cells.
This capillary change is often spontaneously reversible if venous
flow is reestablished or if the development of collateral circulation is efficient.

C. Veins. The abnormal permeability of retinal venous walls
has been demonstrated in many vascular diseases: venous hyperpressure
ischemic capillaropathies; inflammatory vasculitis. The breakdown
of the barrier is shown by wall staining and leakage. In late
stages of angiography, the vein lumen becomes less fluorescent
(depending on blood concentration) but the walls become hyperfluorescent. The vein appears as two hyperfluorescent lines framing
a less fluorescent lumen. The diameter of the vein, appears then
much larger than its diamter in red free light.

Leakage is slow and moderate and results in lage stages, in
cloudy masking of the vein. It extends rarely to more than one or
two venous diameters of the vein itself.

There are many causes for these wall changes. The alteration
is more severe when several factors are associated but each of them
is sufficient to produce wall staining and leakage:

   -Ischemic change in arterial occlusion without vein occlusion
    (hypertensive retinopathy). Ischemia appears to be a main
    cause of damage to the blood retinal barrier and plays a
    major role in retinal vascular disease by making the vascular
    endothelium vulnerable to other and further influences.
   -Venous hyperpressure in R.C.V.O.
   -Ischemia with hyperpressure, like in diabetic retinopathy
    with venous dilatation and venous loop.
   -Inflammatory changes in peripheral periphlebitis.
   -Ischemia, hyperpressure, and inflammation in Behcet's disease
    with inflammatory venous occlusion.

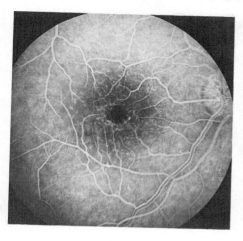 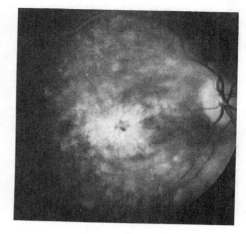

a   b

Figure 14

D. Tissue damage due to breakdown of the inner blood ocular
barrier (alteration of the retinal vascular endothelium).
Hyperpermeability of the retinal vessels results in retinal edema,
hemorrhages and, later on, hard exudates. Retinal edema becomes
clearly visible by dye leakage and late hyperfluorescence. It is
always present when there are hemorrhages and/or exudates.
Fluorescein angiography demonstrates capillary dilatation and
leakage but does not always allow to understand why the resulting
edema is sometimes cloudy and diffuse and sometimes of cystoid
character. One may evoke the role of the volume of extravasated
fluid, of the duration of the change in the blood-retinal
barrier and the size of the molecules and, maybe, alteration of
R.P.E.

Angiographic aspect of cystoid macular edema is well known
(Fig. 14a, b):
   -Partial blockage of choroidal background fluorescence in early
    phases;
   -Dilatation and abnormal visibility of macular capillaries;
   -Intraretinal dye leakage from the deep perifoveal capillaries;
   -Dye pooling in cystoid spaces;
   -Papillary hyperfluorescence is frequently associated in
    aphakia.

In Irvine-Gass syndrome, the cause of breakdown of B.R.B. is
still controversial; for some authors the cause could be essentially
mechanical due to vitreous traction before the complete posterior
vitreous detachment. But for the majority of authors, intraocular
inflammatory disease might be the most significant contributing
factor.

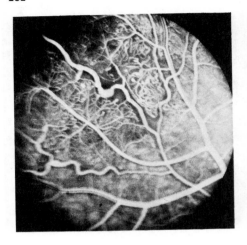
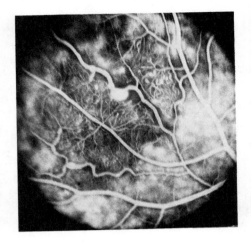

a   b

Figure 15

Fluorescein angiography shows that leakage is coming from perifoveal capillaries. But pigment epithelium seems also changed. According to Tso, after experimental aphakia in monkeys, macular capillary endothelial cells and macular pigment epithelium are abnormally permeable to horseradish peroxydase.

The role of the passage of aqueous humor towards the vitreous remains controversial but it seems that the incidence of macular edema is lower in patients after extra-capsular extraction than intra-capsular extraction.

Cystoid macular edema may occur as a complication of many retinal vascular disorders as diabetic retinopathy, retinal vein occlusion, retinal telangiectasia and uveitis with retinal vasculitis.

Cystoid edema may be very extensive far beyond the macula. In the periphery, capillary dilatation is sometimes less evident and the role of the barrier breakdown of pigment epithelium in the genesis of this cystoid edema has to be mentioned.

E. Abnormal vessels in the fundus. In vascular developmental defects such as those of Coat's disease and angiomatosis retinae, there is profuse fluorescein leakage but not always. This is probably directly related to the degree of alteration of endothelial vascular cells (Fig. 15a,b).

Collateral channels (arterio-venous or veno-venous) appear by remodeling of the preexistent vascular bed with dilatation and

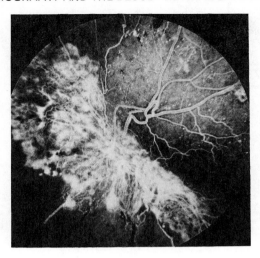

Figure 16

progressive change of some retinal capillaries after vascular
obstruction.   Their wall structure is maintained due to rapid
proliferation of their endothelial cells.

Collateral channels do not leak.   Collateral channels seem
to be less altered than other capillaries because they have to
drain the blood towards an area of less resistance without stasis.

New vessel proliferations are originating by budding on venous
walls or pre-existant capillaries and outside of the normal capillary bed.   They spread out at the border of the ischemic retinal

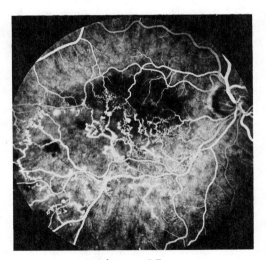

Figure 17

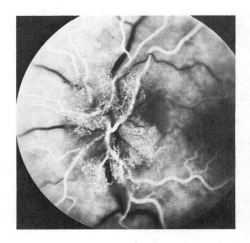
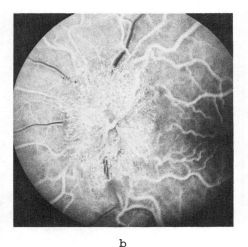

a   b

Figure 18

areas.   Their walls are completely abnormal, they have no mural
cells, their basal membrane is very thin and the walls present
fenestration and poorly developed junctional complexes (Fig. 16)

During angiography, there is an early, rapid and extensive
leakage from these new vessels and their anastomotic arcades.

Nevertheless, some collateral channels allow dye leakage and
intraretinal exudation (Fig. 17).

On the other hand, "intraretinal" new vessels may not leak.
Their histologic structure is quite the same as those of normal
capillaries except at their end, where endothelial cells without
tight junctions are proliferating.

BREAKDOWN IN THE BLOOD-OCULAR BARRIER AT THE LEVEL OF THE DISC

Papilledema.   Edema of the optic nerve may occur from a number
of primary and secondary disorders of the optic nerve.   Fluorescein
angiogram demonstrates characteristic changes which include pronounced dilatation and leakage of the superficial and intra-
capillary disc capillaries and late staining of the disc (Fig.18a,b).

Late hyperfluorescence can be explained by necrotic tissue
staining.

Fluorescein is leaking in the disc from neighboring choriocapillaris through the border tissue of Elschnig and staining the
intracellular material.

PATHOLOGY OF THE BLOOD-RETINAL BARRIER

Mark O.M. Tso, M.D.

University of Illinois Eye and Ear Infirmary

1855 West Taylor Street, Chicago, Illinois

The primary sites of the blood-retinal barrier are the endothelium of the retinal capillary and the retinal pigment epithelium (RPE). Yet, these two types of cells are very different. Embryologically, the endothelium of the retinal capillary is of mesodermal origin, but the RPE derives from neuroectoderm. Structurally, the retinal capillary is of the continuous type.[1] The apices of the endothelial cells of the retinal capillary are in direct contact with the bloodstream, and the villi of the endothelial cells are believed to be specialized for transport function. Endothelial cells are joined to each other by a zonula occludens type of cell junction. In contrast, the RPE is not in direct contact with the bloodstream. Nutrients from the choroidal circulation pass through the fenestrated endothelium of the choriocapillaris and Bruch's membrane to reach the base of the RPE. The basal plasmalemma of the RPE cells develops numerous infoldings to facilitate the transport function. The RPE cells are joined to each other by zonula adherens and zonula occludens types of cell junctions. Physiologically, while the endothelial cells are specialized for transport function, the RPE serves as the metabolic warehouse for the retina and provides support for photoreceptor cells in addition to its function as the blood-retinal barrier for the outer retina.

Both the endothelium of the retinal capillary and the RPE are noncycling cells under normal conditions, that is, there is no proliferation or replacement of cells in the normal phsiologic state. Deem, Futterman, and Kalina[2] have shown that when tritiated thymidine is supplied to the normal endothelial cells of the retinal capillary, there is essentially no uptake of thymidine, suggesting that endothelial cells do not normally multiply.

When injury such as needling of the lens produces an inflammatory
reaction in the eye, proliferation of endothelial cells, as
manifested by tritiated thymidine uptake, is observed.[2] The
multiplication of cells seems limited only to endothelial cells of
postcapillary venules and no excessive proliferation is seen. The
RPE cells also are noncycling, and mitosis is rarely, if ever,
seen in the normal retina. However when injured, the RPE may
multiply and develop nodular proliferation.[3] Because endothelial
cells of the retinal capillary and the RPE are very different
embryologically, structurally, and physiologically, they behave
distinctly in pathologic conditions of the blood-retinal barrier.

PATHOLOGY OF THE ENDOTHELIUM OF THE RETINAL CAPILLARY ASSOCIATED WITH DISRUPTION OF THE BLOOD-RETINAL BARRIER

In diseases, the cell junctions or the plasmalemma of the
endothelial cells may be injured, resulting in disruption of the
blood-retinal barrier. These pathologic alterations may be
conveniently described into five categories.

1. Disruption of Cell Junctions

In various diseases, the zonulae occludentes between the
endothelial cells may be opened and macromolecules may leak from
the intravascular compartment. In cystoid macular edema after
cataract extraction, disruption of the blood-retinal barrier at
the retinal blood vessels, resulting in leakage of fluorescein is
commonly observed clinically. To study the mechanisms of disruption of blood-retinal barrier in this condition, lens extraction associated with vitreous loss was performed in the normal
rhesus monkey.[4] Postoperatively horseradish peroxidase was injected intravenously to detect the retinal vascular leakage. By
electron microscopy, the tracer material was observed to pass
between endothelial cells presumably due to disruption of tight
cell junctions and, extended from the lumen of the blood vessels
to the perivascular space (Fig. 1).

Wallow and Engerman studied the blood-retinal barrier in an
Alloxan-induced diabetic dog with a five-year history of poorly
controlled diabetes.[5] They observed that the endothelial cell
junctions of the retinal capillary were opened and that horseradish peroxidase passed between the endothelial cells to the
perivascular space.

2. Increase of Pinocytotic Activity

Pinocytotic activity and vesicular transport are commonly
observed in the normal endothelium of the skeletal muscles, but

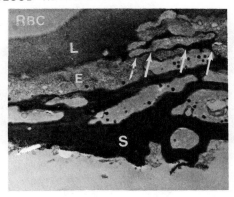

Figure 1. Disruption of blood–retinal barrier at a retinal blood
vessel of a rhesus monkey who had lens extraction with vitreous
loss. Horseradish peroxidase leaks from the lumen of the capillaries and infiltrates the basement membrane of the endothelial
cells. Tracer material is seen passing between endothelial cells
(white arrows) presumably as a result of opening of cell junction.
RBC, red blood cell; L, lumen; E, endothelial cell; S, extravascular interstitial space.

few vesicles are seen in the endothelium of the normal retinal
capillary.[6] An increased number of vesicles containing horseradish peroxidase was observed in the endothelial cells of retinal
capillary of monkeys that had lens extraction associated with
vitreous loss[4] (Fig. 2). At the abluminal side of the endothelial
cells, vesicles filled with tracer material also communicated
freely with the extravascular interstitial space. Tracer material
infiltrated the basement membrane of the endothelial cells and
pericytes. Similarly, increased pinocytotic activity was observed
in retinal capillary of cats with retrolental fibroplasia[7] and in
monkeys with ocular hypotony secondary to cyclocryotherapy.[8] However, how much the increased pinocytotic activity quantitatively
contributes to the disruption of blood–retinal barrier is unknown.

3. Focal Attenuation of the Cytoplasm of Endothelial Cells

In the eye, capillaries of the fenestrated type are normally
seen only in the choroid and the ciliary body. Macromolecules
may transverse these fenestrations which are covered by thin
diaphragms. In disease conditions, fenetrated blood vessels have
been seen in the iris of patients with rubeosis iridis[9,10] or
with diabetic retinopathy.[11] It has been proposed that these
fenestrations are the locus leakage in human intraocular
neovascularization.

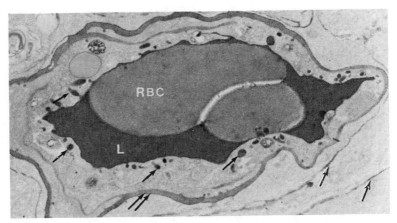

Figure 2.   Disruption of blood-retinal barrier at the retinal
vasculature of a monkey which had lens extraction with vitreous
loss.   Numerous vesicles are seen in the lumenal and ablumenal
side of the endothelial cells of a retinal blood vessel.   Horseradish peroxidase infiltrates the basement membrane of the
endothelial cell and pericytes (double arrows) as well as the
extracellular interstitial space (black and white arrows).   L,
lumen; RBC, red blood cells.

     We also have observed focal attenuation of cytoplasm in the
endothelium of vitreous neovascularization in kittens with retrolental fibroplasia[7] (Fig. 3).   Even though diffuse leakage of
fluorescein has been observed in these capillaries, fenestrated
capillary are uncommonly observed.

          4. Failure of Formation of Tight Cell Junctions

     In a horseradish peroxidase tracer study of kittens with
retrolental fibroplasia,[7] we have observed leakage of tracer
material between adjacent endothelial cells of retinal or vitreous
new blood vessels (Fig. 4).   These cell junctions frequently
appear open.   It seems logical to assume that these cell junctions
are not formed properly since these blood vessels are new proliferations.   It must, however, be pointed out that it is difficult to differentiate failure of formation of tight cell junctions
from disruption of tight cell junctions.

          5. Necrosis and Decompensation of the Endothelial Cells

     In some retinal vasculopathies the endothelial cells are
decompensated.   This allows tracer material to pass through the

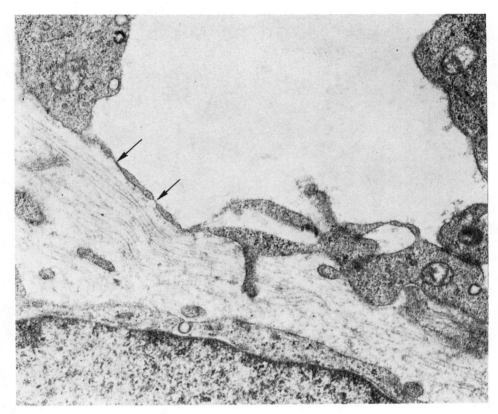

Figure 3. Blood vessels in the vitreous of a kitten with retrolental fibroplasia. Noteworthy is focal attenuation (arrows) of
the cytoplasm of a endothelial cell.

plasmalemma into the cytoplasm of the cells and subsequently into
the perivascular interstitial space (Fig. 5). The tracer may
diffuse in the ground substance of the cytoplasm of the endothelium. The endoplasmic reticulum is frequently dilated, and
mitochondria appear irregular. We have observed this pathologic
alteration in endothelial cells of retinal capillary of monkeys
that had lens extraction with vitreous loss[4] and in retinal
capillary of kittens with retrolental fibroplasia. Endothelial
cell degeneration in the latter disease was previously described
by Ashton et al[12] and our observation of passage of horseradish
peroxidase into these cells confirms the severe pathologic state
of these blood vessels.

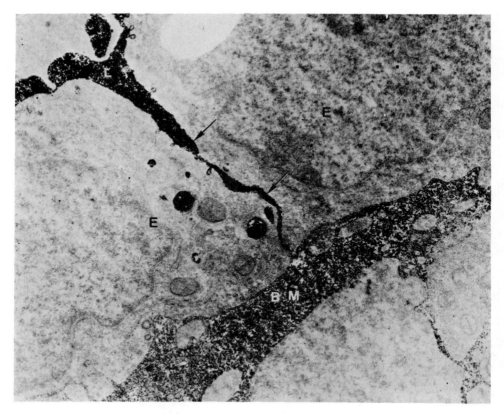

Figure 4. Disruption of blood-retinal barrier at a retinal blood
vessel of a kitten with retrolental fibroplasia. Tracer material
(arrows) passes from the lumen (L) between endothelial cells (E)
into the basement membrane (BM) of the endothelial cells, pre-
sumable as a result of failure of formation of normal tight cell
junctions.

PATHOLOGY OF RPE ASSOCIATED WITH DISRUPTION OF THE BLOOD-RETINAL BARRIER

The condition of the blood-retinal barrier at the RPE depends
on the integrity of the plasmalemma and the cell junctions of
these cells and the pathologic changes of pigment epithelium or
its cell junctions may be conveniently described in four
categories.

1. Dissolution of Cells

In severe injury to the RPE, acute necrosis leads to dissolution of the cells. In a collaborative study with Dr. Sohan

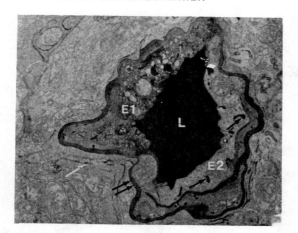

Figure 5. Decompensation and necrosis in an endothelial cell (E1) of a retinal blood vessel in a monkey who had lens extraction with vitreous loss. The endoplasmic reticulum is dilated. Horseradish peroxidase infiltrated the plasmalemma and the ground substance of the cytoplasm of the endothelial cell. The basement membrane (double arrows) of the endothelial cells and the pericytes are infiltrated by tracer material. A number of vesicles (single arrow) filled with tracer material is also present. L, lumen of blood vessel, E2, endothelial cell which is not decompensated.

S. Hayreh, we have observed that six hours after occlusion of the short posterior ciliary artery, some of the RPE cells in the posterior retina of the rhesus monkey showed dissolution and disappears from Bruch's membrane (Fig. 6). As a result, outer segments of photoreceptor cells were in direct apposition to Bruch's membrane.

Two days after the posterior pole of the rhesus monkey is exposed to the light of an ophthalmoscope (American Optical) for one hour,[13,14] dissolution of the RPE was observed in the center of lesion and the outer segments approached bare Bruch's membrane. In both instances, during the acute phase of the disease, no macrophages were observed in the subretinal space. The necrotic RPE was quickly removed and disappeared from Bruch's membrane. The exact mechanism by which the necrotic cells were removed from the subretinal space is not yet determined. In horseradish peroxidase tracer studies, of these severe cases of pigment epithelial injury, the tracer substance passed from the choriocapillaris through the bare Bruch's membrane into the subretinal

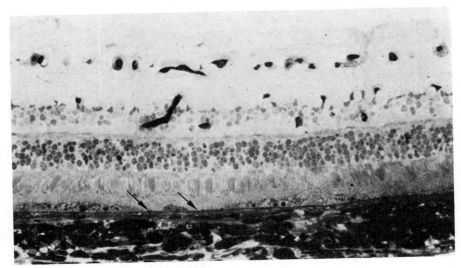

Figure 6.   Dissolution of the retinal pigment epithelial cells, six hours after occlusion of the short posterior ciliary artery. RPE cells (arrows) disappear from Bruch's membrane and photoreceptor outer segments are in direct contact with Bruch's membrane. Note the absence of macrophages in the subretinal space. No retinal detachment is observed.

space and traversed the external limiting membrane into the interstitial space of the outer nuclear layer. Yet no retinal detachment was seen.

2. Necrosis of Cells

When the RPE is necrotic the blood-retinal barrier is broken. Tracer substance passes through the pigment epithelium and accumulates in the subretinal space. The necrotic cells appear freely permeable to horseradish peroxidase, and the cytoplasm of these cells does not seem to retain tracer material (Fig. 7).

There are several forms of necrosis of the RPE. After the retina is exposed to bright light, coagulative necrosis may be seen in the RPE. The cells are shrunken and the plasmalemma appears discontinuous. The cytoplasm is granular and the mitochondria disintegrated (Fig. 8). In contrast, liquefactive necrosis is observed in RPE in eyes suffering from ischemia. Swelling of the RPE cells is noted, the cytoplasm of the RPE becomes watery, and the plasmalemma appears discontinuous. The

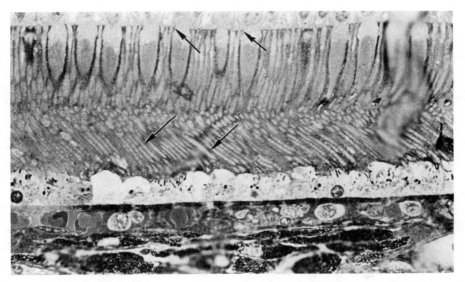

Figure 7. Liquefactive necrosis of retinal pigment epithelium of rhesus monkey six hours after short posterior ciliary artery was occluded. Noteworthy is the marked swelling of cells. Horseradish peroxidase (arrows) infiltrates the subretinal space and is temporarily stopped by the cell junctions of the external limiting membrane.

mitochondria are broken up into lamellar bodies with vesicle formation. In both types of necrosis, the RPE is freely permeable to tracers. In spite of the extensive necrosis of the pigment epithelium, the cell junctions between adjacent pigment epithelial cells appear to be present (Fig. 8).

3. Disruption of Cell Junctions

The disruption of tight cell junctions as a sole pathologic alteration in the disruption of the blood—retinal barrier is uncommonly observed because the RPE cells appear to be more susceptible to injury than their cell junctions in most diseases. In a study of proliferative changes of the RPE over malignant melanoma, we have noted that cell junctions between the RPE cells appear to be open and the adjacent cells do not appear necrotic[15] (Fig. 9). Horseradish peroxidase has also been observed to pass between the RPE into the subretinal space presumably due to disruption of the cell junctions in a monkey which had lens extraction.[4]

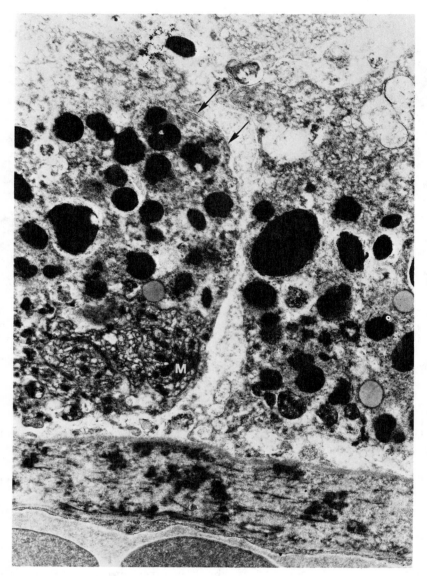

Figure 8.   Coagulative necrosis of retinal pigment epithelium
after having been exposed to the indirect ophthalmoscope light
for one hour.   The cytoplasm of the cells appears granular.   The
mitochondria (M) are broken up.   The plasmalemma is discontinuous.
Cell junctions are, however, still present between adjacent cells
(arrows).   Horseradish peroxidase was injected intravenously into
this animal but the tracer material passes through Bruch's membrane and pigment epithelium rapidly so that no horseradish peroxidase reaction product is seen in the necrotic cells.

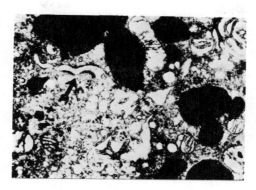

Figure 9. The retinal pigment epithelium of a patient with malignant melanoma. Note the opening of cell junctions (arrow) between adjacent proliferative pigment epithelial cells.

4. Decompensation of Cells

In certain pathologic states, the RPE appears decompensated but not necrotic. The cells are mildly edematous, the endoplasmic reticulum is dilated, and the mitochondria are irregular, but the plasmalemma is continuous and the cell junctions frequently remain intact. When horseradish peroxidase is administered intravenously, the tracer material passed into the cytoplasm of these decompensated cells (Fig. 10). In a mildly decompensative phase, the tracer substance may not enter the nuclear or the mitochondrial matrix. In a more severely decompensative phase, the tracer material passes from the cytoplasm through the apices of these cells into the subretinal space (Fig. 11). We believe that these cells are injured but are not necessarily necrotic. They are typically seen in chronic retinal diseases. In the retina of a rhesus monkey that has undergone lens extraction with vitreous loss, decompensation of RPE is observed in the posterior pole where tracer material passes through the plasmalemma and remains in the cytoplasm.[4] Similar injury is observed in the pigment epithelium of a rhesus monkey that has developed ocular hypotony secondary to cyclocryotherapy.[13]

CONSEQUENCES AFTER DISRUPTION OF THE BLOOD-RETINAL BARRIER

After the blood-retinal barrier is broken at the pigment epithelium, tracer material infiltrates the retina by an extracellularly or an intracellularly routine. After passing through the RPE cells or their cell junctions, the tracer material extends into the subretinal space. Some tracer material is temporarily stopped by the zonulae adherentes of the external limiting'

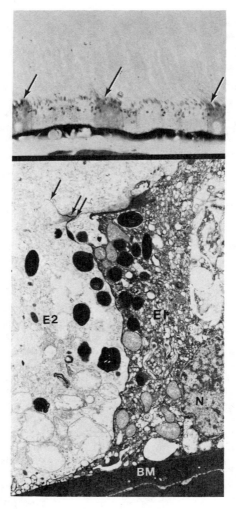

Figure 10. The retinal pigment epithelium of a monkey which had
lens extraction showing horseradish peroxidase permeated the
cytoplasm of three cells (upper figure). Tracer material infiltrates the cytoplasm of cell E1 but spares cell E2. N, nucleus;
BM, Bruch's membrane.

membrane. Even though these cell junctions are not tight cell
junctions, they are capable of impeding diffusion of the subretinal horseradish peroxidase. In cases of severe disruption of
the blood-retinal barrier, tracer material passes through the
external limiting membrane to the interstitial space of the outer
nuclear layer.

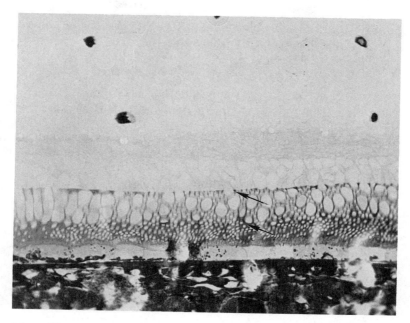

Figure 11. The retina of rhesus monkey which had been exposed to the light of an AO indirect ophthalmoscope of 1½ hours. The animal was sacrificed 24 months later. The retinal pigment epithelium is still decompensated and horseradish peroxidase is observed in the subretinal space. Note the integrity of the photoreceptor cells in spite of the history of decompensation of the pigment epithelium for 24 months.

Some of the tracer material also extends from the subretinal space into the cytoplasm of photoreceptor cells. The cone cells appear to be more frequently involved than the rod cells.[4] Similarly, the cone pedicles at the outer plexiform layers are more frequently impregnated with tracer material than the rod spherules. The cytoplasm of some of the cells at the inner nuclear layer may be also filled with tracer material. Occasionally, ganglion cells are infiltrated with tracer. While the mechanisms of passage of tracer material in these cells are unknown, it is possible that some tracer material passes from the photoreceptor cells transsynaptically through the bipolar cells to the ganglion cells.

The tolerance of the photoreceptor cells to mild disruption of the blood-retinal barrier at the RPE is remarkable. We have observed by fluorescein angiography that the blood-retinal barrier at the pigment epithelium in the retina of a monkey appeared leaky for 3 years and 10 months after having been exposed to the light of an indirect ophthalmoscope. The disruption of the barrier was subsequently confirmed by horseradish peroxidase study. Yet histologically, no degeneration of the photoreceptor cells was observed, even though there was mild retinal edema at the outer plexiform layer.

REPAIR OF THE DISRUPTION OF THE BLOOD-RETINAL BARRIER AT THE RPE

Even though the cells of the RPE are noncycling and do not proliferate under normal conditions, they have a great capability for regeneration and proliferation after injury.

1. Regeneration and Recovery of the RPE

After a necrotic lesion has been inflicted, the normal RPE cells surrounding the lesion flatten and migrate to reline Bruch's membrane. Mitosis and proliferation may be observed in the RPE cells in the vicinity of the lesion. Tight cell junctions develop between these newly formed RPE cells. Even though some of the cells may be devoid of pigment granules and may appear thin or atrophic, they may still re-establish their function as a blood-retinal barrier (Fig. 12).

2. Placoid Proliferation of the RPE

Following a severe injury, the RPE may undergo placoid proliferation. The proliferated RPE cells appear spindly and have been described as being under "fibrous metaplasia".[13,14] Electron microscopic examination of these proliferated cells shows that they produce basement membrane, join to the adjacent cells with cell junctions and retain some of the epithelial characteristics to the RPE.[13,14] The innermost layer of cells in placoid proliferation remains cuboidal and restore relationship with the photoreceptor outer segments. The RPE cells at placoid proliferation tend to remain decompensated for a longer time but some may eventually recover their blood-retinal barrier.

3. Failure of Regeneration of RPE

However, if the retinal lesions are large and the cells adjacent to the necrotic area are severely decompensated, proliferation of RPE may not occur. Glial cells from the retina may grow over Bruch's membrane without regeneration of RPE in the lesion. As a result, there is a permanent loss of blood-retinal barrier and a chorioretinal scar develops.

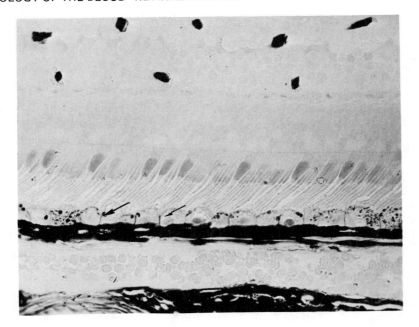

Figure 12. Recovery of the RPE barrier in the retina of monkey after having been exposed to the light of an indirect ophthalmoscope for 1½ hours. The RPE is depigmented but the cell junctions are reformed (arrows) and no horseradish peroxidase is observed in the subretinal space.

4. Chronic Decompensation of the RPE

In still other lesions, the RPE cells remain chronically decompensated and the blood-retinal barrier is continuously being disrupted. Yet, no necrosis provides stimulus for proliferation of the adjacent pigment epithelium. In such conditions, decompensation of pigment epithelium may last for many months, resulting in eventual retinal edema and decompensation of the photoreceptor cells. Therefore, it is most important in such disease states to produce acute necrosis in these cells by argon laser or xenon-arc photocoagulation so that the surrounding healthy pigment epithelium is stimulated to proliferate and reline Bruch's membrane. The blood-retinal barrier may then be reformed and chronic retinal edema will be prevented.

From the Georgiana Theobald Ophthalmic Pathology Laboratory, University of Illinois Eye and Ear Infirmary, Chicago. This investigation is supported in part by Public Health Service Grants EY01903 and EY01904 and 1P30EY01792 and EY703802. Dr. Tso is a Research to Prevent Blindness—William Friedkin Scholar, 1976-1977.

REFERENCES

1. Rapoport, S.: Blood-Brain Barrier in Physiology and Medicine. Raven Press, New York, New York. 1976, p. 212.
2. Deem, C.W., Futterman, S., and Kalina, R.E.: Invest. Ophthalmol. 13:580, 1974.
3. Tso, M.O.M., and Albert, D.M.: Arch. Ophthalmol. 88:27-38, 1972.
4. Tso, M.O.M., and Shih, C.Y.: Invest. Ophthalmol. 16:381-392, 1977.
5. Wallow, I.H.L., and Engerman, R.L.: Invest. Ophthalmol. 16:447, 1977.
6. Shiose, Y.: Jap. J. Ophthalmol. 14:73, 1970.
7. Tso, M.O.M., Shih, C.Y., and Patz, A.: ARVO Meeting, Sarasota, Florida, 1977.
8. Tso, M.O.M., and Shih, C.Y.: Exp. Eye Res. 23:209-216, 1976.
9. Tanigushi, Y., and Sameshima, M.: Acta Soc. Ophthalmol. Jpn. 75:1685, 1971.
10. Goldberg, M.F., and Tso, M.O.M.: Ophthalmol. (AAOO) 85:1028-1041, 1978.
11. Taniguchi, Y.: Jpn. J. Ophthalmol. 20:19, 1976.
12. Ashton, N., Tripathi, B., and Kight, G.: Exp. Eye Res. 14:221, 1972.
13. Tso, M.O.M., Fine, B.S., and Zimmerman, L.E.: Am. J. Ophthalmol. 73:686, 1972.
14. Tso, M.O.M.: Invest. Ophthalmol. 12:17, 1973.
15. Wallow, I.H.L., and Tso, M.O.M.: Am. J. Ophthalmol. 73:914, 1972.

RETINAL EDEMA: POSTULATED MECHANISM(S)

Paul Kenking, Roy W. Bellhorn and Burton Schall

Department of Ophthalmology
Montefiore Hospital & Medical Center/Albert Einstein
College of Medicine, Bronx, New York, U.S.A.

Retinal edema has been recognized and described by ophthalmologists and ophthalmic pathologists for more than a century (Duke-Elder, 1941, 1967). The advent of fluorescein angiography as a practical clinical procedure has revealed that retinal edema is very common, and a major cause of visual disturbance in many conditions (Table 1). In spite of this veritable explosion in clinical knowledge, little has been written about the mechanism(s) of retinal edema. It is generally recognized that the edema follows some derangement of either the blood-retinal (BR) or retinal pigment epithelial (RPE) "barrier". While there is some information of a general nature concerning these barriers, little is known about the quality and quantity of materials which normally traverse the barriers in order to nourish the retina, and even less about the composition of edema fluid.

Retinal edema can be simply defined as an excess of fluid within the retinal tissue. With this broad definition, the edema could be intra or extracellular, or both. At the outset, we stress that retinal edema is not a disease entity, but rather a sign occurring in the course of many disorders. A variety of clinical and histopathological pictures have been described and these will be considered.

In order to understand the mechanism(s) of retinal edema it is necessary to consider data from many sources including anatomy, physiology, clinical ophthalmology and ophthalmic pathology, as well as material dealing with the parallel situation in the brain.

Let us consider the anatomy of the retina. The retina appears on routine histologic cross section to be a relatively thin tissue bounded externally by the retinal pigment epithelium and internally by the vitreous body. It is attached to the rest of the central ner-

Table 1. Human Conditions with associated Edema of the Retina*

CONDITION	POSTULATED MECHANISM(S)	NOTES
Diabetes mellitus	Breakdown of BRB and/or RPEB (? 2:osmolarity alterations; physical damage to junctions)	May be modified by photocoagulation.
Retinal vein Occlusion	Intraluminal pressure plus hypoxia/hypercapnia causing retinal endothelial damage.	Repaired by development of collaterals. Photocoagulation may be beneficial.
Aphakic CME	? secondary to low grade inflammation with inflammatory products causing breakdown of BRB.	May clear spontaneously or improve with steroids.
Epinephrine plus Aphakia	" " " " " +direct damage of retinal vessels by Epinephrine. ? increased pinocytic activity.	Reverses on ceasing epinephrine drops.
Nicotinic Acid	?	Reverses on ceasing excess nicotinic acid.
Hereditary Macular Edema	?	A familial condition.
Papilledema	Increase in interstitial fluid from disc region to surrounding retina, especially macula. ? breakdown of optic nerve head vessel "barrier".	Decreases when papilledema reverses. Macular exudates in "wing" or "star" are late findings.
Retinal Telangiectasis (Coat's, Leber's, Von Hippel's)	Increase in retinal interstitial fluid secondary to leakage from the retinal vascular malformation. ("exaggerated macular response").	Destroy malformation and edema and exudation often resolve.
Pigmentary Retinal Degeneration(s)	? increased fluid leaking into retina through abnormal RPE. Most prominent in macula as CME.	
Malignant Melanoma or Choroidal Nevus	? breakdown of RPE barrier with fluid accumulation in Henle's layer.	
Choroidal Hemangioma	" " "	
Choroidal Metastasis	" " "	
Laser Photocoagulation	" " "	

BRB = blood retinal barrier; RPEB = retinal pigment epithelial barrie
CME = cystoid macular edema; *This is not an all inclusive listing.

vous system by the axons of ganglion cells which form the nerve fiber layer. The alternating layers of cells and cell processes are
easily discerned even under low power. Special stains reveal that
the neural elements are held in a framework of vertically arranged
glial elements, mainly Muller cells. Expansions of the innermost
portion of the Muller cells form the basement membrane known as the
inner limiting membrane of the retina. The outer limiting membrane
consists of zonulae adherentes which link the inner segment of rods
and cones to Muller cells and Muller cells to each other.

The retina thins as it extends peripherally but the thinning
is not uniform. For example, the macula is thick because of its
large ganglion cell population but centrally it thins containing
only cones, their cell bodies and the obliquely arranged fibers
(Henle's layer) of the outer plexiform layer.

Intraretinal vessels occupy the inner half of the retina to
the inner nuclear layer. Capillary networks are present except in
the central macula and at the far retinal periphery. Relatively discrete capillary networks can be defined in the nerve fiber-ganglion
cell layer, and in the inner nuclear layer. A specific capillary
plexus, termed the radial peripallary capillaries (RPC), is present
in the nerve fiber layer adjacent to the optic nerve head (Henkind,
1967).

Ultrastructural and Golgi stain analysis of the retina reveals
that it is composed of neural elements with complex horizontal and
vertical intercommunications and with the neuropil enmeshed in a
framework of glial elements. The tissue appears, in routinely fixed
E.M. preparations, to be very compact. According to Hogan et al
(1971) Muller cells fill out all the retinal area not occupied by
neurons except for the inner retina where astrocytes also participate as "space occupying" cells. Indeed, these authors state, "Because of close contact of the Muller cells with other retinal cells
it is evident that there is little extracellular space in the retina". They acknowledge that there is a gap between adjacent cells
which may measure up to 200 A. In the nerve fiber layer they note
that not all axons are surrounded by glial tissue and, in some bun-
dles, many of the axons lie close to one another without any intervening glial tissue.

At this point it is appropriate to bring up the question, does
the normal retina possess a functional extracellular space ? Most
workers seem to accept a view that the normal retina contains little
or no extracellular space. They appear to agree with the idea of
Sjostrand (1961) that, "the glial elements in the retina, the Muller's cell, and the neural glia in the central nervous system, represent the "extracellular space". Indeed, DeRobertis and Gerschenfeld (1961) conceived of the astroglia as the water-ion compartment

involved in the selection and transport of metabolites and fluid in the brain, (and presumably, the retina). It appears that Smelser and colleagues (1965) were the only investigators to take a contrary view, and their work, though little remembered, is crucial to our concept. They injected Thorotrast (thorium dioxide in aqueous dextrin) into the vitreous humor of cats and were able to detect its presence within 6 hours throughout the retina between the internal and external limiting membranes, and mainly in the extracellular space. None penetrated the external limiting membrane. Some particles did enter the basement membrane around retinal vessels and were transported across the endothelial cells suggesting "no obvious blood-retinal barrier in this direction".

They conclude that the intercellular space in the retina is available for diffusion of even particulate matter and that such clefts are important in retinal nutrition and possibly in pathological processes.

In our opinion, the normal retina possesses a functioning extracellular space, and such a space has characteristics which allow us to understand the process(es) of retinal edema.

Klatzo (1967) in his major paper dealing with brain edema, noted that one could not depend solely upon electron microscopy of routinely fixed material to provide correct answers about edema localization. He also discussed the situation of extracellular space in the brain and pointed out that physiologic data strongly suggested the existence of an appreciable and functionally active extracellular space, and that some anatomic studies confirmed the presence of such a space. For example, Van Harreveld et al (1964, 1965) using a freeze-substitution technique found in mouse cerebellar tissue an extracellular volume of 23.6% if they processed the tissue within 30 seconds of decapitation, but only a 6% volume if decapitation was delayed up to 8 minutes. This is a far different result from the 3-5% extracellular volume postulated by analysis of immersion or perfusion fixed material. Furthermore, the work of Sumi (1969) clearly demonstrated that fixation techniques are crucial in determining the extent of the extracellular volume of the brain, particularly in the immature animal. This investigator showed that considerable extracellular space was present in the newborn cerebral cortex, but the extent of the space could be easily modified by changes in the osmolarity of the glutaraldehyde fixative. Sumi stated, "Following immersion fixation the extracellular space was somewhat narrower. The most marked decrease in the extracellular space was noted after immersion fixation in isotonic fixative". With maturation the extracellular volume of the brain progressively decreased.

Thus, 1) the method of fixation, 2) the tonicity of the fixative, 3) the time after removal of the tissue until fixation, and 4) the age of the tissue, are all crucial elements in any study of extracellular space in the central nervous system. No studies have been conducted on retinal tissue with regard to these four factors.

With regard to the extracellular volume of the retina there has been little physiologic study although there are numerous studies conducted on brain tissue of various species. Cheek and Holt (1978) in a recent major review of the subject concluded that the distribution of chloride gave the most accurate assessment of the brain ECV. They reported values of 24.8% in the cerebrum and 23.6% in the cerebellum of adult rhesus monkeys. Inulin and other polysaccharides apparently do not penetrate the perivascular space and thus may not fully measure the ECV. However, even these substances show an ECV of 10% or more in adult animals. Similarly, Vernadakis and Woodbury (1965) found a brain interstitial space in the rat of 15% in mature animals compared to 22% in neonates. Other physiological studies support the concept of a significant ECV in the brains of all species studied, and the size of the space is apparently age-dependent.

If the data obtained for brain can be extrapolated for retina then there must be a considerable retinal ECV and this fits well with observed clinical data.

We believe that the retinal extracellular space is a system of interconnected pathways of varying dimension and present throughout the retinal tissue between the internal and external limiting membranes (fig. 1). This is consistent with the view of Brightman and Reese (1969) who state, "Therefore, the interspaces of the brain are generally patent, allowing intercellular movement of colloidal materials", and the study of Smelser et al (1965).

Topographical differences in the patterns of clinical retinal edema are due to anatomical factors such as the richness of intercommunication between adjacent cells at any one level-apparently complex in the nuclear layers and sparse in the nerve fiber and inner portion of the outer plexiform layer and the distance of the neuropil from the retinal vascular bed.

We must examine more closely the retinal vessels, for much of the retinal edema seen clinically is derived from them. The gross angioarchitectural pattern of the intraretinal vessels has been described. Now, we concentrate on the ultrastructure. All retinal vessels are lined by a continuous layer of non-fenestrated endothelium. The adjacent endothelial cells are held together by "tight" junctions, and these junctions are felt to be barriers to many substances. The presence of this type of endothelial lining in retinal and brain vessels is apparently responsible for the blood-retinal (BR) and blood-brain (BB) barriers. Whether both barriers are identical is not known, and the recent study by Laties et al (1979) suggests that retinal vessels may be more resistant to certain insults than are cerebral vessels. Pinocytotic vesicles have been noted

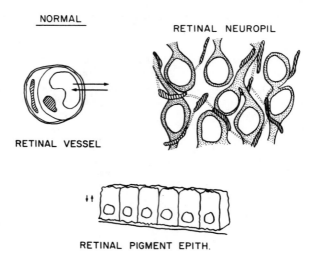

NORMAL

RETINAL NEUROPIL

RETINAL VESSEL

RETINAL PIGMENT EPITH.

Fig. 1. Schematic drawing showing relationship of retinal vessels, retinal pigment epithelium and the retinal neuropil. The extracellular space in the retina is indicated by cross hatched lines.

in retinal capillary endothelium by many authors, but Au and Bellhorn (1977) morphometrically demonstrated that they may well have a role in transport of material across the vessel. The nonluminal surface of the endothelium is lined by a continuous basement membrane whose thickness increases with age. Intramural pericytes also lie within this basement membrane and, in man, there is normally a 1:1 ratio between them and endothelial cells. With regard to retinal arterioles, they contain some muscularis even out to their terminal branches. Of some interest is the fact that all retinal vessels lack nervous innervation. In spite of lacking innervation, the larger retinal vessels can certainly constrict and dilate and this is felt to be on the basis of an autoregulatory mechanism.

Analogous to the blood-retinal barrier is the barrier provided by the retinal pigment epithelial cells (RPE). Tight junctions between the cells of the RPE exclude many of the larger molecules which circulate in the choroid after readily crossing the choriocapillaris. One could readily imagine that a physical break in either the RPE or retinal vessel endothelium would permit ingress of blood derived fluid into the retinal substance, and such breaks may account for some cases of retinal edema.

What materials cross the normal blood retinal and RPE barriers ?

Blood gases, amino acids, and some lipids certainly enter the retina. Glucose is actively transported rapidly into the retina from either the retinal or choroidal circulation provided it is D and not L glucose (Dollery, Henkind and Orme, 1971). Larger protein moities are generally excluded from the normal retina. There is some evidence from studies of the brain that the blood-brain barrier is not absolute and this may be true for the BR and RPE barriers as well. For example, Westergaard and Brightman (1973) demonstrated transport of protein (ferritin and horseradish peroxidase) across some vessels of the surface of mouse brain as well as some of the vessels in the neuropil itself. The vessels involved in this transport were cerebral arterioles and neither capillaries nor venules, and the pathway for the transport was by vesicles within the arteriolar endothelium, and not across intercellular junctions. Møllgard and Sørensen (1974) feel that the term "blood-brain barrier" should be substituted by the designation, "selective permeability of cerebral vessels". They have studied the permeability properties of the brain and found that tight junctions between endothelial cells of brain capillaries are permeable to Alcian blue which has a molecular weight of 1390 and a Stoke-Einstein radius of 8 Å. Bellhorn et al (1977) have shown that normal rat retinal vessels are impermeable to fluorescein iso-thiocyanate (FITC) labeled dextrans of effective diffusion radius of 12 to 85 Å, but anterior segment vessels are permeable to the smaller size dextrans (Benjamin et al, 1977). Further studies will probably elucidate the barrier and the permeability properties of retinal and brain vessels. Obviously, all portions of the vascular tree will have to be considered, not only the capillary bed.

Having briefly reviewed the anatomy and physiology of the BR and BB barriers let us consider some of the pathological responses of the microvasculature. Here we introduce the concept of retinal vascular lability or plasticity. One generally views the retinal vascular bed as a rather static entity. There is evidence, however, that is not so. First of all, the embryonic development of the retinal vessels reveals enormous plasticity and modeling (Henkind and de Oliveira, 1967; Ashton, 1969). Once maturity is reached the gross alterations in the vascular bed are relatively minor with the exception of some marked changes at the retinal periphery (Glatt and Henkind, 1979). This is true for the healthy individual, but what happens in retinal vascular disease ? A number of discrete retinal vascular entities have been examined clinically and pathologically and some have been duplicated experimentally (Table 2). Most have associated retinal edema because of some alterations in the BRB.

The pathogenetic mechanisms responsible for the various retinal vascular alterations are, with the exception of collaterals and neovascularization, really not understood (Henkind and Wise, 1974; Henkind, 1978). It should be clear, however, that the ready accessibility of the retinal circulation should make it a prime site for any-

Table 2. Clinically Visible Retinal Vascular Entities

ENTITY	PATHOGENESIS	FLUORESCEIN FINDINGS	LIGHT & ELECTRON MICROSCOPY
Neovascularization	Liberation of a biochemical factor generated by hypoxic retinal tissue, TAF, or inflammation+diseased vessel.	Irregular vessels either intra or extraretinal, profuse leakage unless "fibrotic" stage develops.	Poorly formed endothelial junctions, sparse basement membrane, possible fenestrae in endothelium.
Collaterals	Follow vascular occlusion. Collaterals arise within existing capillary bed.	Tortuous intraretinal channels of varying size do not leak except in early stage.	Mature vessels approximating wall characteristics of arterioles or venules, normal endothelium.
Shunts	Congenital or developmental arteriovenous communication. May represent faulty remodeling during fetal life.	Dilated intraretinal channel. Rapid flow without leakage.	Variably enlarged vascular channel. Normal vessel wall.
Microaneurysms	Unknown. May relate to developmental structural weakness associated with certain diseases.	Small dilations arising from capillaries or terminal arterioles or venules. Almost always adjacent to area of capillary bed nonperfusion. May or may not leak.	Best seen on "digest". May have decreased intramural pericytes or abnormal endothelial cells, sometimes acellular.
Macroaneurysms	Unknown. More common in elderly hypertensive individuals. ?embolic origin.	Generally single arterial aneurysmal dilation fills with fluorescein. Marked surrounding leakage and hemorrhage and exudation.	Dilated, thick-walled arteriole with marked fibroglial reaction in wall. Protein and lipid exudate in surrounding retina.
Telangectasia	? Congenital or developmental dilation of a portion of the retinal vascular bed.	A wide spectrum of possible alterations with dilated tortuous capillaries predominating. Increased stain and leakage of dye.	Abnormal endothelium and vessel wall infiltrated with plasma, platelets and RBC's.

one studying microvascular alterations in the central nervous system.

Another way to look at the breakdown of the BR or BB barriers is to examine the fine structural alterations seen in various conditions. While this has been attempted to a small degree in the retina, more work has been conducted on the brain. Hirano (1974, 1976) has been particularly interested in this subject. He lists five alterations which may be of consequence in disruption of the normal blood-brain barrier: 1) alteration of the intercellular junction; 2) alteration of pinocytotic function; 3) diffuse infiltration of endothelial cells; 4) endothelial fenestration and: 5) presence of tubular bodies.

Disruption of the intercellular junction may result in massive outpouring of the vascular contents including red blood cells, but such disruption has not been clearly demonstrated in brain or retinal pathology. However, Wallow and Engerman (1974) suggest that such separation may occur in diabetic retinopathy. Perhaps the junctions are only transiently disrupted as speculated by Hockley et al (1979) in their study of experimental branch vein occlusion, and as suggested by Rapoport et al (1976) and Brightman et al (1973) from their studies of cerebral tissue subjected to hyperosmotic arterial infusions. According to Rapoport (1976) the blood-brain barrier is reestablished minutes to hours after various insults. It is also possible that rather than junctional separation, the endothelial cell is itself transiently disrupted or tunnel-like openings may develop through it. The latter route has been demonstrated as a pathway for lymphocytes to leave cerebral vessels (Barringer and Griffith, 1970; Barringer and Nathanson, 1972). We have noted inflammatory cell cuffing around retinal veins in experimental vein occlusion (Kohner et al, 1970), but did not determine how the cells left the vessels.

As we mentioned previously, retinal vessels do have some normal pinocytotic vesicles and according to Hirano (1974) pinocytotic activity greatly increases in conditions lowering the blood-brain barrier. There is, however, little but speculation that an increase in pinocytosis occurs in any specific retinal disease process. Hockley et al (1979) briefly note peroxidase "may have escaped from the capillaries via endothelial pinocytotic vesicles" in experimental branch vein occlusion, and Essner et al (1979) have considered transcellular vesicular transport as a mechanism of increased permeability of retinal capillaries in the RCS rats with inherited retinal degeneration. Tso and Shih (1976) in their experimental model of ocular hypotony, noted the presence of HRP in the basement membrane of vessels and adjacent tissue. Pinocytotic vesicles, some filled with reaction product, were prominent.

Diffuse infiltration of endothelial cells with fluorescein has been noted on many occasions in various retinal vascular disorders.

This is manifest by persistent "staining" of a vascular segment long after the fluorescein has completed its circuit through the retina. Often the fluorescein appears to leak into the adjacent retinal tissue. Peroxidase staining of brain endothelial cells has been noted under experimental conditions most notably after electroshock (Hirano, 1974).

Hirano (1974) points out that in most experimentally induced alterations of the blood-brain barrier endothelial fenestration is absent. However, he has noted fenestrations in various natural and experimental neoplasms within the brain. Fenestrated capillaries presumably of retinal origin have been noted in urethan-induced retinopathy in pigmented rats (Bellhorn et al, 1973). These capillaries were actually upon or within the layer of disturbed pigment epithelium, while the capillaries in the inner retina appeared normal. Similarly, fenestrae have been found in capillaries of retinal origin which get incorporated into the RPE in phototoxic retinopathy in rats (Bellhorn et al, 1977). Such fenestrae were not described in the retinal degeneration that spontaneously develops in RCS rats (Essner et al, 1979), possibly because the vessels had not yet been incorporated into the RPE. The fact that retinal capillaries can become fenestrated, particularly when they are associated with retinal pigment epithelium is strong evidence for the lability of retinal endothelium. Hirano (1974) has also demonstrated that fenestrated vessels can derive from nonfenestrated ones in the brain. He feels that it is most reasonable to assume that, rather than transforming already developed vessels, whatever the stimulus is changes the developmental pattern of vessels which arise to nourish the new environment.

Tubular bodies (Weibel-Palade) of endothelial cells are normally absent in cerebral vessels but are quite prominent in pathological conditions. They have been noted to be increased in number in the choroid in Behcet's disease by Matsuda and Sugiura (1970). However, these authors did not study the retinal vessels. Whether such bodies have any role in altering retinal or brain vascular permeability is unknown.

Much less is known about the potential alterations in the RPE with regard to pathogenetic mechanisms of leakage. What is clear is that the RPE cells are tightly bound to one another. In some clinical situations the RPE is lifted off Bruch's membrane in a continuous sheet, and fluid fills the sub-RPE space but does not penetrate into the neural retina. Sometimes, serous fluid leaks through the RPE and merely causes a localized serous neural retinal detachment. In cases with major RPE disruption, hemorrhage and edema pour first beneath and then into the neural retina, the classic example being disciform macular degeneration. We are now appreciating more subtle RPE alterations, and it may be that the elegant studies of Cunha--Vaz and colleagues (1975; 1979) on diabetic individuals are revealing permeability of the RPE barrier. Support for this view comes from the fluorescein study of the RPE in streptozotocin diabetes in rats. In some cases, fluorescein was noted to penetrate the RPE as forward as the external limiting membrane of the retina with no leakage noted from intraretinal vessels (Kirber et al, 1978). The locus of the "leak" was not clear. Grimes and Laties (1979) using the same model have demonstrated by stereology an increase in surface ares of basal surface of RPE cells and suggest that this may account for the increase in permeability.

Let us now turn to the subject of retinal edema and examine the "facts".

Retinal edema is almost always a secondary phenomenon which occurs in the course of many ocular and systemic disorders. It is usually secondary to whatever causes disruption of the BR or RPE barriers and can be considered analogous to the "vasogenic" brain edema of Klatzo (1967). In such cases the retinal edema is predominantly extracellular, though intracellular swelling of neurons and glia may occur secondarily.

In ischemic conditions intracellular neuronal swelling predominates and apparently is partially due to blockage of axoplasmic flow. The cotton wool spot seen in many diseases such as hypertension, diabetes, and collagen diseases is an excellent clinical example of such intracellular swelling, and the experimental production of such lesions has been studied in depth (Ashton et al, 1966).

Retinal edema is, at least in its early stages, reversible provided the inciting pathology is eliminated.

Retinal exudation is related to retinal edema and most such exudation is a product of edema residue. However, not all retinal edema leads to exudate formation. If the edema fluid contains little protein or lipid, then exudate is absent or mild; but if it is rich in such components then exudation may be prominent.

There are specific anatomic regions within the retina where edema tends to be most prominent, these include the macula and Henle's layer in particular; the nerve fiber layer, mainly in the peripapillary region; the outer plexiform layer; less frequently the inner nuclear layer; and possibly, the retinal periphery. What makes these areas particularly prone to collect edema fluid ?

If edema fluid in the retina was basically localized to the glia compartment as believed less than two decades ago, (Duke-Elder and Dobree, 1967), then we could not explain the clinical and histopathological findings in a rational manner. For example, in the nerve fiber layer, the glia is sparse and edema is common and the same seems to hold true for Henle's layer. Furthermore, the very nature of the Muller cell which extends the full width of the retina from inner to outer limiting membrane would mandate a "full-thickness" edema - unless one postulated that only a portion of a cell would be involved in the process - highly unlikely !! It is worth noting that, only recently, the view that cerebral edema is localized to the glial compartment has been supplanted by the idea of extracellular edema (Klatzo, 1967).

In disregarding a glial hypothesis we remain cognizant of the fact that retinal glia can be involved in various disease processes and may, under certain circumstances, swell.

In our opinion, the retina normally contains an extracellular space which can be thought of as a complex network of intercommunicating channels of various diameters. Broader spaces exist in Henle's (and in the rest of the outer plexiform layer) and the nerve fiber layer. Raviola (1967) who has studied the outer plexiform layer by freeze fracture in animals, has noted an enlarged intercellular cleft between horizontal and bipolar cells.

We imagine that the network of intercellular space exists in three dimensions, from the disc head to the periphery and from the internal down to the external limiting membrane. Outside of the nerve fiber layer and the outer plexiform layer, especially Henle's layer, all of the extracellular channels are relatively narrow, but possibly larger than the 200 Å spaces seen by conventional EM studies. Narrow channels might inhibit flow of material and might become clogged by particulate matter, i.e., red blood cells. Thus, hemorrhages from the deep capillary bed would remain close to the seat of bleeding in the inner nuclear layer. Clinically, retinal hemorrhages in this locale tend do be of the "dot and blot" variety, and do not tend to spread vertically or horizontally. Edema fluid, passing through an altered BR barrier would have an easier transit and tend to accumulate in the larger available spaces closest to the site of leakage. Thus, edema fluid escaping from the superficial capillaries, especially the RPC's, tends to collect in the nerve fiber layer. Clinically, the nerve fibers are noted to be delineated as widely separated. In such a case, the edema spread is mainly in a horizontal plane primarly in the superior and inferior temporal fibers, and often sparing the papillo-macular bundle. The deeper retinal layers may or may not be spared depending upon the degree of leakage.

A condition that has often puzzled clinicians, is the so-called idiopathic stellate maculopathy of Leber, which develops in younger patients who have optic disc swelling, either papilledema or papillitis. In such patients, the exudative star is not seen initially, but it develops as the disc swelling regresses. In such cases, fluorescein angiography has revealed fluorescein leakage from the disc but not from the vessels of the macula nor the underlying pigment epithelium (Gass, 1977). We propose the following explanation: edema fluid leaking from the disc, travels centripetally along the paths of the retinal extracellular space in the papillo-macular bundle of nerve fibers. This is a rather compact bundle of fibers and, presumably, the extracellular space is composed of relatively narrow channels and, thus little separation of the nerve fibers is noted. But, when the fluid enters the broader spaces of Henle's layer, it may accumulate and dilate the spaces. Presumably, most of the excess fluid is resorbed by normal macular capillaries. The fluid leaking from the disc is probably rich in lipid and protein components because, in papillitis and papilledema, hemorrhage in the peripapillary region is not uncommon and, certainly if red blood cells can extravasate other molecules can presumably do so. The higher molecular weight lipid and protein material is probably not readily resorbed by the macula capillaries, and it precipitates out in the extracellular space as exudate. The macula star is always more prominent in the nasal portion of the macula region and, indeed, sometimes this only appears as a so-called macular wing. Apparently, in such cases, the fluid has not percolated through the entire macular region but only in the area closest to the disc.

Analogous situations where edema pours into the macular region from distant loci are also well known. For example, in retinal macroaneurysms or in branch vein occlusion, edema fluid from the damaged vessel(s) appears most prominent in the macular region rather than immediately adjacent to the lesion. Often as the lesion resolves exudates accumulate in the macula in a pattern often pointing to the initial lesion.

The most dramatic form of macular involvement from a distant site occurs in telangiectatic peripheral retinal vascular abnormalities including entities such as Coats' disease, Leber's disease, and Von Hippel's disease. In such cases, particularly, when there is a temporal retinal vascular malformation, one often finds macular edema and/or exudation with the intervening retina between the macula and the vascular abnormality clinically normal. The late Dr. George Wise, who coined the term, "exaggerated macular response" (Wise and Wangvivat, 1966) felt that the peripheral vascular abnormality somehow shunted blood away from the macula and led to hypoxia which caused a breakdown of the macular vessels. There is no evidence, however, that this occurs. Instead, we suspect that the very "leaky" vessels of the angiomatous malformation pour protein-rich fluid into the surrounding retina, and this fluid traverses the retinal extravascular pathways. When the fluid reaches the macula, some of it may be resorbed but not the lipid and protein. Clinical support for this mechanism is provided by the observation that destruction of the angiomatous malformation leads to the "drying out" of the macula region; the macular edema disappears, leaving behind the residual exudation.

Cystoid macular edema occurs in numerous conditions and, simply reflects the fact that retinal extravascular fluid accumulates in Henle's layer. Let us consider some examples of this condition. Aphakic cystoid macular edema is thought to be secondary to intra-ocular inflammation causing increased permeability of the small vessels in the region of the macula. The exact type of blood-retinal barrier breakdown is not known but since there is never an accompanying hemorrhage, one can assume that there is no disruption either of the endothelial cells nor their junctions. There is, however, sufficient damage to allow fluorescein-labeled material, i.e., presumably some protein, to enter into the retinal extravascular space. Since exudate is rarely seen, only small molecular weight protein and/or lipid passes the BRB. The outpouring of fluid is greater than the capillary bed ability to drain it away. The classic "petaloid" appearance seen on angiography may suggest that the edema fluid is limited to the central macula region. Careful analysis of the angiograms reveals a much more diffuse edema with extension into the surrounding retina.

In the clinical situation of central serous choroidopathy, fluid from the choroicapillaris penetrates the RPE barrier in one or several spots and then separates the RPE from the sensory retina. In mild cases it seems that the subretinal edema fluid does not extend beyond the outer limiting membrane. In advanced cases it breaks through this physical barrier and enters the outer plexiform layer thereby causing cystoid edema, but rarely any exudate. If the pigment epithelium remains permeable, permanent cystic changes develop and macrocysts and holes may form.

In recent years it has been appreciated that a number of patients with retinitis pigmentosa or other retinal degenerations will develop cystoid macular edema. This, in spite of the fact that the pathology is most evident equatorally and not in the macula region itself. It is still not clear whether the RPE has increased permeability, or whether there is an alteration in the BRB in the macula which is responsible for the outpouring of fluid.

An important study of experimental ocular siderosis by Watanabe (1974) showed marked edema in Henle's layer but no obvious abnormal permeability of the intraretinal vessels. The major finding on histology was an alteration in the RPE, the presumed site of fluorescein leakage. Similarly, Tso and Fine (1979) in their study of the primate foveola after injury by argon laser, noted the very late production of edema in Henle's layer. This occurred four years after the laser burn and developed concomitantly with RPE edema. They suggest that decompensation of the retinal pigment epithelium is the cause of some cases of cystoid retinal edema.

Diabetes mellitus is perhaps the most common disease with associated retinal edema. It is only within the past decade that clinicians have appreciated the importance of macular edema as a cause of visual disturbance in diabetes (Patz et al, 1973). In most cases, fluorescein will demonstrate microvascular abnormalities at the border of the edematous area. These are the seat of the leakage. If leaking vessels are present elsewhere than the macula, edema is less obvious clinically but can be suspected for there is almost always a ring of exudate at the border of the affected area. The exudates form mainly in the outer plexiform layer, the same strata in which the edema fluid collects.

Virtually all instances of so-called circinate retinopathy can be shown on fluorescein angiography to be centered about a zone of leaking intraretinal micro-circulation, with the exudate collecting at the border between normal and abnormally perfused retina. If the circinate ring is centered on the fovea then there is ophthalmoscopically visible edema centrally, due to the fluid accumulation in Henle's layer. In eccentric rings the edema is less obvious by ophthalmoscopy, but clearly seen on angiograms.

We have not considered every possibility in the spectrum of retinal edema. For example, we have not discussed the shimmering appearance of the infant and childhood fundus, but suggest that one possiblity not heretofore considered is that it may reflect the presence of a larger retinal extracellular fluid-filled space in the young compared with the aged individual. Similarly, the fact that retinal edema tends to be more florid in younger than older individuals may indicate the presence of a larger extracellular space in the former. We have not dwelled on the presence of fluid-filled spaces at the periphery of the retina, especially the temporal retina. These may be instances of physiologic trapping of fluid in the extracellular spaces of the outer plexiform layer beyond the periphery of the retinal circulation - a situation somewhat analogous to the avascular central macula. Nor have we touched upon the pseudoedemas, those conditions in which edema of the retina is suspected on clinical grounds due to a "wet" appearance on ophthalmoscopy-conditions such as chloroquine retinopathy and preretinal macular gliosis-but where fluorescein angiography and histopathology do not reveal edema pockets.

We could continue discussing other entities associated with retinal edema, but these would add little to our thoughts concerning the mechanism(s) of retinal edema.

EPILOGUE

The subject, Mechanism of Retinal Edema, was chosen for us by Professor Cunha-Vaz. We had not spent any particular time studying the topic nor conducted any research and readily accepted the notions extant in various texts and articles. It was only as we probed beneath the accepted generalities that we realized the state of our ignorance. No unifying thread appeared that would unite the findings of various disciplines. Furthermore, if one accepted the available anatomic "evidence" then the clinical pictures of retinal edema made little or no sense, and yet they had to be explained.

Thus, we have deduced, from sifting through our own related data and experiments, through examination of clinical and histopathological material and through scrutiny of the available brain and retinal literature, a concept which satisfies us with regards to the mechanism of retinal edema. What we propose has not been seen by anatomists, except Smelser et al (1965), has not been proven by physiologists, has not been enunciated by pathologists, and remains unsuspected by clinicians.

Can it be that the retina harbors a complex network of interlinked, intercommunicating, extracellular channels ? Channels which in health act as extravascular conduits enabling the materials penetrating the blood-retinal and RPE barriers to reach neural elements and facilitating removal of unwanted metabolic products. Channels which in situations of altered permeability of BRB or RPEB carry excessive fluid (edema) of varying composition-depending essentially upon the character of the barrier breakdown. Channels which, because of their differing dimensions in different parts of the retina may distend and trap fluid. The fluid, if rich in high molecular weight proteins and lipids, may "coagulate" in the extracellular space as exudate. Such is our concept - we shall now try to prove it and fully expect others to challenge and try to disprove it.

REFERENCES

Ashton, N. (1969): The mode of development of the retinal vessels in man. In J.S. Cant (ed.). The William Mackenzie Centenary Symposium on the Ocular Circulation in Health and Disease. Mosby, St. Louis, p. 7.

Ashton, N., Dollery, C.T., Henkind, P., Hill, D.W., Paterson, J.W., Ramalho, P.S. and Shakib, M. (1966) Brit. J. Ophthal., 50:281.

Au, Y.K. and Bellhorn, M.B. (1977) Invest. Ophthal. Vis. Sci. Suppl. 1977, p. 147.

Barringer, J.R. and Griffith, J.F. (1970) Jl. Neuropath. Exp. Neurol. 29:89.

Barringer, J.R. and Nathanson, N. (1972) Jl. Neuropath. Exp. Neurol. 31:172 (abstract).

Bellhorn, M.B., Bellhorn, R.W. and Poll, D.S. (1977) Exp. Eye Res., 24:595.

Bellhorn, R.W., Bellhorn, M.B., Friedman, A.H. and Henkind, P. (1973) Invest. Ophthal., 12:65.

Bellhorn, R.W., Bellhorn, M.B. and Benjamin, J.V. (1977) Invest. Ophthal. Vis. Sci.,Suppl. 1977, p.53.

Benjamin, J.V., Bellhorn, M. and Bellhorn, R.W. (1977) _Invest. Oph-
    thal. Suppl. 1977_, p. 56.
Brightman, M.W., Hori, M., Rapoport, S.I., Reese, T.S. and Wester-
    gaard, F. (1973) _J. Comp. Neurol._, 152:317.
Brightman, M.W. and Reese, T.S. (1969) _J. of Cell Biol._, 40:648.
Cheek, D.B. and Holt, A.B. (1978) _Pediat. Res._, 12:635.
Cunha-Vaz, J.G., Faria de Abreu, J.R., Campos, A.J. and Figo, G.M.
    (1975) _Brit. J. Ophthalmol._, 59:649.
Cunha-Vaz, J.G., Goldberg, M.F., Vygantas, C. and Noth, J. (1979)
    Tr. Am. Acad. Ophth., 86:264.
DeRobertis, E.D.P. and Gerschenfeld, H.M. (1961) Submicroscopic
    morphology and function of glial cells. Di H.C. Pfeiffer and
    J.R. Smythies (eds.) _Intern. Rev. Neurobiol. New York_, Acade-
    mic Press. Vol. 3, p. 1.
Dollery, C.T., Henkind, P. and Orme, M.L'E. (1971) _Diabetes_, 20:519.
Duke-Elder, W.S. (1941) Textbook of Ophthalmology. _Vol. 3_. Diseases
    of the Inner Eye. London, Kimpton, p. 2588.
Duke-Elder, W.S. and Dobree, J.H. (1967) _System of Ophthalmology._
    Vol. X. Diseases of the Retina. London, Kimpton, p. 121.
Essner, E., Pino, R.M. and Griewski, R.A. (1979) _Invest. Ophthal._
    Vis. Sci., 18:859.
Gass, J.D.M. (1977) _Stereoscopic Atlas of Macular Diseases. Diagno-
    sis and Treatment. 2nd Edit_. St. Louis. C.V. Mosby, p. 376.
Glatt, H. and Henkind, P. (1979) _Microvasc. Res._, 18:1.
Grimes, P.A. and Laties, A.M. (1979) _Invest. Ophth. Vis. Sci. Suppl._
    1979 (abstract) p. 17.
Henkind, P. (1967) _Brit. J. Ophthal._, 51:115.
Henkind, P. (1978) _Amer. J. Ophthal._, 85:287.
Henkind, P. and de Oliveira, L.F. (1967) _Invest. Ophthal._, 6:520.
Henkind, P. and Wise, G.N. (1974) _Brit. J. Ophthal._, 58:413.
Hirano, A. (1974) Fine structural alterations of small vessels in
    the nervous system. In J. Cervos-Navarro (ed.) _Pathology of_
    Cerebral Microcirculation. Berlin. Walter de Gruyton, p. 203.
Hirano, A. (1976)Further observations of the fine structure of pa-
    thological reaction in cerebral blood vessels. In J. Cervos-
    -Navarro (ed.) _The Cerebral Vessel Wall_. New York. Raven Press.
    p. 41.
Hockley, D.J., Tripathi, R.C. and Ashton, N. (1979) _Brit. J. Ophthal._
    63:393.
Hogan, M. Alvarado, J.A., Weddell, J.E. (1971) _Histology of the Hu-
    man Eye: An Atlas and Textbook_. Phila. W. B. Saunders, p. 393.
Kirber, W.M., Nichols, C.W., Laties, A.M. and Winegrad, A.I. (1977)
    Invest. Ophthal. Vis. Sci. Suppl. 1977, p. 225.
Klatzo, I. (1967) Jl. _Neuropath. Exp. Neurol._, 26:1.
Kohner, E.M., Dollery, C.T., Shakib, M., Henkind, P., Paterson, J.W.,
    de Oliveira, L.N.F. and Bullpitt, C.J. (1970) _Amer. J. Ophth.,_
    69:778.
Laties, A.N., Rapoport, S.I. and McGlinn, A. (1979) _Arch. Ophthal._
    97:1511.
Matsuda, H. and Sugiura, S. (1970) _Invest. Ophthal._, 9:919.

Møllgard, K. and Sørensen, S.C. (1974) The permeability of cerebral capillaries to a tracer molecule, Alcian blue, with a molecular weight of 1390. In J. Cervos-Navarro (ed.) Pathology of Cerebral Microcirculation. Berlin. Walter de Gruyton, p.228.

Patz, A., Shatz, H. Berkow, J.W., Gittlesohn, A.M. and Ticho, U. (1973) Trans. Amer. Acad. Ophth. Oto., 77:34.

Rapoport, S. (1976) Modification of cerebrovascular permeability by hypertonic solutions and conditions which alter autoregulation of cerebral blood flow. In J. Cervos-Navarro (ed.) The Cerebral Vessel Wall. New York, Raven Press, p. 215.

Raviola, E. (1976) Invest. Ophthal. , 15:881.

Sjostrand, F.S. (1961) Electron microscopy of the retina in Smelser, G.K. (ed.) The Structure of the Eye. New York, Academic Press., p. 1.

Smelser, G.K., Ishikawa, T. and Pei, Y.F. (1965) Electron microscopic studies of intraretinal spaces: Diffusion of particulate materials. In J.W. Rohen (ed.) The Structure of the Eye. II Symposium. Stuttgart. Shattauer-Verlag, p. 109.

Sumi, S.M. (1969) J. Ultrastructural Res., 29:398.

Tso, M.O.M. and Fine, B.S. (1979) Invest. Ophthal. Vis. Sci., 18:447

Tso, M.O.M. and Shih, C.Y. (1976) Exp. Eye Res., 23:209.

Westergaard, E. and Brightman, M.W. (1973) J. Comp. Neurol., 152:17.

Van Harreveld, A., Collewijn, H. and Malhotra, S.K. (1966) Am. J. Physiol. 210:251.

Van Harreveld, A., Crowell, J. and Malhotra, S.K. (1965) J. Cell Biol. 25:117.

ACUTE HYPERTENSION AND EXPERIMENTAL DIABETES: EVALUATION OF THEIR EFFECTS ON BLOOD-OCULAR BARRIERS

A.M. Laties, P.A. Grimes, S.I. Rapoport
Department of Ophthalmology, Scheie Eye Institute, University of Pennsylvania, School of Medicine and *Laboratory of Neurosciences, National Institute on Aging, Gerontology Research Center, Baltimore City Hospitals

For the past several years we have been engaged in a series of studies on the effects of stress on the blood-ocular barriers. A variety of stresses have been studied -- including osmotic shock,[1] acute hypertension,[2] drug reactivity,[3] experimental diabetes,[4,5] and carbon dioxide inhalation.[6] For the measurement of barrier status, chief reliance has been placed on the localization of fluorescent dyes in freeze-dried tissue by darkfield microscopy. When appropriate, brains of the same animals have also been evaluated. In special instances, electron microscopy after the prior administration of horseradish peroxidase has been performed.

Accuracy of localization and ease of tissue handling have been the chief reasons for relying on fluorescence microscopy. Given today's freeze-dry equipment, it is a straightforward matter to freeze-dry an entire eye or, for that matter, if a little patience is exercised, to freeze-dry an entire brain. Further, after vacuum infiltration with paraffin, quite extensive tissue regions can be studied in single section. Thus the entire posterior segment can be in view in one tissue section, permitting comparison of a stress effect starting at one ora serrata and inspecting the tissue in continuous fashion to the other.

Fluorescein has proved to be a useful tracer. It is relatively nontoxic. Its yellow fluorescence can readily be differentiated from the blue autofluorescence of most tissues. In addition, its fluorescence is intense, thus making the method sensitive, even permitting low power inspection. In turn, this allows rapid and accurate evaluation of large numbers of tissue sections. When needed, the same tissue section can be viewed with an oil objective to define cell boundaries and the like. The details of this method have been previously published.[1]

The use of fluorescein as a marker dye in experimental studies yields a bonus: the results can be compared directly to those of clinical studies in humans using the same dye. One obvious but important difference exists, however. In fluorescein angiography the view is necessarily en face; in tissue sections the viewing plane depends on the plane of the section but allows a wide choice. In sagittal sections, for instance, a clear delineation of pigment epithelium from retinal blood vessels is readily made, permitting independent evaluation of barrier qualities of each.

I.   ACUTE HYPERTENSION

Acute hypertension can be induced in a number of ways. Carotid infusion of isotonic saline alone or in conjunction with intravenous administration of aramine (metaraminal 0.2 - 0.4 mg/kg intravenously) provides a predictable elevation of systolic blood pressure. Experiments have been performed both on adult rhesus monkeys and on 400 gm Wistar rats. A brief summary of experimental detail is given in Table I.

Table I: Effect on blood-brain barrier of experimental hypertension in macaque monkey.

EXPT NO.	ARAMINE DOSE MG/KG	CAROTID INFUSION 3.8 ML/SEC FOR 15 SEC	BLOOD PRESSURE, MM HG INITIAL	MAXIMUM	BARRIER CHANGES
ANIMALS KILLED 30 MIN AFTER TREATMENT					
1	0.4	NO	90	160	OCCASIONAL CAPILLARY LEAKAGE
2	0	YES	70	175	STAINING RIGHT SUPERIOR CENTRAL GYRUS
3	0	YES	120	190	STAINING MIDDLE CEREBRAL ARTERY
4	0.3	YES	90	250	STAINING RIGHT SIDE, MIDDLE CEREBRAL ARTERY DISTRIBUTION
5	0.4	YES	90	300	OVERALL RIGHT-SIDED STAINING
ANIMALS KILLED 2 DAYS AFTER TREATMENT					
6	0.3	YES	80	200	GROSS BILATERAL STAINING, MOTOR WEAKNESS, DECREASED ACTIVITY
7	0.4	YES	90	310	GROSS BILATERAL STAINING, COMA

In order to facilitate evaluation, experimental animals were given two marker dyes intravenously, Evans blue and fluorescein, before being killed. Since Evans blue binds avidly to protein and looks blue in daylight, it can be readily seen in fresh brain sections. The remarkably brilliant yellow fluorescence of fluorescein can

Table II: Effect of acute hypertension in the monkey on the blood-
            retina barriers.

ACUTE HYPERTENSION: MONKEY

BLOOD-RETINA BARRIER VERSUS BLOOD-BRAIN BARRIER

B.P.	RETINAL BLOOD VESSELS	PIGMENT EPITHELIUM
160	INTACT	INTACT
175	INTACT	INTACT
190	INTACT	INTACT
200	INTACT	INTACT
250	INTACT	INTACT
300	INTACT	INTACT
310	INTACT	INTACT

be visualized in tissue sections with the darkfield of a fluorescence microscope more easily than can the reddish fluorescence of
Evans blue bound to protein. Thus, each dye offers advantages for
specific purposes. They do not interfere with each other. When
both are present in the same locale, the fluorescence is orange.
As shown in Table I, an acute rise of systolic blood pressure above
160 mm Hg leads to widespread extravasation of protein (Evans blue)
into the brain. Yet, the same blood pressure elevation does not
disrupt the integrity of the retinal blood vessels; they did not
leak fluorescein (Table II). Interestingly, the pigment epithelial
barrier held uniformly throughout its extent in all experimental
monkeys while giving way in 4 out of eight rats. To date the number
of rats studied is too small to indicate a significant difference.
However, the finding does raise the suspicion that in acute hypertension the pigment epithelium is at greater risk than the retinal
blood vessels. Whatever the explanation of the pigment epithelial
leak in the rat may be, it is undoubted that the effect of acute
hypertension on the two vascular beds, brain and retina, differs.
The retinal blood vessels clearly are affected to a much lesser
degree than are those of the brain. Even a hypertensive surge
sufficient to put a monkey into coma, does not disrupt the tight
junctions of the retinal blood vessels.

     Two explanations for this difference, perhaps additive in
nature, can be offered. First, the autonomic innervation differs
between brain and eye. In the brain, a dense innervational network
supplying the great vessels at the base of the brain is immediately
succeeded by a sparse but persistent adrenergic innervation to
arteriolar branchings within the hemispheres. For the eye, matters
are more complex: the choroid has a dense innervational network.
So does the central retinal artery as it passes forward into the
optic nerve. The central retinal artery clearly has a density of

adrenergic innervation surpassing that of a similar sized arterial branch in the brain. But all innervation to the central artery ceases just at or just before the optic nerve head. Within the retina, the blood vessels are devoid of all innervation.

Second, there are differences in structure between brain and retinal blood vessels. These are of quantity rather than of kind; concerning as they do the distribution of mural cells (pericytes). In the retina, mural cells are in constant one-to-one ratio to endothelial cells.[7] Everywhere blood vessels have a double envelope. In contrast, the distribution of mural cells in the brain is less predictable. In some areas in the cerebrum they are just as numerous as endothelial cells, while in others, they are much less common, gaps are present (Brightman, 1978, personal communication). If the hypothesis of Cogan and Kuwabara that mural cells buttress the endothelium is indeed true,[8] their constancy in retina might explain the resistance of the vasculature to surges of blood pressure. Lending further support to such an idea is the recent finding that retinal mural cells contain an abundance of actin filaments, as would be expected were the cell playing a supporting or contractile role.[9]

II. EXPERIMENTAL DIABETES MELLITUS

The assertion by Cunha-Vaz et al in 1975 that penetration of fluorescein into the posterior vitreous humor could be measured in angiographically normal human diabetics opened new vistas for all in diabetes research.[10] Soon thereafter the finding was confirmed by Krupin et al.[11] Both research groups spoke of the disturbance in the blood-retina barrier. However, a specific locus of barrier breakdown was not described. Waltman measured a complementary pattern of excess fluorescein in the acqueous humor as well. Shortly thereafter, rats made diabetic by the injection of streptozotocin were shown to have similar findings.[12]

These publications stimulated us to undertake tissue distribution studies of fluorescein in the rat; they are still in progress. Several findings, some negative, some positive, have already been made. In the completed experiments we gave streptozotocin in a standard dose (65 mg/kg) intravenously, following an overnight fast. Hyperglycemia in the range of 375 - 500 mg/dl at 48 - 72 hours after injections was accepted as evidence that the animals were indeed diabetic. The rats were killed three to five weeks after streptozotocin administration. For fluorescein studies, 0.25 ml of a 10% solution was injected into the femoral vein two minutes before the animals were killed. After immediate enucleation, the eyes were quick-frozen. Freeze-drying, tissue embedding, and sectioning were done as previously described.

A total of 35 eyes from 20 rats with streptozotocin-induced diabetes of 4 weeks' duration were examined. In not a single instance did the dye leak from a retinal blood vessel. In all respects the blood vessels were indistinguishable from those of controls. Nor could any stain of neural retina such as might occur by diffusion of fluorescein from the adjacent vitreous humor be seen. There was however one distinct difference from the control series. In one-half of the diabetic rats, the pigment epithelium of the retina was altered. In these instances it had a yellow stain, varying from the just discernible to the vivid. Whatever its intensity, when present, the color was uniform in individual cells and was present in all pigment epithelial cells. The entire cell layer had the same general appearance. No dye was seen to radiate from these cells into the adjacent photoreceptor layer.

It is generally held that weight gain can be used as an approximate index of the severity of streptozotocin-induced diabetes in young rats: the more severe the diabetes, the less the gain.[13] For this reason we divided the rats into two groups, those gaining more and those gaining less than 60 gms in 4 weeks. There is a clear tendency by this measure for those who were severely affected to show a pigment epithelial abnormality: 8 of 11 of the low gainers had fluorescein staining of the pigment epithelium versus 2 out of 9 of the high gainers. In addition, six eyes from four insulin-treated rats from an accessory series were also studied. Each of these eyes was normal in all respects.

Horseradish Peroxidase Studies

Both to define the extent of the pigment epithelial abnormality and to be reassured that the negative result for the retinal blood vessels would stand up to an independent and sensitive test, a second protocol was undertaken. In another, 6 diabetic rats after induction of deep pentobarbital anesthesia (50 mg/kg ip) with diphenhydramine hydrochloride and methysergide maleate (1 mg/kg iv) were injected to forestall vascular permeability breakdown by horseradish peroxidase. Five minutes later, horseradish peroxidase (200 mg/kg) dissolved in 1 ml of .85% sodium chloride solution was given intravenously. Ten minutes later, the rats were killed and the eyes enucleated. They were immediately immersed in a solution of 3% glutaraldehyde and 0.5% formaldehyde. Fixation and histochemical processing were done by a standard method.[14]

To light microscopic observation of the resulting tissue sections, there apparently were inclusions in the pigment epithelial cytoplasm, irregularly rounded aggregates of reaction product being visible. However, this observation was misleading. When viewed in the electron microscope, the aggregates were all exterior to the cell. The discordance between light and electron microscopic obser-

vations was due to an unusual inward penetration of the fingerlike
basal infoldings. In the diabetic rat, these were markedly elong-
ated. In tissue sections, horseradish peroxidase could readily be
observed in the choroid, Bruch's membrane, and in the area immediately surrounding the pigment epithelial cells. Once the elaborate
infoldings had been observed, it was clear that there had been no
entry of horseradish peroxidase to the epithelial cell cytoplasm.
Nor when retinal blood vessels were carefully studied was any
reaction product visualized outside their lumens. Reaction product
could however be seen extending out as far as the tight junctions
between neighboring endothelial cells.

Proliferation of RPE Basal Surface Membrane

Although a negative study in terms of permeability, the HRP
experiments led to a new and perhaps a more significant finding
than that originally sought: in the diabetic rat the basal surface
membrane of the retinal pigment epithelium had proliferated. Full
details of the stereological procedures by which the surface area
was measured and calculated are published elsewhere.[5] Using carefully prepared photographic montages, the method depends on the
counting of intersects of basal cell surface membrane with the
parallel lines of a transparent overlying grid. When properly
done, membrane length can be accurately calculated. In the present
instance the calculated value was expressed as length of basal cell
membrane per unit length of Bruch's membrane. In turn, this can
quite readily be converted into surface area.

Even before precise measurements were available, it was clear
that the basal membrane was increased in length. Infolded basal
membrane, assuming tortuous configurations, extended deeply into
the retinal pigment epithelium cytoplasm in the diabetic rats
(Figure 1). Since the infoldings were filled with reaction product,
they were clearly outlined. When basal surface measurements were
undertaken, the result was nevertheless startling: on a linear
basis, basal membrane length per length of Bruch's membrane rose
by a third from 8.6 to 11.6 (expressed as a ratio, independent
magnification). In terms of surface area, this works out to an
effective doubling, or put into practical units, for every 1 μm^2
of Bruch's membrane there was now 135 μm^2 of pigment epithelial
basal surface area instead of the former 76 μm^2. Since by our
calculations and those of Lerche[15] the retinal blood vessels have
a total surface area slightly less than Bruch's membrane, this
also means that the basal retinal pigment epithelial surface area
in the diabetic rat exceeds that of the retinal blood vessels by
a factor of 200. Interestingly, within the limits of this study,
there was an as yet undefined but clear tendency for the basal
surface area to increase with an increased duration of diabetes
(see Table III).

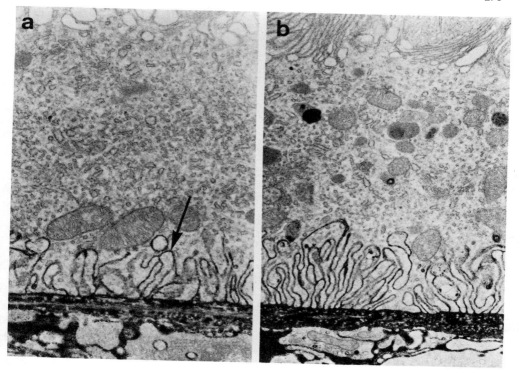

Retinal Pigment Epithelium

Figure 1a: Control retina. Basal infoldings (arrow) can be readily seen. Horseradish peroxidase is within them but has not entered the cell.

Figure 1b: In diabetic rat, basal infoldings are both more elaborate and of greater extent.

SUMMARY

At present, light and electron microscopic methods permit the evaluation of the status of the blood-brain and blood-retinal barriers through the use of marker dyes and test substances. In the present series of studies, fluorescence microscopy of freeze-dried tissues and electron microscopy of liquid-fixed tissues were used to measure barrier integrity under stress. Although this review describes the results of two stresses -- hypertension and diabetes -- information is now available on the effects of several others as well. In the case of acute hypertension in the monkey,

Table III: Basal pigment epithelial surface area increases with
            duration of experimental diabetes.

INTERVAL	$(L_C/L_B)^2$	%INCREASE
CONTROL	75.7	
STREPTOZOTOCIN		
3 WKS	116.6	54
4 WKS	132.3	75
5 WKS	156.3	106
AVERAGE		78

a remarkable difference in susceptibility between brain and retina
was found. In the diabetic rat, the essential nature of the
barriers is retained while unexplained alterations of the basal
surface membrane of the pigment epithelial cell take place.

REFERENCES

1. Laties, A.M. and Rapoport, S.: Arch. Ophthalmol. 94:1086-1091,
    1976.
2. Laties, A.M., Rapoport, S.I. and McGlinn, A.: Arch. Ophthal-
    mol. 97:1511-1514, 1979.
3. Laties, A.M., Neufeld, A.H., Vegge, T. and Sears, M.L.: Arch.
    Ophthalmol. 94:1966-1971, 1976.
4. Kirber, W.M., Nichols, C.W., Grimes, P.A., Winegrad, A.I., and
    Laties, A.M.: (In press, Arch. Ophthalmol.).
5. Grimes, P.A. and Laties, A.M.: (In press, Exp. Eye Res.).
6. Rapoport, S.I., Fredericks, W.R. and Laties A.M.: (In press
    Exp. Eye Res.).
7. Hogan, M.J., Alvarado, J.A. and Weddell, J.E.: HISTOLOGY OF
    THE HUMAN EYE. W.B. Saunders Co., Philadelphia, 1971.
8. Cogan, D.G., Kuwabara, T.: Ocular microangiopathy in diabetes,
    in Kimura, S. and Caygill, W.M. (eds.): VASCULAR COMPLI-
    CATIONS OF DIABETES MELLITUS. St. Louis, C.V.Mosby Co.,
    1967, pp.53-63.
9. Burnside, B. and Wallow, I., personal communication, 1978.
10. Cunha-Vaz, J., Faria DeAbreu, J.R., Campos, A.J. and Figo, G.M.:
    Brit. J. Ophthalmol. 59:649-656, 1975.
11. Krupin, T., Waltman, S.R., Oestrich, C., Santiago, J., Ratzan,
    S., Kilo, C. and Becker, B.: Arch.Ophthalmol. 96:812-814,

1978.

13. Junod, A., Lambert, A.E., Stauffacher, W. and Renold, A.E.:
    J. Clin. Invest. 48:2129-2139, 1969.

14. Karnovsky, M.J.: J. Cell Biol. 35:213-236, 1967.

15. Lerche, W.: Die kapillarisierung der menschlichen retina in
    Rohen, J.W. (ed.): EYE STRUCTURE II. SYMPOSIUM. Schattauer
    Verlag, Stuttgart, 1965, pp. 121-128.

EXPERIMENTAL INNER RETINAL ISCHAEMIA AND THE BLOOD-RETINAL BARRIERS

D.B. Archer, F.R.C.S., and T.A. Gardner

Department of Ophthalmology
The Queen's University of Belfast
Royal Victoria Hospital, Belfast

The blood retinal barriers are remarkably rugged and resilient structures which are designed to protect the internal environment of the highly specialized and cellular retina. The barriers strictly regulate the movement of fluid, protein and metabolites into and out of the retina, thereby maintaining the critical architecture and orientation of the outer retinal receptors.

Both inner and outer barriers can withstand considerable physiological and aphysiological stress and can function adequately despite limited pharmacological insults, e.g. hypertonic and hypotonic solutions, histamine and prostaglandins. They can also resist short periods of hypoxia and ischaemia without significant loss of barrier properties. Even when barrier functions have been disturbed by acute circulatory failure both the retinal pigment epithelium and retinal vascular endothelium exhibit considerable recuperative and regenerative properties so that when circulation is restored there may be a rapid re-establishment of barrier integrity.

In health, the retinal vascular endothelium has a stable cell population with a relatively low turnover rate, e.g. Engerman[1] estimates that in the mouse each endothelial cell renews itself only once every three years. Nevertheless, following injury, stress, or pathological conditions the endothelial cells have a potential to hypertrophy and proliferate to reline denuded regions of vascular basement membrane and to expand to accommodate the increased luminal diameter of collateral vessels.

There are, nevertheless, many stresses and pathological conditions which precipitate either transient or permanent breakdown of one or both retinal barriers, leading to abnormal vascular permeability, altered retinal metabolism and loss of visual functions. The integrity of the retinal vessels, particularly the microvasculature, may be affected by a) distension of the vessel walls, e.g. following acute branch vein occlusion, b) venous stasis and ischaemia, e.g. diabetes and chronic retinal vein occlusion, c) inflammation, either direct, e.g. retinal vasculitis, or secondary to an acute retinitis, e.g. toxoplasmosis, d) various pharmacological agents, e.g. nicotinamide and epinephrine, or e) a defect in the retinal endothelial cells themselves, e.g. telangiectasias, vascular tumours or preretinal neovascularization.

There are few clinical conditions in which all these factors are operational; however, in branch retinal vein occlusion many come into play at one stage or another during the evolution of the disease process. Immediately following occlusion there is acute distension of the involved venous circulation, and this is followed by varying degrees of venous stasis and inner retinal ischaemia according to the order of the vein obstructed and the efficiency of the developing collateral circulation. The liberation of irritative degradation products from the necrotic inner retina excites a chronic inflammatory reaction, and, in long standing branch vein obstruction with extensive ischaemia, preretinal and papillary neovascularization commonly occur. In addition, alterations may also occur at the level of the outer retina secondary to widespread inner retinal ischaemia and venous stasis, occasionally to such an extent that there is a failure of barrier functions.

Branch vein occlusion can be conveniently studied in the experimental animal, particularly the rhesus monkey whose retinal circulation is virtually identical to that of the human.[2,3] Venous occlusion and obstruction can be produced easily by photocoagulation, and, although the alterations which occur in the affected vessels of a healthy monkey may not completely parallel those occurring in an elderly arteriosclerotic individual, useful comparisons and extrapolations can be made. The reminder of this presentation concerns itself principally with the effects of an acute branch retinal vein occlusion and subsequent inner retinal ischaemia on the retinal microvasculature and the retinal pigment epithelium. The formation of subretinal neovascular membranes secondary to retinal vein occlusion will also be briefly discussed.

1. BRANCH VEIN OCCLUSION - ALTERATIONS TO THE RETINAL VASCULATURE

Branch retinal vein occlusions were produced in the rhesus monkey by photocoagulating single or multiple branch veins of varying magnitude using an O'Malley log 2 photocoagulator. Small target size, high intensity burns were used to occlude selected veins without affecting nearby arteries. A technique was established whereby flow was initially arrested with a single, high intensity burn straddling the selected vein, followed by one or more supplementary burns directed downstream to the partially collapsed adjacent segment of the vessel. Occasionally patency was re-established following such treatment and rephotocoagulation was undertaken at a later date. Photocoagulation produced necrosis and atrophy of the nearby retina, retinal pigment epithelium and choriocapillaris, but the choroidal circulation was not significantly affected elsewhere as judged by fluorescein angiography, histopathological analysis and neoprene-latex injection studies.

Immediately following photocoagulation of a major retinal vein there is an acute dilatation of all venous radicals within the distribution of the obstructed vein and an accompanying outpouring of fluid into the retina. Occasional punctate or blotch haemorrhages occur at distended terminal venules although haemorrhage is not a feature of the immediate post-occlusive phase. Concomitant narrowing of the fellow artery occurs, and there is substantial reduction in arterial flow as measured by fluorescein angiography, and radioactive microsphere impaction technique.[5]

Fluorescein angiography in the immediate post-occlusive stages demonstrate marked slowing of the obstructed circulation with pronounced stasis at the junction of the precapillary arteriole and the capillary network (Fig. 1). Many precapillary arterioles have characteristic blunt terminals with little or no filling of the capillary network beyond these points. This angiographic appearance probably represents constriction of the precapillary arteriole and may be an autoregulatory response to the acute rise of pressure in the retinal venous circulation and microvasculature. Eventually dye circulates through the capillary network and dilated venules, and leakage of dye can be appreciated at the terminal venules. The terminal venules are particularly vulnerable as their wide lumina and relatively thin walls have low resistance to sudden increases in intraluminar pressures. A further manifestation of the high capillary pressure within the obstructed capillary bed is the retrograde flow of dye for a short distance into terminal arterioles at the junction of the obstructed and normal circulations (Fig. 2). Capillary collaterals form almost immediately following occlusion and rapidly drain blood from the obstructed to the non-obstructed circulation. They are very efficient and if the area of venous stasis is not too great, they permit full perfusion of the implicated capillary bed. Late phase angiograms demonstrate widespread decompensation of the blood retinal barrier on the venous side of the circulation. It is particularly pronounced at the level of the terminal venules although leakage may be confined in certain areas to the capillary network.

Histological examination of incompetent areas of the microvasculature shows that the terminal venules and venous capillaries are widely dilated and lined by attenuated endothelial cells (Fig.3).

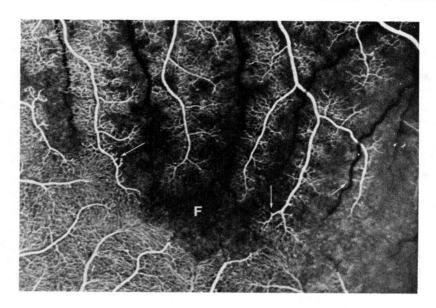

Fig. 1. Mid venous phase fluorescein angiogram of foveal (F) and
macular region of rhesus monkey in which a left supero-temporal vein
has been occluded by photocoagulation. There is marked retardation
of venous return in the territory of the occluded vein and stasis
is particularly pronounced at the level of precapillary arterioles
which have characteristic blunt tips (arrows).

Despite their marked thinning the endothelial cells characteristically remain structurally intact, and there is no evidence of
tearing or dissolution of the plasma membranes or tight junctions.
The endothelial cells, which normally show only minimal vesicular
transport, exhibit increased and intense pinocytotic activities at
all levels within the cells. Fused and often giant pinosomes are
a typical feature, suggesting that such vesicular transport is a
possible route for the extravascular outpouring of fluid (Fig. 3).
It may also be that in the immediate post-obstructive phase when
there is a marked gradient between intraluminar and tissue pressure
contiguous pinosomes fuse across the entire width of the attenuated
endothelial cells thus providing a rapid transcellular route for
bulk fluid flow. As tissue pressure increases with retinal hydra-
tion and intraluminar pressure decreases secondary to collateral
formation the rapid transfer of fluid will correspondingly diminish.

Studies using horseradish peroxidase demonstrate that the

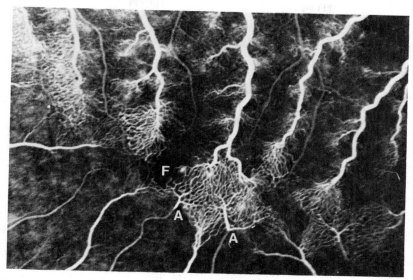

Fig. 2. Late venous phase angiogram of fundus shown in Fig. 1.
Dilated capillary collaterals divert dye across the median raphe into
the non-obstructed venous circulation. There is also retrograde
flow of dye into some nearby arterioles (A) for a short distance.
Dye leakage occurs predominantly at small venules.

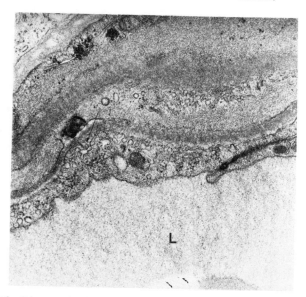

Fig. 3. Endothelium of obstructed post-capillary venule 15 mins.
after photocoagulation. Fused pinosomes are present at the basal
plasma membrane of the endothelial cell (arrow). (Lumen - L).
x 50,000. (Reduced 50% for reproduction.)

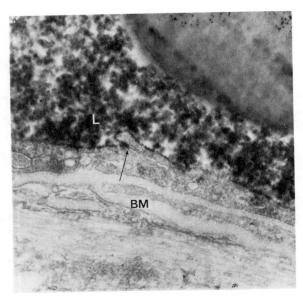

Fig. 4. Obstructed post-capillary venules 15 mins. after occlusion. Peroxidase reaction product is present in the lumen (L) but has not passed the tight junction. Basement membrane (BM) also remains free of product. x 80,000. (Reduced 50% for reproduction.)

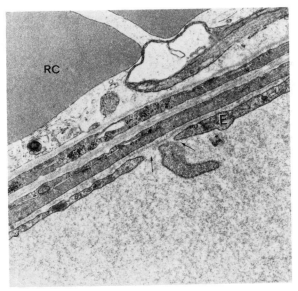

Fig. 5. Breach in endothelium (E) of terminal venule 15 mins. post-occlusion (arrows). Red blood cells are present in the extra-vascular space (RC). x 40,000. (Reduced 50% for reproduction.)

tracer accumulates on the luminal aspect of the tight junctions and
does not penetrate to the basal lamina via the junctional complex
(Fig. 4). Tracer, however, could be identified within pinosomes
in endothelial cells although no significant amounts were identified
at this early stage beyond the vessel wall. Hockley, et al,[4]
demonstrated that by 1½ hours after the acute vein occlusion horseradish peroxidase could be identified in the vascular basement membrane and extra cellular space of the retina, but no tracer transit
was observed via the intercellular junctions. Therefore, it seems
likely that the immediate outpouring of fluid secondary to venous
occlusion occurs through the endothelial cells with pinocytosis
being an important mechanism of fluid transport. It is not clear
what size of molecules pass through the endothelial cells at this
stage, however, it is likely that large molecules can bypass the
more selective endothelial transport mechanism and gain the extravascular space. Following angiography fluorescein accumulates extra-
vascularly in high concentrations and presumably much of this compound is protein bound. It also seems likely that at this early
post-occlusive stage most of the changes can be attributed to an
increased hydrostatic pressure and that hypoxia or anoxia play only
a subsidiary role or no role at all in causing vascular incompetence.

Although the plasma membrane and tight junctions were generally
preserved in the immediate post-occlusive phase, occasional defects
in the vessel walls were detected. Dehiscences were typically found
in terminal venules particularly where red blood cell extravasation
had occurred (Fig. 5). Such dehiscences breached both plasma membranes of the endothelial cells but did not involve junctional complexes. At the zones of cytoplasmic discontinuity plasma membranes
were well defined, exhibiting their typical trilaminar structure.
Such "pores" could provide a convenient route for the extravasation
of large particles, particularly red blood cells, inflammatory
cells and macromolecules. As capillary competence was regained in
most instances within 2 to 7 days, it is likely that the endothelial cells can rapidly repair such cytoplasmic defects and re-
establish barrier properties.

Events which follow the acute phase of vein obstruction are
dictated by the order of the vein obstructed, the formation of
collaterals and whether circulation is re-established at the site
of photocoagulation. In small order vein obstructions with extensive collateral systems oedema resolves within a few days and
intraretinal haemorrhage rapidly absorbs over three to four weeks.
After a few weeks residual preferential collateral channels are all
that remain and these typically remain competent to dye. Some
subtle structural and architectural alterations can always be
detected within the involved retinal microvasculature; however, no
abnormality of the blood retinal barrier is present as judged by
vascular competence during fluorescein angiography.

Monkeys with large order complete vein occlusions frequently develop extensive haemorrhage within the obstructed venous circulation some 12 to 24 hours after photocoagulation. The cause of haemorrhage at this stage is not known, but it probably represents the cumulative effects of hypoxia, anoxia and raised intraluminar pressure. Haemorrhages were often extensive, persisted 7 to 8 weeks and occurred at all levels within the retina, occasionally extending to the subretinal space. Some obstructed veins became sheathed with lymphocytes and acute inflammatory cells, and areas of frank retinal infarction (cotton wool spots) were noted. Once haemorrhage and oedema had resolved, areas of capillary closure could be identified. These were often extensive although once established they did not tend to progress (Fig. 6). Major retinal vessels which traversed areas of capillary non-perfusion often showed structural abnormalities and stained with fluorescein during angiography indicating an abnormality of their endothelial cells.

A wide variety of structural abnormalities were noted in the residual retinal microvasculature, particularly stunted and spike-like venules and arterioles which bordered and projected into areas of non-perfused retina. Microaneurysmal-like dilatations were also common usually representing the remnants of the atrophic capillary bed (Fig. 6). These focal microvascular abnormalities were often hyperfluorescent but in no instance was there any significant or sustained leakage of dye from such vascular abnormalities into the retina. Indeed, despite widespread structural abnormalities of the retinal microvasculature and the presence of vast areas of non-perfused retina, in no instance were we able to achieve chronic intraretinal oedema. Hamilton, et al.[2] report similar findings.

Proliferative as well as atrophic and degenerative changes also took place within the affected microvasculature. Fine capillary-like vessels originated from the venous side of the circulation and randomly infiltrated ischaemic or non-perfused regions of the retina for varying distances. These irregular vessels formed loops and spirals and forged links with fellow adjacent new capillaries. On occasion , they seemed to parasitize residual major ghost vessels but the rate of growth was slow, and they characteristically remained competent to fluorescein apart from their apices which were hyperfluorescent. The new capillary complexes were constantly being remodelled and in some regions showed closure and atrophy. At no time were any of these intraretinal new vessels observed to penetrate the internal limiting membrane or form typical preretinal neovascular fronds.

In subsequent experiments areas of greater inner retinal ischaemia were produced by occluding both major superior temporal and inferior temporal veins. This model had the advantage of producing a well defined watershed between nasal perfused and temporal non-perfused inner retina, and foci of intraretinal neovascularization

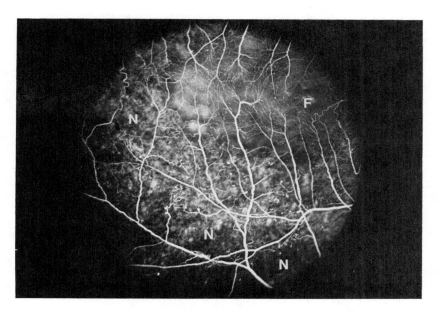

Fig. 6. Venous phase angiogram of posterior fundus (Fovea-F) of
rhesus monkey taken 2 months following photocoagulation of left
inferotemporal vein. Widespread areas of non-perfused retina are
present (N) and microaneurysmal-like dilatations occur in the residual capillary bed. The mottled background fluorescence reflects
pigment epithelial alterations.

that infiltrated ischaemic retina could be easily identified, orientated, and blocked for electron-microscopic evaluation without
involving the adjacent perfused retinal microvasculature.

   Histological studies of experimental intraretinal new vessels
demonstrate that they have the features of a normal retinal capillary for most of their course.[6] They characteristically extend into
the ischaemic retina either via basement membranes of old necrotic
veins and arterioles or within the interstices of the abundant glial
tissue which occupies the scarred inner retina (Fig. 7). Electronmicroscopy demonstrates that the new vessels have normal retinal
capillary features with bulky endothelial cells showing hetero-
chromatic nuclei, numerous mitochondria and well developed golgi
apparatus (Fig. 7). There is usually a fine basement membrane, and
pericytes or their processes are always in evidence. Strands of
redundant basement membrane from old ghost vessels frequently encir-
cle the new vessels and the entire complex is usually encapsulated
by the processes of Mueller cells which themselves have a fine base-

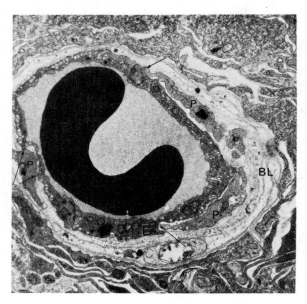

Fig. 7. New intraretinal capillary relining redundant vascular basal
lamina (BL).   Pericyte(P)-endothelial cell (E) contacts or junctions
are common (arrows). x 20,000.   (Reduced 50% for reproduction.)

ment membrane.   The endothelial cells for the most part are joined
by well defined intercellular junctions.   There appears to be an
important spacial relationship between the pericytes and the endothelial cells and not infrequently cell to cell contacts are established that penetrate the basement membrane between the endothelial
cell and the pericyte (Fig. 7).   Towards the growing end of the
capillary the endothelial cells show a corresponding increase in
the density of cellular inclusions.   The cell junctions in this
region are poorly defined; however, membranous densifications in the
region of cellular apposition indicate that some form of assembly
is in progress.   At this stage the basal lamina which ensheaths both
endothelial cells and pericytes is tenuous and incomplete, and the
voluminous endothelial cytoplasm has in places reduced the lumen to
a convoluted slit-like structure.   The endothelial cell organelles
are remarkable both in concentration and development (Fig. 8).
Mitochondria are large and numerous and encompassed by extensive,
sometimes dilated cisternae or rough endoplasmic reticulum which
are filled by a finely granular, homogeneous material.   The golgi
apparatus in these cells occupy a large volume of the cytoplasm and

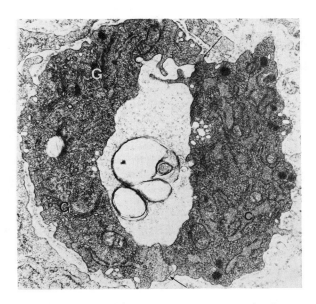

Fig. 8. New intraretinal capillary sprout proximal to growing tip.
The elaborate golgi complexes, dilated rough endoplasmic reticulum
cisternae (C) and tenuous cell junctions characterize this region
of the vessel. x 40,000. (Reduced 50% for reproduction.)

are highly active in the production of both smooth surfaced and
coated vesicles. Weibel-Palade bodies are common and could often
be seen close to their origin within the golgi saccules.[7] Pinocytotic vesicles, many of which show fusion with one another, are
much in evidence at both major cell surfaces although this activity
varies greatly from cell to cell. These cells, as noted previously,
are in close contact with pericytes and translaminar zones of contact are common. The morphological evidence is that these are new
endothelial cells which are actively metabolizing, synthesizing
and proliferating.

     At the growing tip of the capillary the endothelial cells are
loosely approximated with poorly defined intercellular junctions
and without an established lumen. Many of these apical cells have
numerous processes which interdigitate and link up with fellow
cellular prolongations, occasionally forming a primitive lumen.
Pericyte processes are also present in considerable numbers and may
be difficult to differentiate from processes of endothelial cells;
however, the identification of Weibel-Palade bodies is always a

valid and helpful marker for an endothelial cell.[8] The advancing
tips of the new intraretinal vessels are surrounded and preceded
by clusters of phagocytes which actively engulf extraneous debris
thereby aiding the progress of the proliferating endothelial cells.
Also in the vanguard of the advancing new vessels are processes of
pericytes which show subplasma membrane densifications and grow in
tandem with the processes of endothelial cells. Redundant acellular
basement membranes of former retinal vessels are parasitized not
only by endothelial cells and pericytes but also by other cells
such as phagocytes and the processes of Mueller cells (Fig. 9).

Intraretinal neovascularization or revascularization is a well
known clinical phenomenon and can be easily identified in young
patients with branch retinal vein thrombosis where non-perfused
areas of retina develop. As in the experimental model the new intraretinal vessels develop from the retinal venous bed that surrounds
the zone of ischaemic retina and may arise from capillaries, venules
or veins. The new vessels range in calibre from 20 to 50 μ's and
are usually identified as linear capillary-like outgrowths which
bifurcate in a typical wide-angle fashion, intertwine with adjacent
retinal vessels and ramify within areas of retina known to be avascular, e.g. the fovea or capillary free zones of arteries. The new
vessels remain competent to fluorescein for the most part although,
as in experimental models, the leading edge of the new capillary is
generally hyperfluorescent and dye may even extravasate for a short
distance into the adjacent retina.

It is unlikely that the new intraretinal vessels fulfill any
significant metabolic function within the retina they infiltrate;
however, they do not appear to have any adverse affect on the retina
and are not generally associated with significant intraretinal
oedema or haemorrhage.

The exact mechanism of intraretinal neovascularization is not
known but a process of endothelial and pericyte budding and proliferation would seem most likely with basement membrane of residual
necrotic vessels providing convenient, if not preferential pathways
of low resistance. The almost normal structure of these newly formed
capillaries and their competence during fluorescein angiography is
in striking contrast to the poorly constructed and incompetent
vessels found in preretinal neovascularization, and the exact relationship between these two forms of vessel growth has yet to be
defined. Perhaps the dense glial tissue and residual basement membranes into which many of these new intraretinal vessels grow
restrict the rate of proliferation of endothelial cells and favour
the formation of well organized vessels. By the same token the
absence of restraining influences in the preretinal space may account
for more rapid growth and extension of endothelial cells in this
area leading to the formation of more primitive preretinal tubes.

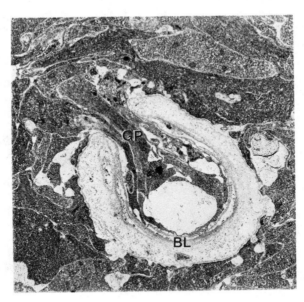

Fig. 9. Glial processes (G) infiltrating redundant vascular basal lamina (BL). x 12,000. (Reproduced 50% for reproduction.)

We conclude therefore that intraretinal neovascularization is a process of revascularization of ischaemic inner retina by capillary-like vessels. The process is slow, incomplete and without obvious functional benefit to the retina. The new vessels that develop are mature in structure with well defined junctional complexes and are, for the most part, competent to fluorescein. The vast majority of these new vessels remain within the retina and do not appear to be the normal precursors of preretinal neovascularization.

The stimulus responsible for the proliferation of endothelial and pericyte cells and the formation of new intraretinal vessels is not known, although in view of their characteristic tendency to infiltrate ischaemic retina it might be argued that hypoxia and anoxia are important factors. To determine whether the ischaemic inner retina which had been infiltrated by new vessels was hypoxic or anoxic, oxygen tension measurements were made in the immediate vicinity of perfused and non-perfused retina using an oxygen microelectrode.[9] The oxygen microelectrode was introduced into the rhesus monkey eye through a pars plana incision and readings taken 100 μ's

above the internal limiting membrane over areas of normal and ischaemic retina where new intraretinal sprouts had formed. No significant difference in oxygen tension was found between normal and non-
perfused inner retina indicating that the intact choroidal circulation was capable of furnishing the oxygen requirements of the
now atrophic and relatively acellular inner retina.

2.   BRANCH VEIN OCCLUSION - ALTERATIONS AT THE OUTER RETINA

In experimental vein occlusion significant structural alterations also occurred at the level of the outer retina. Some of the
changes occurred at or near the site of vein occlusion and were
clearly secondary to the effects of photocoagulation; however, some
structural alterations occurred remote from photocoagulation marks
and appeared to be a response to, or a direct consequence of, the
inner retinal ischaemia.

Subtle alterations in the retinal pigment epithelial cells and
outer receptors occurred in those regions bordering the territory
of the vein occlusion, particularly where a watershed existed between perfused and non-perfused retina. Mild retinal pigment epithelial alterations were also detected in areas of normally perfused
retina where subretinal accumulation of fluid had probably occurred
following the acute vein occlusion.

Profound alterations to both the retinal pigment epithelial
layer and retinal receptors occurred in those regions where there
was marked inner retinal ischaemia and necrosis, and in some regions
there was total absence of the retinal receptors. Alterations in
the retinal pigment epithelial layer were easily observed and took
the form of irregular areas of depigmentation, pigment mottling and
clumping. Drusen-like bodies were frequently seen, and where the
internal limiting membrane was defective pigment accumulation
occurred on the surface of the retina. In affected regions fluorescein angiography demonstrated a generalized hyperfluorescence
consistent with alterations to the pigment epithelial cells. Only
in rare instances, however, was there any breakdown of the retinal
pigment epithelial barrier with extravasation of dye into the subretinal space or outer retina.

Histological changes occurring at the retinal pigment epithelium
included atrophy, depigmentation, proliferation, migration and phagocytosis and membrane formation.

a)   Depigmentation and Atrophy

Depigmentation and atrophy of the retinal pigment epithelial

cells were the commonest alteration in the outer retina subsequent
to severe inner retinal ischaemia. The more severely affected cells
had degenerate and pyknotic nuclei, ruptured mitochondria and accumulations of autophagosomes. In some areas the retinal pigment epithelial cells were absent or replaced by the processes of Mueller
cells. Despite atrophy and degeneration of pigment epithelial cells
their basal lamina typically remained intact.

b)   Proliferation

     Retinal pigment epithelial proliferation was also a common
phenomenon and occurred both in the vicinity of photocoagulation
marks and beneath ischaemic inner retina. Reduplication of the
retinal pigment epithelial layer was not infrequent. A second layer
of pigment epithelial cells formed with their apical portions closely
approximated to the processes of the original pigment epithelial
cells. The basal lamina of the newly elaborated pigment epithelial
cells in such instances was oriented towards the neuro-retina (Fig.
10). The newly formed pigment epithelial cells generally had a full
complement of cytoplasmic organelles and characteristic spindle-
shaped pigment granules.

     Excessive proliferation of pigment epithelial cells in some
regions led to the formation of intraretinal pigment epithelial
mounds which were highly pigmented and often occupied the full thickness of the residual retina. Occasional giant cells were identified
in the vicinity of the photocoagulation marks and were characterized
by multiple nuclei incorporated within a complex cytoplasmic syncytium (Fig. 11). The nature of these giant cells was not clear
although it is possible that they originated from the retinal pigment epithelial layer. They differed strikingly from the typical
Langhan's giant cells in that they lacked a common cytocentrum,
having their golgi complexes located about individual nuclei. The
plasma membrane displayed an elaborate microvillous border and much
of the cell cytoplasm was occupied by numerous large mitochondria.

c)   Migration and Phagocytosis

     Pigment epithelial migration occurred commonly in the neigh-
bourhood of photocoagulation marks and to a lesser extent beneath
ischaemic retina. The migrating pigmented cells appeared to bud off
the free edges of the residual pigment epithelial cells and infiltrated the ischaemic and necrotic retina. These migrating cells had
no basement membrane but possessed typical spindle-shaped melanin
granules which were unrelated to secondary lysosomes and were therefore interpreted as primary or native granules. These altered
retinal pigment epithelial cells actively phagocytosed the debris

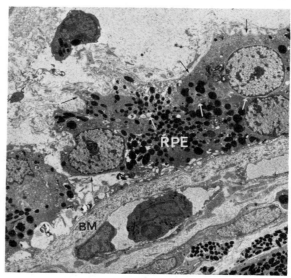

Fig. 10. Discontinuous retinal pigment epithelium (RPE) showing
reduplication. Note apposition of cell apices (white arrows) and
presence of basal lamina at both retinal and choroidal aspects of
pigment epithelial cells (black arrows). Bruch's membrane (BM)
remains intact. x 50,000. (Reduced 50% for reproduction.)

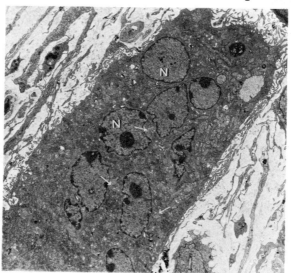

Fig. 11. Giant cell in subretinal space. Multiple euchromatic nuclei
(N) with prominent nucleoli are embedded in a cytoplasmic syncytium
which shows large aggregates of mitochondria, many individual golgi
complexes (white arrows) and an elaborate microvillous border.
x 5,000. (Reduced 50% for reproduction.)

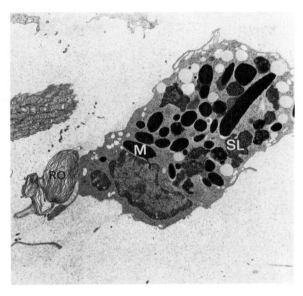

Fig. 12. Phagocytosis of rod outer segment (RO) by migrating pigment
epithelial cell.   Native melanin granules (M) may be seen in the
cytoplasm which also contains many secondary lysosomes (SL).
x 12,000.   (Reduced 50% for reproduction.)

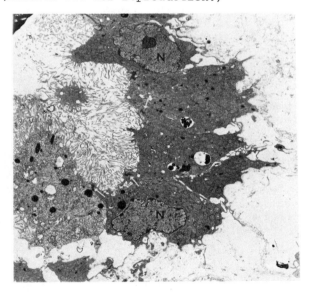

Fig. 13. Subretinal pigment epithelial membrane.   Cells are joined
by desmosomal junctions (white arrows) and have lost much of their
native pigment.   Microvillous border is orientated towards neural
retina. x 5,000.   (Reduced 50% for reproduction.)

in the subretinal space and were frequently observed engulfing remnants of degenerate outer receptors (Fig. 12).

Defects in the internal limiting membrane were found both in the
vicinity of photocoagulation marks and overlying ischaemic and necrotic retina particularly where superficial retinal haemorrhage had
occurred. At such locations the migrating retinal pigment epithelial
cells gained the preretinal space.

d)   Membrane Formation

Intraretinal pigment epithelial membrane formation was occasionally observed in the vicinity of photocoagulation marks. The membranes were formed of pigment epithelial cells either loosely approximated or secured by well defined desmosomal junctions. The pigment epithelial cells had well defined basement membranes and melanin granules and maintained a uniform polarity with their apical
processes directed towards the retinal receptors (Fig. 13). Pigment epithelial membranes were also identified on the surface of the
retina where the internal limiting membrane was defective.

The reaction of the retinal pigment epithelium to stress and
disease has been well documented and responses such as proliferation,
migration and membrane formation have been noted in experimental
retinal detachment and laser photocoagulation burns.[10,11] A response of the retinal pigment epithelium to disease of the inner retina has also been noted in experimental vein occlusion although to
a much lesser degree than that observed in the above experiments.[4]
Why such profound structural alterations occur in the outer retina
secondary to inner retinal ischaemia is not clear, particularly in
the absence of any observable alterations to the choroidal circulation. It is possible that the accumulation of intraretinal and
subretinal fluid and blood following the acute venous occlusion
resulted in damage to the outer retinal receptors and provoked a
retinal pigment epithelial response. Alternatively, the liberation
of toxic degenerative products from the necrotic inner retina may
also have adversely affected the outer retina. Transynaptic degeneration of the neuro-retina may also have followed necrosis and
atrophy of the ganglion cell layer. Whatever the mechanism, it seems
clear that alterations to the inner retina, if severe enough, have
a significant influence on outer retina structure and barrier functions.

3.   BRANCH VEIN OCCLUSION - SUBRETINAL NEOVASCULARIZATION

A third alteration which took place at the level of the outer
retina in monkeys with ischaemic inner retina was the formation of

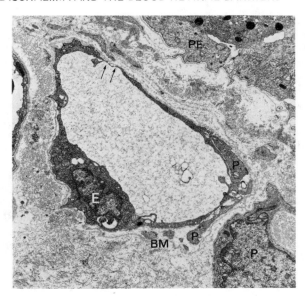

Fig. 14. Established subretinal neovascular capillary.   Fenestrae
are present in the endothelium (arrow) and both endothelial cells (E)
and pericyte processes (P) are surrounded by a fine basement membrane
(BM). A pericyte of adjacent capillary and pigment epithelial cells
(PE) are also present. x12,000. (Reduced 50% for reproduction.)

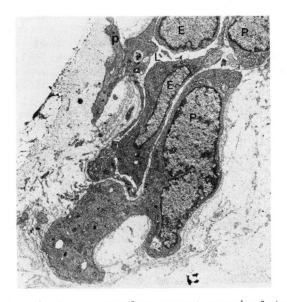

Fig. 15. New subretinal neovascular sprout proximal to growing tip.
The lumen (L) is narrow and convoluted, and the endothelial cells (E)
are ensheathed by pericyted (P) or their processes.   x 8,000.
(Reduced 50% for reproduction.)

subretinal fibrovascular membranes. The neovascular membranes were
identified in the region of photocoagulation scars and infiltrated
for varying distances beneath the ischaemic and necrotic retina.
In no instance did the neovascular fronds extend beneath normal retina. Most neovascular fronds remained in the neighbourhood of the
photocoagulation scars although some new vessels infiltrated the
retina for several disc diameters and developed well defined afferent
and efferent trunks. Fluorescein angiography revealed that the neovascular network were grossly incompetent although the major arterial
and venous radicals did not leak dye to any significant degree.

Histologically the new vessels were identified in the subretinal space and as far as we could detect did not infiltrate beneath
the retinal pigment epithelium. The overlying retinal receptors
were atrophic and the ischaemic inner retina was largely replaced
by glial cells. The retinal pigment epithelium in the vicinity of
the proliferating new vessels showed a wide range of changes including proliferation, atrophy and intraretinal membrane formation.

Ultrastructural examination showed that established neovascular
fronds were composed of capillaries having patent lumina, and perfused with a plasma-like substance containing red blood cells. The
capillaries had a well defined endothelial layer, certain cells of
which exhibited 50 to 60 nanometer fenestrae (Fig. 14). The endothelial cells also had a regular basement membrane and were surrounded by pericyte cells or their processes.

At the advancing front of the neovascular complexes numerous
capillary sprouts were present. The endothelial cells of these more
primitive vessels were bulky and characteristically demonstrated a
well developed rough endoplasmic reticulum (Fig. 15). These endothelial cells were only loosely approximated and frequently reduced
the lumen of the vessel to a mere slit-like cavity. The endothelial
cells were characteristically sheathed by numerous active pericytes
and their processes, and cell to cell contact was common.

The precise factors leading to the formation of subretinal neovascular fronds subsequent to branch retinal vein occlusion are not
clear; however, the important features in each instance were intense
photocoagulation marks, widespread inner retinal ischaemia and alterations at the level of the retinal pigment epithelium and retinal
receptors. The mechanism of new vessel growth appears to be one of
capillary budding with both endothelial and pericyte cells playing
an active role. As the new capillaries develop the endothelial
cells form junctional complexes, fenestrations appear in their cytoplasm and pericytes become much less obvious.

REFERENCES

1. Engerman, R.L., Pfaffenbach, D. and Davis, M.D. Laboratory Investigation 17:738, 1967.

2. Hamilton, A.M., Kohner, E.M., Rosen, D., Bird, A.C. and Dollery, C.T. Brit. J. Ophthal. 63:377, 1979.

3. Archer, D.B., Ernest, J.T. and Maguire, C.J.F. (1976). Proceedings of the Third William Mackenzie Symposium, J.S. Cant, Ed., Kimpton:London, P.P. 226-242, 1974.

4. Hockley, D.J., Tripathi, R.C. and Ashton, N. Brit. J. Ophthal. 63:393, 1979.

5. Rosen, D.A., Marshall, J., Kohner, E.M., Hamilton, A.M. and Dollery, C.T. Brit. J. Ophthal. 63:388, 1979.

6. Archer, D.B. Trans. Ophthal. Soc. U.K. 96:471, 1976.

7. Sengel, A. and Stoebner, P. J. Cell Biol. 44:223, 1970.

8. Weibel, E.R. and Palade, G.E. J. Cell Biol. 23:101, 1964.

9. Ernest, J.T. and Archer, D.B., Invest. Ophthal. and Vis. Sci. (in Press).

10. Machemer, R. and Laqua, H. Amer. J. Ophthal. 80:1, 1975.

11. Wallow, I.H.L. and Tso, M.O.M. Amer. J. Ophthal. 75:610, 1973.

ACKNOWLEDGEMENTS

We wish to thank the Royal National Institute for the Blind for their support and Miss R. Lynch for secretarial assistance.

EXPERIMENTAL RETINAL ANGIOGENESIS

Daniel Finkelstein, M.D. and Arnall Patz, M.D.

The Wilmer Institute, Johns Hopkins Hospital

Baltimore, Maryland 21205

The subject of angiogenesis, although not directly relevant to this symposium, does demonstrate a method of manipulation of retinal vessels that results in the loss of the blood-retinal barrier.

Experimental angiogenesis is of more than passing interest to the clinician. The clinically apparent neovascularization that occurs in the cornea, on the iris, from the retinal vessels, and from the choroidal vessels accounts for the greatest cause of severe ocular morbidity in the United States today and is a significant cause of visual loss in other countries.

It is appropriate to begin this presentation with a discussion of certain common clinical entities associated with retinal neovascularization, not only because of the clinical magnitude, but also because of what they teach us regarding mechanisms of retinal angiogenesis in general. These clinical subjects emphasize our immediate need to understand mechanisms of angiogenesis to establish research directions toward the eventual control of neovascularization.

Retinal neovascularization is defined as the growth of retinal vessels in a configuration different from that of normal retinal vessels, with that abnormal configuration lying in a plane anterior to that of the normal retinal vessels, often extending into the vitreous cavity. In addition to a loss of the blood-retinal barrier and the consequent leakage of fluorescein dye, these blood vessels frequently bleed into the vitreous cavity, obscuring vision. Additionally, a fibrous or glial tissue often grows with the vessels to a degree that traction and distortion of the retina may occur, producing irreparable retinal damage.

Retinal neovascularization may occur at the optic nerve head
or in the peripheral retina and is clinically documented by fundus
photography and fluorescein angiography.

The neovascularization of proliferative diabetic retinopathy
is always preceded by the appearance of capillary non-perfusion
and the presumably consequent retinal ischemia in those areas that
are non-perfused. It seems that the more capillary non-perfusion
is present, the greater is the likelihood for the development of
neovascularization. From this observation, the hypothesis has
developed that retinal ischemia leads to the production of a
biochemical substance, "angiogenesis factor", or "vasoproliferative
factor" that may diffuse away from the area of retinal ischemia
toward adjacent retinal vessels and initiate retinal neovascularization. This hypothesis has received circumstantial support in
the treatment of neovascularization by photocoagulation, a technique
of coagulating retinal tissue that is often followed by the regression of the retinal neovascularization. The photocoagulation
treatment is not directed toward the coagulation of the abnormal
retinal neovascularization itself, but is directed rather toward
the surrounding, presumably ischemic, retinal tissue. It is
presumed that photocoagulation destroys, or changes, ischemic retina
that may be producing a neovascular stimulating factor in such a
way that the production of the stimulating factor is reduced or
eliminated.

Although photocoagulation therapy in the management of
diabetic neovascularization has been demonstrated to be quite
efficacious in many stages of proliferative diabetic retinopathy,
it nevertheless does produce some loss of visual function and at
times may be associated with ocular complications. There is,
therefore, a continued need for the investigation of other
possible methods for controlling retinal angiogenesis. Additionally,
photocoagulation sometimes cannot be performed because of advanced
disease or media opacities.

There are several disease entities in addition to diabetic
retinopathy that support the "working hypothesis" that ischemic
retina produces an angiogenesis material. These other diseases
include retrolental fibroplasia and branch vein occlusion, both of
which have suggested, through their clinical appearance, other
features of the hypothesized angiogenesis mechanisms.

Retrolental fibroplasia may be produced experimentally by
placing certain newborn animals in high oxygen concentration at
birth so that their retinal vessels, which have not yet completely
grown to vascularize the retina in the far periphery, will become

irreversibly occluded. When the animal is then returned to room air, the neovascularization in the far periphery of retrolental fibroplasia is seen to develop, possibly from an angiogenesis material liberated by the peripheral ischemic tissue. As the initial oxygen exposure is increased, vascular closure occurs more posteriorly, with the resultant neovascularization similarly located more posteriorly. With prolonged exposure to oxygen, the capillary bed near the disc is also closed and disc neovascular- ization may result. These experimental models of retrolental fibroplasia that can be produced in the newborn kitten and puppy mimic the human disease quite closely and represent the best animal models to date for retinal neovascularization that resemble a human condition. The experimental model of retrolental fibroplasia has provided initial animal studies of angiogenesis, particularly in the demonstration of a vitreal protein whose concentration follows in direct proportion to retinal vessel growth. The animal model of retrolental fibroplasia may also provide a bioassay system for the testing of inhibitors of angiogenesis as they become available in the future.

It is this clinical background that has held the "working hypothesis" of an angiogenesis factor in some prominence over the past twenty-five years. And it is with this clinical background in mind that several laboratories have begun a biochemical and physiological search for possible retinal angiogenesis activity.

Retinal branch vein occlusion is a common retinal vascular disease which resembles a localized form of diabetic retinopathy in that similar vascular changes including non-perfusion occur in the segment of the retina that is affected by an occlusion of the vein in that segment. Again, the neovascularization that occurs appears to be related to the quantity of non-perfusion of the retina that exists. Additionally, it appears that the neovascularization can occur at a point distant from the non-perfused retina, such as from the optic nerve head or occasionally the surface of the iris, suggesting further that the proposed angiogenesis factor represents a diffusable substance. This concept is supported by the photo- coagulation therapy of neovascularization in branch vein occlusion in which it appears that photocoagulation of the involved retina can produce involution of the neovascularization that is at some distance from the photocoagulation itself.

It is this clinical background that has held the "working hypothesis" of an angiogenesis factor in some prominence over the past twenty-five years. And it is with this clinical background in mind that several laboratories have begun a biochemical and physiological search for possible retinal angiogenesis activity.

In our laboratories, this investigation began with a development of a consistantly produced animal model of retrolental fibroplasia in newborn puppies and newborn kittens. This animal model has provided a bioassay system to investigate certain mechanisms that may be related to angiogenesis. For example, we have performed vitrectomies on a number of newborn puppies with experimental retrolental fibroplasia to determine whether vitrectomy seems to have the same beneficial effect in producing regression of neovascularization as vitrectomy does in proliferative diabetic retinopathy. We have not been able to demonstrate this beneficial effect in experimental retrolental fibroplasia, but the technical difficulties in performing a vitrectomy on a newborn puppy eye may have prevented as adequate a vitrectomy as needed.

In beginning to look for an angiogenesis material as a pilot series of experiments, vitreous was removed from animals with experimental retrolental fibroplasia, the vitreous was concentrated, and the concentrate injected into the vitreous cavity of littermates who did not have experimental retrolental fibroplasia. The experiment was performed to determine whether a transferrable and diffusible factor produced by ischemic retina in RLF might be present in the vitreous and demonstrable in this sort of a bioassay testing procedure. No induction of angiogenesis was seen in the retina of the littermates that were injected. The experimental method suffers from the ability to present a possibly significant quantity of the proposed angiogenesis material, as well as other technical difficulties.

Biochemical studies of the vitreous of newborn animals and those with experimental retrolental fibroplasia demonstrated, however, a vitreous protein whose concentration was proportional to the growth of retinal vessels, suggesting that this protein could be related in etiologic fashion to angiogenesis.

In the early 1970's, we became aware, through the publications of Folkman and colleagues, of tumor angiogenesis factor, a substance produced by solid tumors that could induce neovascularization at a distance from the tumor itself. Folkman and colleagues had demonstrated that an avascular tumor nodule placed in a corneal pocket may induce limbal neovascularization toward the tumor nodule some millimeters away presumably through diffusion of an angiogenesis material. Interestingly, through a similar bioassay technique, they were able to demonstrate an inhibition of this tumor angiogenesis mechanism by a substance extractable from neonatal cartilage.

We became interested in tumor angiogenesis factor because of the possibility that its action on retinal vessels might provide some clues regarding mechanisms of retinal angiogenesis in general. We initiated a series of experiments in collaboration with Dr. Folkman and his colleagues (Steven Brem, Henry Brem, and Robert Langer) to determine whether tumor angiogenesis factor might produce retinal vessel neovascularization. These studies were undertaken not because we felt that tumor angiogenesis factor might be the active substance in proliferative retinopathy, but rather to begin to learn something of mechanisms of retinal neovascularization in general.

In order to test the effect of tumor angiogenesis factor on retinal vessels, we used a model system with the rabbit as the experimental animal. Although the rabbit retinal vessels may have distinct differences from those of man, the rabbit was chosen because of the availability of a homologous, transplantable rabbit tumor, the V_2 carcinoma. The rabbit V_2 carcinoma was used as a continuous source of tumor angiogenesis factor, with nodules of rabbit V_2 carcinoma injected into the vitreous cavity of the rabbit. Following the injection of this tumor suspension, isolated nodules of tumor could be seen to grow slowly in the vitreous as avascular spheroids and stalks, slowly growing over a period of many weeks toward vascularized retina. We had hoped to see the rabbit retinal vessels begin to undergo neovascularization as a response to the tumor angiogenesis factor presumably being elaborated by the tumor nodules, with this retinal neovascularization growing up anterior to the plane of the retina into the vitreous cavity toward the growing nodules of tumor. In this way, we would be able to demonstrate that retinal vessels were able to undergo neovascularization in response to a diffusible angiogenesis material. Unfortunately, this type of retinal growth did not occur, but retinal neovascularization only occurred after the tumor infiltrated the vascularized retina proper. Other bioassay systems that monitor TAF action, such as the corneal model, were able to show the action of tumor angiogenesis factor at a distance; therefore, we concluded that a possibility might be that vitreous could interfere with the angiogenic mechanism in our test system, just as it is known that cartilage contains an inhibitory substance. It was for this reason that we performed the intravitreal tumor implantation again in the rabbit, this time following vitrectomy. Unfortunately, following vitrectomy, the tumor grows quite rapidly to infiltrate the vascularized retina with too short a period of observation prior to the infiltration to observe the possible angiogenic effect.

The experiments were performed again using irradiated rabbit V_2 carcinoma, a preparation of tumor that is known to produce tumor angiogenesis factor while the tumor cells themselves are not capable of tissue invasion. This bioassay system also did not produce retinal neovascularization.

At the suggestion of Dr. Paul Henkind, we produced a branch vein occlusion in several rabbits prior to tumor placement in the vitreous, following his concept that an angiogenesis factor may only be active upon retinal vessels that are previously damaged. Again, we saw the tumor invade retina before we could observe any retinal neovascularization occurring from the damaged retinal vessels.

In the mid 1970's, tumor extracts containing partially purified tumor angiogenesis factor became available to us through the courtesy of Dr. Folkman and his colleagues. Because there were indications that this tumor angiogenesis factor may not be strongly antigenic, we examined the effect of tumor angiogenesis factor on retinal vessels in the rhesus monkey. The tumor angiogenesis factor was placed in a slow release polymer of ethylene vinyl acetate. In this way, we were able to present 300 ug of partially purified tumor angiogenesis factor in a slow release polymer pellet with the knowledge that it would be released slowly over a three-week period after the pellet was placed in the vitreous cavity of the rhesus monkey. We placed these polymer pellets containing tumor angiogenesis factor through a pars plana incision directly onto the surface of the monkey optic nerve head. The surgical technique was not difficult and induced little trauma. Control experiments with empty polymer pellets on the optic nerve head demonstrated that no neovascularization was induced nor was any clinically apparent inflammatory response evident.

The advantage of using such a TAF containing polymer pellet in the monkey was multifold. First, the problem of tumor infiltration was circumvented. Additionally, the pellet provided a direct contact with the retinal vessels with an opportunity of breaking the overlying internal limiting membrane in the process of placing the pellet on the surface of the optic nerve head. Importantly, we were able to explore a retinal vascular system more like that of the human's.

We found that the pellets placed on the surface of the rhesus nerve head remained in good contact and, over a period of several months, disc neovascularization resulted as evidenced by vessels growing over the surface of the pellet from the optic nerve head. Fluorescein angiography demonstrated this disc neovascularization and demonstrated the loss of the blood-retinal barrier as late fluorescence typical of human retinal neovascularization.

We did recognize, however, that tumor angiogenesis factor represented a heterologous protein for the rhesus monkey so that further controls were performed with the slow release polymer pellets in the rhesus monkey containing rabbit serum. We did not expect to see disc neovascularization from the resulting antigenic inflammation because retinal neovascularization is seen extremely rarely, if at all, in human situations associated with retinal inflammation. Nevertheless, when we performed these control experiments we were surprised to find that disc neovascularization did occur. Consequently, we cannot determine from the TAF experiment in the monkey what portion of the resulting disc neovascularization may have been secondary to inflammation and what portion may have been secondary to the tumor angiogenesis factor itself.

Recently, Glaser and co-workers in our laboratories have identified a substance from retina that stimulates endothelial cells in tissue culture and stimulates neovascularization in the chick chorioallantoic membrane. Studies are in progress to purify and characterize this substance with further documentation of its possible physiologic role in retinal neovascularization.

For the future bioassay of possible angiogenesis substances, we await the ideal experimental model that will not be subject to the problems of inflammation. For example, the ideal situation might be the experimental production of retinal neovascularization in one eye of a rhesus monkey with the extraction of possible angiogenesis materials from the retina and vitreous of that monkey and the transferal of that substance to the vitreous and retina of that monkey's other eye, to avoid problems of antigenic inflammation.

The response of the retinal vessels of the rabbit to rabbit intravitreal tumor implantation suggested that adult vitreous might be acting as an inhibitor to that angiogenesis model. For that reason, vitreous extracts were bioassayed for possible inhibitory activity through the corneal bioassay technique that had been popularized by Folkman. According to this methodology, a corneal pocket was produced in the rabbit followed by the placement of lyophilized vitreous closest in the pocket to the limbus with placement of the source of tumor angiogenesis factor just central in the corneal pocket to the proposed vitreous inhibitor. When compared to control experiments, it was clear that vitreous was acting as an inhibitor of TAF induced vascularization, similar to the effect shown by extracts of neonatal cartilage.

These basic laboratory investigations of angiogenesis and its inhibition represent a new line of investigation regarding the clinical problem of retinal angiogenesis. Although the presence of a retinal angiogenesis material must remain hypothetical, there is an accumulating weight of circumstantial evidence from clinical and basic observations that encourages us to pursue this subject further.

DISEASES AFFECTING THE INNER BLOOD-RETINAL BARRIER

Morton F. Goldberg, M.D.

University of Illinois
Eye and Ear Infirmary
1855 West Taylor Street, Chicago, Illinois 60612

The inner blood-retinal barrier (I-BRB) is affected by a surprising array of ocular diseases, often with deterioration of vision. These retinal vasculopathies can be classified[1,2] within the following eight categories: stretching of the vascular wall; hypoxia; metabolic (chemical, physiologic, and pharmacologic) alterations; inflammatory processes; tapetoretinal dystrophies and retinoschisis; trauma; developmental vascular anomalies; and preretinal neovascularization. This report will provide clinical examples of diseases within each of these major pathogeneses. Frequently, the categories overlap, and may have an additive effect on disturbances of permeability. Thus, disruption of the I-BRB is often multifactorial, and a single disease affecting the retinal vasculature may be classified under more than one category. Diabetic retinopathy, for example, is such a disease, and, because of its complexity and prevalence, is discussed separately.

Methods of examination include ophthalmoscopy, fluorescein angiography, fluorophotometry, and histology. Simple ophthalmoscopy is often sufficient to detect breakdown of the I-BRB. When severe, loss of vascular competence in the retina is manifested by hemorrhages, perivascular sheathing, and dense collections of exudates and edema fluid. When moderate, vascular incompetence may require fluorescein angiography for the detection of staining, leaking, and pooling of dye. When mild, breakdown of the I-BRB may be detectable only by vitreous fluorophotometry[1] or by microscopic tracer techniques, such as electron microscopic visualization of horseradish peroxidase or other markers.

I.   STRETCHING

Extension, without rupture, of the retinal vascular endothelium can be sufficient to render the I-BRB incompetent. If the process involves a large number of vascular tributaries, considerable retinal dysfunction can occur, with edema, hemorrhage, and even neovascularization. If the process is localized to one or only a few vascular segments, visual disability is unlikely to occur, unless the macular region is involved by edema, exudates, or hemorrhage, or by associated ischemia or tractional distortion.

Stretching of the endothelial membrane occurs in two major forms: traction from without and distention from within. Examples of the former include premacular fibrosis and vitreous tug syndromes. Examples of the latter include retinal macroaneurysms, both central and branch vein occlusion, and hypertensive retinopathy.

A.   Traction from Without

Premacular fibrosis. Also known as cellophane maculopathy, surface wrinkling retinopathy, epiretinal membrane formation, or contraction of the internal limiting membrane, premacular fibrosis is usually acquired in older life and is usually idiopathic. Similar processes occur in the form of congenital preretinal fibrosis, macular pucker associated with retinal detachment, subretinal fibrosis, and reaction to photocoagulation, trauma, inflammation, or retinal vein obstruction.[3] Ophthalmoscopically, one observes a glistening, watered silk fundus reflex, often with minimal but definite tortuosity of the surrounding vessels. The vessels may also be abnormally straightened (Fig. 1). The macula is the most common area of the posterior pole to be affected. As contracture of the preretinal tissue proceeds, traction lines may become more obvious. Connections between the contracting tissue and the vitreous are almost never observed. Ultrastructural studies[4] have shown retinal glial cells migrating onto the anterior surface of the retina through breaks in the internal limiting lamina.

Over a prolonged period of time, intraretinal edema and, occasionally, even small hemorrhages and microaneurysms appear, because of localized traction on small retinal vessels. The leakage responsible for macular edema may not be seen angiographically, presumably because the rate and amount of leakage are below the resolving capacity of the angiographic system. On other occasions, however, retinal capillary leakage is easily documented angiographically (Fig. 1).

There is no known effective treatment, but, possibly for those cases characterized by a marked reduction of central acuity, surgical stripping of some membranes might be considered. Interestingly,

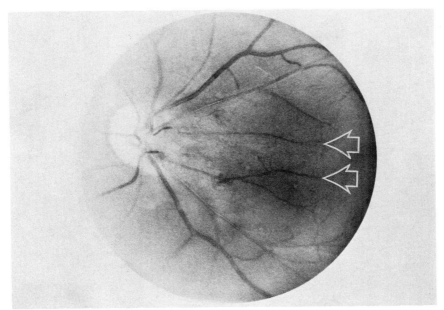

Fig. 1A. Premacular fibrosis of left eye (red-free view in 1974). Note straightening and temporal dragging of papillomacular vessels (arrows).

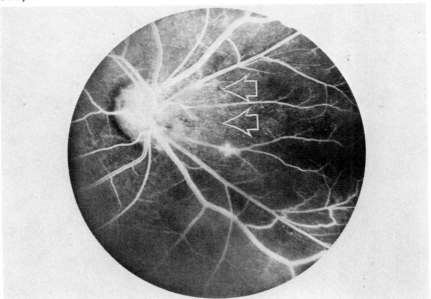

Fig. 1B. Venous phase of angiogram in 1974 shows minimal leakage from papillomacular vessels (arrows; cf Fig. 1D).

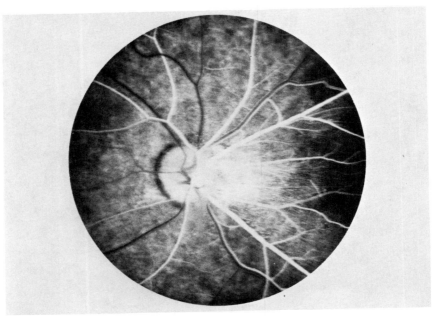

Fig. 1C. Premacular fibrosis in 1979.   Leakage is noted in early
venous phase of angiogram.

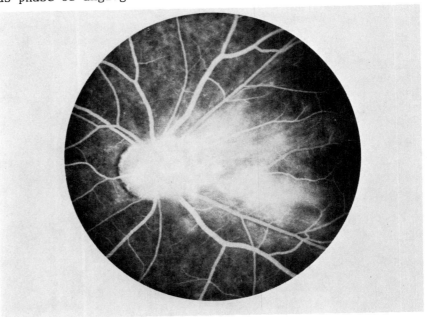

Fig. 1D. Late venous phase of angiogram in 1979 shows marked leakage
(cf Fig. 1B).

spontaneous peeling of such membranes has been observed, especially after peripheral fundus photocoagulation.[5]

Vitreous tug syndromes. Localized tugging of vitreous on the macula has been implicated "in a small percentage of eyes"[6,7] having cystoid macular edema (CME) after cataract extraction. It should be emphasized that most eyes with CME do not have actual adherence of the vitreous to the macula. Yet, there exists, nonetheless, a specific syndrome of localized vitreomacular tugging, occurring in otherwise normal-appearing eyes (either with or without surgical aphakia). The syndrome is characterized by focal, minimal leakage of fluorescein and moderate to severe, although sometimes transient, reduction of visual acuity (Fig. 2). In such cases, careful biomicroscopy, with fine resolution and high magnification, is necessary to detect the vitreomacular adhesion and traction. Pigment epithelial leakage is the major source for macular edema, but retinal capillaries may leak as well.

B. Distention from Within
    Retinal macroaneurysms. These localized vascular outpouchings of arteriolar walls should be distinguished from two other aneurysmal disorders of the retinal vasculature; namely, capillary microaneurysms (seen in a large variety of diseases, including diabetic background retinopathy) and large aneurysms of venous radicles (observed following occlusion of retinal veins).

Macroaneurysms generally affect the main retinal arterioles within the first three orders of bifurcation. Patients are usually elderly with systemic hypertension and generalized arteriosclerotic vascular disease. Similar aneurysms may simultaneously affect the cerebral circulation. Macroaneurysms occur without pathologic sequelae or, if stretching of the endothelium is severe enough, may actually cause rupture and hemorrhage into the vitreous, retina, or subretinal space[8] (Fig. 3A and B). In less severely affected aneurysms, fluorescein angiography shows staining of the aneurysmal wall, often with late leakage of dye into the retina. The centrifugal flow of plasmoid fluid away from the macroaneurysm frequently results in heavy deposits of circularly arranged, hard, lipid-like exudates (Fig. 3C and D), which may involve the macula through contiguous spread, or which may be so extensive that they suggest an adult Coats-like syndrome. The center of the macula may also become involved by an area of perifoveal capillary leakage that is geographically separate from the macroaneurysm. This intramacular leakage may directly contribute to accumulation of macular lipid or edema.[8]

The phenomenon of an extramacular vascular anomaly giving rise to deposition of intramacular lipid is more well known and occurs with, for example, Coats' disease and von Hippel-Lindau disease. An occult migration of lipid-containing plasma from the peripheral vascular le-

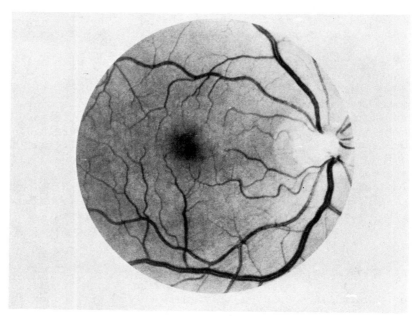

Fig. 2A. Vitreous tug syndrome (red-free view; no definite ophthalmoscopic abnormalities are seen); (cf Figs. 2B and 2C).

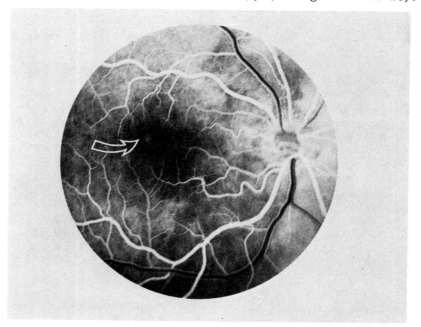

Fig. 2B. Early venous phase of angiogram shows small area of leakage at site of vitreo-macular adherence (arrow).

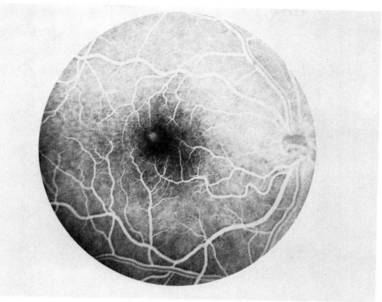

Fig. 2C. Later venous phase of angiogram shows slight increase in hyperfluorescence. The pigment epithelium appears to be a major source for the leakage. Capillaries may also contribute.

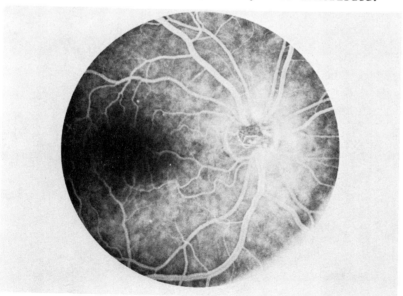

Fig. 2D. Late venous phase of angiogram (obtained 8 weeks after Fig. 2A–C) shows no leakage following spontaneous detachment of posterior hyaloid from macula.

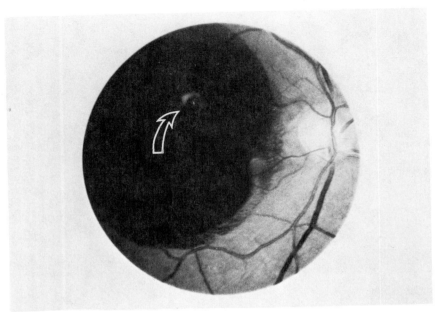

Fig. 3A. Arteriolar macroaneurysm (arrow) with surrounding hematoma (red-free view).

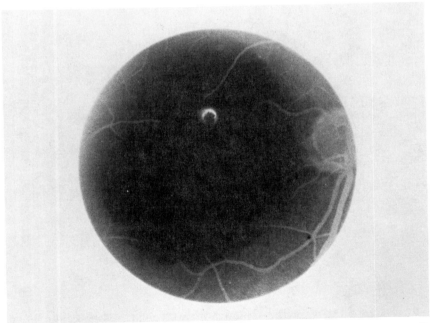

Fig. 3B. Venous phase of angiogram shows staining of aneurysmal wall and slight peri-aneurysmal leakage.

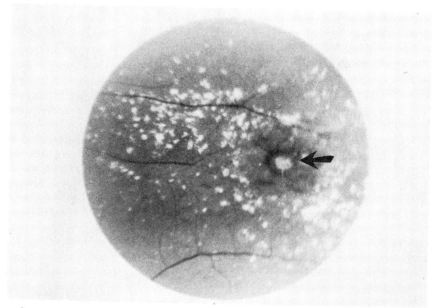

Fig. 3C. Arteriolar macroaneurysm (arrow) with surrounding hard exudates (red-free view).

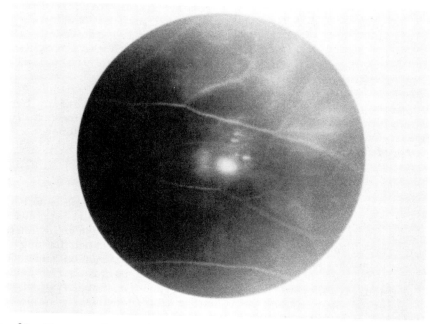

Fig. 3D. Venous phase of angiogram shows staining of macroaneurysm and leakage into surrounding retina.

sion into the macula has often been invoked to explain the preferential involvement of the macula in these disorders. Because intramacular capillary abnormalities have been observed not only in association with macroaneurysms but also in von Hippel-Lindau disease,[9] it is reasonable to suggest that the macular lipid so often observed in association with peripheral vascular anomalies may, in at least some cases and at least partially, originate from local, intramacular capillary lesions. Why these capillaries leak is presently unknown.

Therapeutic obliteration of macroaneurysms is uncommonly required, because macular lipid accumulation may not occur, because gross disruption of the I-BRB in the form of hemorrhage is relatively uncommon, and because thromboses and involution may ensue spontaneously. Therapy by photocoagulation should probably be instituted when exudates involve or when hemorrhage threatens the visual axis.

Retinal vein occlusion. Branch retinal vein occlusion (BRVO), a common disabling human disorder, has been widely studied in both clinical[10-13] and experimental[14-16] settings.

The pathogenesis of BRVO varies, but many patients have evidence of arteriosclerosis and systemic hypertension.[13] The importance of retinal arteriovenous crossings cannot be overemphasized, and the great number of these anatomic configurations in the superotemporal quadrant probably explains the disproportionately high incidence of BRVOs occurring in this location. The proximity of BRVOs to the macula accounts for frequent damage to this vital structure, through mechanisms of edema, hemorrhage, ischemia, or traction. It is noteworthy that almost 50% of patients with BRVOs have final visual acuity of 20/50 or less.[13]

Fluorescein angiography is invaluable in understanding the course of clinical events in BRVO (Fig. 4A and B). Diffuse intraretinal leakage of dye is the hallmark of this disorder. Evidence of capillary nonperfusion is also commonly present and may foretell the development of preretinal neovascularization, with even a worse breakdown of the I-BRB.

Archer et al[11] classified human cases of different severity into four categories: (1) those having unimpaired arterial perfusion with competence of the microvasculature's BRB; (2) those having unimpaired arterial perfusion but breakdown of the BRB; (3) those having either focal or extensive areas of impaired arterial perfusion and, also, incompetence of the BRB; and (4) those having particularly severe arterial insufficiency with areas of surrounding breakdown of the BRB. Retention of recovery of visual acuity depends, in less severely affected groups, on either absence of or recovery from the macular edema that is a direct consequence of an incompetent I-BRB. Mechanisms of repair of the I-BRB are very poorly understood. In the more

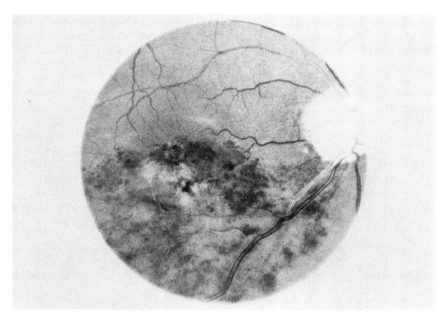

Fig. 4A. Branch retinal vein occlusion with innumerable hemorrhages (red-free view).

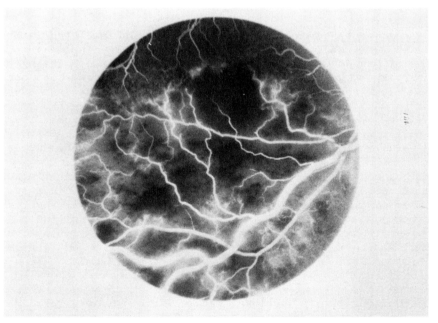

Fig. 4B. Early venous phase of angiogram shows fluorescein emanating from venous radicles.

severely affected groups, loss of vision is related to ischemia of
the macula or induced neovascularization, with its complications of
vitreous hemmorrhage, retinal traction, or retinal detachment.

In addition to demonstrating capillary leakage and nonperfusion,
fluorescein angiography may highlight the precise point of venous obstruction as a localized area of hyperfluorescence associated with
focal breakdown of the I-BRB.[13,17] Low-velocity collaterals and microaneurysms often develop, and these, as well as venous segments
traversing ischemic retinal zones, may show fluorescent staining of
their walls and minimal to moderate perivascular leakage. Transudation, if pronounced, causes CME, and may, if particularly severe,
cause serous detachment of the macula.[13] Circinate retinopathy may
also occur, possibly because of chronicity of the leakage or possibly
because of a difference in the size of leaking sites.

Elimination of both macular edema and preretinal neovascularization constitutes the major therapeutic goal. Evidence for the effi-
cacy of photocoagulation in eliminating neovascularization is widespread, although the mechanism of this treatment is poorly understood.
As yet, no definitive evidence exists that photocoagulation or any
other therapeutic modality can predictably eliminate macular edema
and preserve or improve visual acuity. To this end, a collaborative,
prospective, randomized photocoagulation trial is currently underway
in the United States.

The acute features of human BRVO have been simulated in monkeys
by experimental occlusion of one or more retinal veins.[14,15] Within
minutes of venous occlusion, venous dilation, delayed filling of the
adjacent artery, and delayed emptying of the occluded vein occurred.
The dependent venous and capillary radicles showed an increase in permeability and leakage of dye that took place primarily from the venu-
lar ends of the capillaries. During the subsequent weeks, there were
secondary arterial and venous changes, including leakage of dye from
those veins and arteries crossing hypoxic zones of ischemic retina.[14]

Light and electron microscopic studies of these experimentally
occluded vessels indicated that the rapid, almost immediate onset of
increased capillary permeability was purely functional, and that no
structural damage to the capillary wall could be identified. Although
morphologic sites of leakage or rupture could not be identified anato-
mically, some erythrocytes were seen lodged between the capillary endothelium and its basement membrane. Other extraluminal blood cells
were found adjacent to apparently normal capillaries. Hockley et al
speculated that initial leakage probably occurred through temporarily
disrupted endothelial junctions (intercellularly) or through rapidly
repaired areas of focal capillary "rhexis."[15] They also postulated
increased activity of endothelial pinocytotic vesicles.

An alternative or additional, and possibly more attractive, speculation for the leakage would involve transcytoplasmic intracellular passage of red blood cells and presumably plasma as well, because junctional complexes between retinal endothelial cells seem remarkably resistant to disruption. Ample studies of endothelia from a wide variety of vascular and lymphatic tissues have shown that direct transcytoplasmic endothelial passage of both white and red blood cells can occur without actual rupture (rhexis) and without leaving any ultrastructural evidence of membrane bound vacuoles or of damage to the endothelial cells whose cytoplasm has been traversed.[18]

In the monkey studies cited, endothelial damage was documented microscopically only after about six hours. Eventually, if the process progressed, there was complete loss of capillary endothelial cells and pericytes. Glial cells, growing into acellular capillary tubes, effected permanent capillary closure in the most severe instances.[15]

One is forced to conclude from the available evidence that the precise mechanism underlying early incompetence of the I–BRB in BRVO is still unknown. Nonetheless, it is clear that outflow obstruction causes a rise in intraluminal pressure, which, in turn, produces retinal edema and even hemorrhage. Stagnant flow then causes hypoxia and overt damage to endothelial cells, leading to additional loss of both formed and unformed elements of the blood.[16] As intraluminal viscosity rises, flow is reduced further, until complete shutdown occurs with necrosis of the entire capillary wall. This course of events has been called a "progressive ischemic capillaropathy."[16]

Central retinal vein occlusions. Considerable controversy attends the pathogenesis of central retinal vein occlusion (CRVO)[16,19–21] (Fig. 5A and B) and the putative role of arterial ischemia in the production of typical fundus lesions. This forum will be used not to settle this controversy but to illustrate an aneurysmal variant that we have observed in long-standing cases of CRVO as well as BRVO (Fig. 6). In distinction to macroaneurysms of the retinal arteries and classic microaneurysms of the retinal capillaries, these large postocclusive aneurysms are found at or near the end of small venous radicles. They appear to be the result of increased hydrostatic pressure within the lumina of small venous vessels.

To choose an appropriate name for these lesions is difficult in view of existing terminology, but they are conveniently called large microaneurysms or macro-microaneurysms. Fluorescein angiography reveals these lesions to be considerably larger than microaneurysms and approximately the same size or slightly smaller than macroaneurysms. They are associated with considerable breakdown of the I–BRB and thus may cause extensive circinate retinopathy. In this respect, they resemble the classic forms of both arteriolar macro-

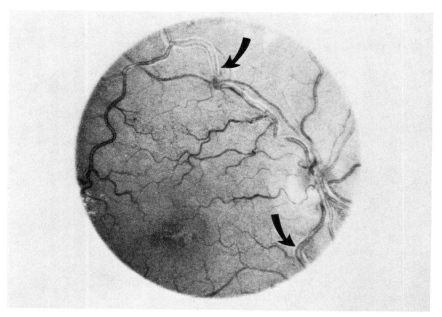

Fig. 5A. Central retinal vein occlusion long after resolution of hemorrhagic stage (red-free view). Note sheathed, dilated and tortuous veins (arrows; cf Fig. 5B).

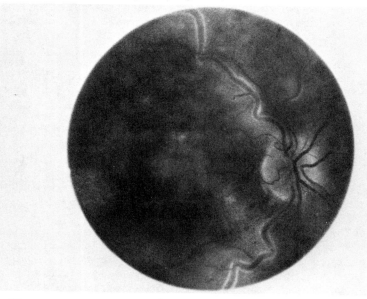

Fig. 5B. Late venous phase of angiogram shows staining of and perivascular leakage from retinal veins (cf Fig. 5A). Diffuse, irregular staining of macula is also present.

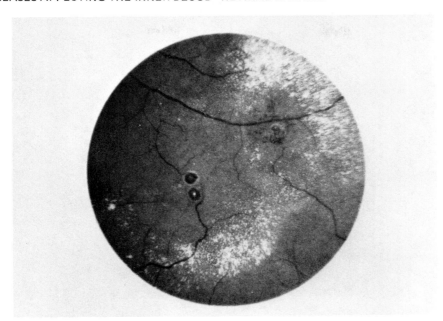

Fig. 6A. Post-occlusive venous macro-microaneurysms (red-free view). Note circinate retinopathy (courtesy of Lee Jampol, M.D.).

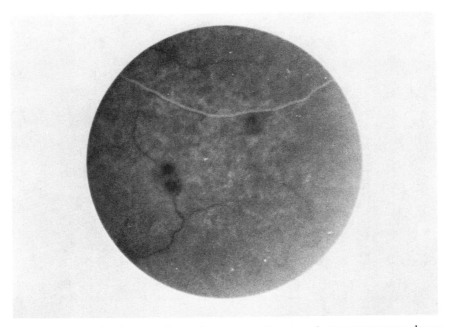

Fig. 6B. Arterial phase of angiogram.   Macro-microaneurysms have not yet filled.

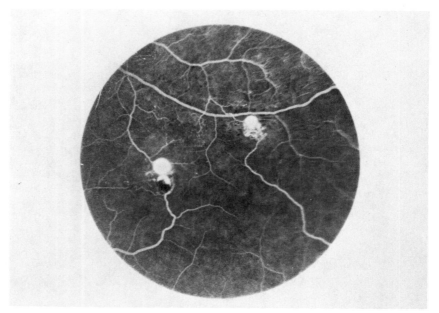

Fig. 6C. Mid-venous phase of angiogram shows early filling of macro-microaneurysms.

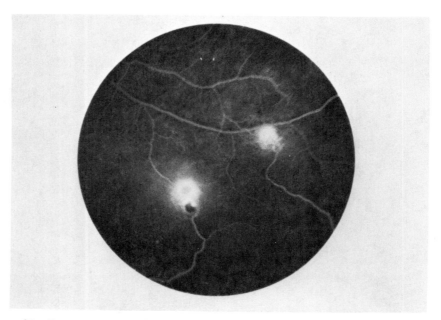

Fig. 6D. Late venous phase of angiogram shows peri-aneurysmal staining.

aneurysms and capillary microaneurysms. Obliteration of these leaking aneurysms can be effected by photocoagulation if the macula is threatened by edema or the encroachment of hard exudates.

Hypertensive retinopathy. This disorder has considerable importance, because breakdown of the I-BRB and ultimate closure of retinal arterioles have prognostic implications for the life of the patient.[22] Forty years ago, Keith, Wagener, and Barker pointed out that 90% of patients with malignant hypertension would be dead within one year of diagnosis, if therapy were not instituted. Because retinopathy is often an early sign of an impending malignant phase of the hypertension,[23,24] an understanding of its pathogenesis is clearly desirable.

This problem has been studied experimentally in the monkey, using the Goldblatt model of renal hypertension.[24] The earliest and most characteristic abnormality was the presence of profusely leaking punctate spots on arteries and terminal arterioles, both on the disc and elsewhere in the retina (Fig. 7A). Arteriolar and capillary closure as well as leakage occurred in areas of cotton wool spots. These findings have also been observed in hypertensive humans. Diffuse leakiness (Fig. 7B) may also occur. Insudation of lipohyaline material was microscopically detected in the walls of precapillary arterioles. This abnormal material resulted in displacement or replacement of the smooth muscle cells. Except for the appearance of occasional arterioles with extensive necrosis, where breaks within endothelial cell' cytoplasm were found, there was no obvious explanation for the pathogenesis of the plasma insudation.

As in the analogous experimental studies of BRVO (see above), the precise mechanism for passage of plasma and blood cells across the vascular endothelium (in this case, that of the arteriole) remains unexplained. As in experimentally produced BRVO, disruptions of the (arteriolar) intercellular junctions were rare, as were breaks in the nonjunctional endothelial cytoplasm. Thus, an explanation for many of the arteriolar leaking spots observed with fluorescein angiography is missing, and there currently is insufficient evidence to choose among the possibilities of increased pinocytosis, disrupted intercellular junctions (although they appeared remarkably normal), intimal degeneration or necrosis, and so on. In the case of capillaries, extremely focal necrosis and degeneration involving single endothelial cells were occasionally observed in the presence of an otherwise intact vascular lining.

Garner et al proposed a sequence of events beginning with arteriolar constriction, which is thought to be an autoregulatory compensation for increased intraluminal pressure.[24] This constriction may result in occlusion of precapillary arterioles and necrosis of vascular smooth muscle. The endothelium appears normal at this stage.

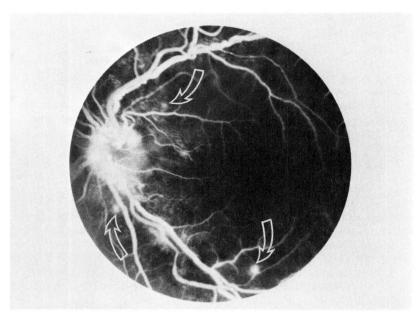

Fig. 7A. Systemic hypertension. Note punctate hyperfluorescence
(arrows); (courtesy of Lee Jampol, M.D.).

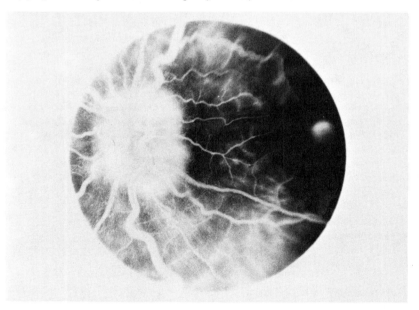

Fig. 7B. Systemic hypertension. Note diffuse leakage from disc and
smaller retinal vessels. Serous detachment of macula is also
present.

Secondly, dilation of constricted arterioles is thought to ensue, because of weakening of the arteriolar wall, with insudation of plasma through defective (? stretched) endothelium into the unsupported arteriolar wall. This stage is characterized by the leaking points observed on fluorescein angiography. Finally, progressive plasma insudation and additional muscle necrosis are thought to eventuate in further vascular occlusion and the typical picture of fibrinoid necrosis, with mural infiltration of plasma and fibrin. The ischemic and, thus, hypoxic events that develop appear to have a profound additive effect on the ongoing breakdown of the I-BRB.

C. Distention in the Absence of I-BRB Incompetence

Simple distention of the vascular lumen does not invariably lead to breakdown of the I-BRB. Some arteriolar macroaneurysms do not leak, for example. Cavernous hemangioma[25] and arteriovenous communications (cirsoid or racemose aneurysm) of the retina[2] are two other examples. It would presumably aid the understanding of the diseases characterized by disturbed permeability if one could explain why the I-BRB remains intact (or regains its competence) in these and some other retinal vasculopathies. Rapidity of distention and level of intraluminal pressure are presumably important factors.

II. HYPOXIA

A. Decreased Oxygenation

Reduction of oxygen content within retinal vessels can, if it is sufficiently severe, produce incompetence of the I-BRB. Retinal hemorrhages in severely anemic patients, in carbon monoxide poisoning, and in healthy mountain climbers at high altitudes are attributed to this pathogenesis. Reduction of oxygen content may be even more profound focally, and localized zones of retinal hypoxia may contribute substantially to breakdown of the I-BRB in segments of vessels found in proximity to such hypoxic areas. In BRVO, and in diabetic retinopathy, for example, it has been noted that both arteries and veins may show staining of only those segments that traverse localized hypoxic zones of retina. When the zones of hypoxia are broader, either in BRVO or in CRVO, incompetence of the I-BRB may be so extensive that massive erythrocytic extravasation occurs, resulting in a "blood and thunder" ophthalmoscopic appearance.[26]

B. Emboli

Embolic events involving the retinal vasculature may irreversibly reduce retinal function because of ischemic infarction. During the evolution of retinal branch arteriole occlusion, for example, an interesting pattern of hyperfluorescent beads may be seen along or at the ends of embolized arteriolar branches (Fig. 8).[27,28] This pat-

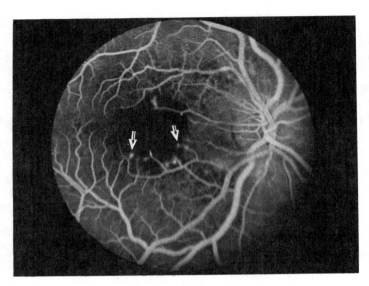

Fig. 8A. Embolic maculopathy in sickle cell anemia. Hyperfluorescent
"beads" are seen at ends of occluded arterioles (arrows). Reprinted
from Ref. 27.

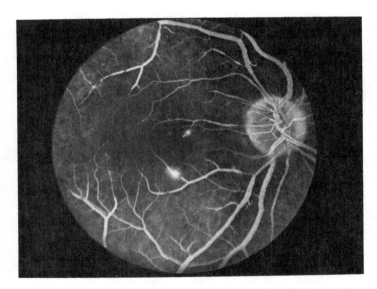

Fig. 8B. Two weeks after Fig. 8A was obtained, 2 hyperfluorescent
areas appear on small arterioles where earlier angiogram showed
filling defects (cf Fig. 8A). Distal arteriolar segments do not leak.

tern may take two forms. In the first,[28] there is simply a pooling of dye in a plasma lake between two stationary columns of blood. The arterial wall in this location is slightly stained, indicating some decompensation of the I-BRB. In the second,[27] there is more intense focal staining of the arteriolar wall with some perivascular leakage of dye occurring either at the site of total obstruction or at the site of a previously occluded arteriole whose embolus has fragmented and moved downstream (Fig. 8B). In both situations, damage to the vascular endothelium at the site of embolization has occurred, presumably from local hypoxia, but possibly from other mechanisms as well. The latter form of hyperfluorescence has been observed clinically in sickle cell anemia and in intravenous drug abusers[29] as well as experimentally in pigs whose eyes have been subjected to microsphere embolization.[30] Electron microscopy of these embolized pig retinas failed to show specific, early defects in the endothelium, other than ill-defined shrinkage, condensation, and degeneration of endothelial cells.

It is of great interest that long distal segments of formerly obstructed retinal arterioles characteristically do not show fluorescein leakage once flow returns (Fig. 8B),[27,30] perhaps because intraluminal pressure is insufficient to overcome even a defective I-BRB;[26] because the endothelial barrier recovers fully; or because the endothelium is relatively resistant to hypoxia, except where locally damaged by an embolus or thrombus. Conversely, only minimal or moderate hypoxia can result in marked fluorescein leakage across a relatively long segment of defective vascular endothelium, if an increase in intraluminal pressure is also present. Thus, these two pathogenic events—hypoxia and stretching (see above)—appear to have additive, deleterious effects on the I-BRB, which generally appear greater than those due to either process alone. Hypoxia also seems to exacerbate the effects of a variety of chemical mediators, which ordinarily have only a minimal decompensatory influence on the I-BRB.[1,31]

Breakdown of the I-BRB under hypoxic circumstances is generally reversible, once the underlying cause is eliminated, but vision may not return if ischemic infarction of the macula has occurred.

III. METABOLIC (CHEMICAL, PHYSIOLOGIC, AND PHARMACOLOGIC) ALTERATIONS

It should be obvious that many clinical disorders of the retinal vasculature (and their appropriate therapies) are modulated by the physicochemical and physiological properties of the endothelial barrier. Nonetheless, profound ignorance pervades our understanding of both normal and abnormal mediators of the I-BRB function. Fundamental understanding of carrier-mediated transport along the retinal vascular endothelium, for example, is severely limited.

Studies to date have shown that the I-BRB is remarkably resistant to disruption, even by such strong chemical mediators as histamine,[31] serotonin, and selected prostaglandins.[1,2] Interestingly,
if the I-BRB is subjected to prostaglandins plus simultaneous ischemia[1] or to large, nonphysiologic doses of prostaglandins,[32] massive breakdown of the barrier function can be easily achieved.
Marked leakage of fluorescein, retinal hemorrhage, and even exudative retinal detachment have occurred in rabbit eyes subjected to
intravitreal injections of a large variety of prostaglandins. Limited ultrastructural studies[32] have shown absence of endothelial
cells in some areas, cytoplasmic degeneration of residual cells,
and apparent loss of continuity of intercellular junctions. These
effects may be entirely nonspecific, in view of the heavy dosages
employed.

A pharmacotoxic effect on the macular vasculature has been
demonstrated for topically applied epinephrine, which, on occasion,
can cause visually symptomatic CME in aphakic eyes.[33] Nicotinic
acid may cause a similar maculopathy. The incidence and pathogenesis
of these conditions are unknown.

Sustained, extensive investigative efforts are clearly needed
in these important areas.

IV. INFLAMMATION

Inflammatory processes generally result in a dramatic increase
of permeability in affected vessels. Ultrastructural studies of inflammation in nonocular tissues have shown that intercellular junctions are most prone to disruption in venules; those of capillaries
remain remarkably intact.[34,35] Similar studies have not been done in
the human retina, but both infectious and noninfectious inflammatory
processes are known to result in either widespread or localized
breakdown of the I-BRB. The pathogeneses are largely unknown, but
may involve toxins, enzymes, immune complex deposition, and so on.
Angiography reveals that the process along the endothelial membrane
can involve all elements of the vascular tree or can actually be confined to either the capillaries, the arterioles, or the venules

A. Infectious Processes

In the case of infectious diseases, the extravascular passage
of both plasma and blood cells is often so extensive that sheathing
of larger vessels becomes ophthalmoscopically visible. In less severe cases, fluorescein angiography is required to show the permeability abnormality. Protozoans, viruses, bacteria, and fungi are
all known to render the I-BRB dysfunctional.

Toxoplasma. In toxoplasmic retinochoroiditis, individual medium-sized vessels may demonstrate sheathing and, in quiescent phases, perivascular pigmentation. These vascular changes are not as characteristic as the necrotizing patches of retinochoroiditis that typify toxoplasmosis, but occur in about 3.5% or more of cases.[36]

Cytomegalovirus. Viral infection of the retina may also cause either diffuse or localized vasculitis (Fig. 9). Cytomegalic inclusion disease, for example, is characterized initially by whitish patches of retinal necrosis associated with extensive sheathing of adjacent arterioles and venules.[37] With time, confluent and extensive patches of retinal hemorrhage occur. The ophthalmoscopic appearance may then simulate a BRVO. Histologic studies have confirmed the presence of cytomegalic inclusion bodies in retinal vascular endothelial cells, and it has been postulated that this endothelial involvement provides a source for new, distant foci of retinal infection.[38] Desquamation of arteriolar endothelial cells apparently also results in subendothelial hemorrhage and accumulations of serofibrinous material that are thought by de Venecia et al to narrow further the blood column and cause an ophthalmoscopically visible white, cord-like appearance. The vaso-occlusive process may be severe enough to cause branch retinal artery occlusion.[39]

Herpes viruses. Herpes simplex virus[40] may cause extensive hemorrhagic necrosis of the retina with occlusions of major peripapillary vessels. These vessels have been histologically shown to have fibrinoid necrosis and obstruction of their lumina by endothelial cells and debris.[40]

Microscopic studies of herpes zoster ophthalmicus have also shown dramatic evidence of vasculitis and perivasculitis,[41] and clinical studies have yielded evidence of retinal arteriolitis.[42]

Bacteria and fungi. Bacterial and fungal endophthalmitis have a particularly devastating effect on the integrity of the I-BRB. Torrential outpouring of white cells can completely obscure the involved vessels' blood columns, and simulate total vascular occlusion. A variety of proteolytic enzymes, toxins, chemotactic agents, and other vasoactive substances presumably participate in this florid reaction to the presence of microorganisms near or in the retina.

Tuberculosis. Tuberculous infection causes a less immediate effect on the retinal blood vessels than do pyogenic organisms, but the ultimate consequences may include local vascular occlusion, retinitis proliferans, vitreous hemorrhage, and retinal detachment (Fig. 10). Although the terms Eales' disease and retinal vasculitis were once considered synonymous, recent opinions suggest that Eales' disease is an idiopathic, possibly heterogeneous disease with closure of the peripheral retinal vasculature (and attendent complications).[43] Nonetheless, in the older literature histologic documentation can be found for the presence of tubercle bacilli around

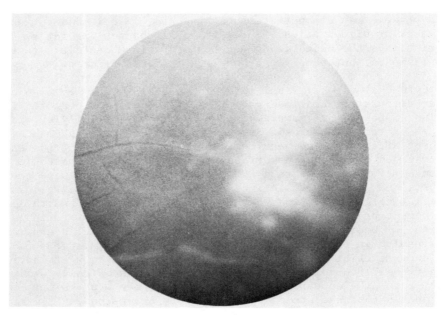

Fig. 9. Cytomegalic inclusion disease. Note widespread breakdown
of I-BRB (courtesy of Lee Jampol, M.D.).

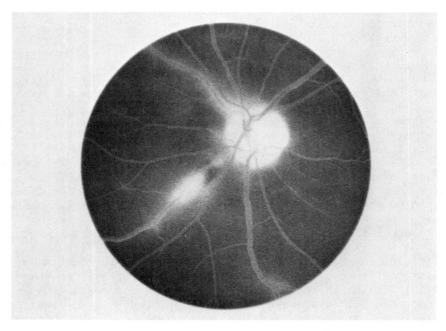

Fig. 10. Retinal phlebitis in patient with pulmonary tuberculosis.

some affected retinal veins.[44]

Syphilis. Syphilitic infection of the retinal blood vessels ranges from gummatous involvement to a relatively benign condition known as retinal periarteritis[45] or segmental periarteritis. In this latter condition, ophthalmoscopically visible lesions include yellow refractile deposits along the arteriolar tree (Fig. 11). Angiography shows no interference with arteriolar flow and no intraluminal filling defects or mural staining. These findings suggest that the abnormalities predominately affect the outer aspect of the arteriolar wall, rather than its endothelium, and that the I-BRB is compromised to a minimal extent, if at all (at least in the healed, quiescent phase of this disorder). Syphilis has also been implicated in the causation of CME, with typical leakage from perifoveal capillaries.[46]

B. Noninfectious Processes

Occlusive retinal arteriolitis. As in the case of syphilitic periarteritis, preferential inflammation of the arteriolar wall occurs in a rare disorder known as occlusive retinal arteriolitis.[47] The etiology is unknown. Ophthalmoscopic examination shows segmental periarteriolar sheathing and cuffing (Fig. 12). Angiography reveals occlusion of arterioles with mural staining and leakage. Neovascularization may ensue.[47]

Phlebitis. Phlebitis of the retinal vasculature is observed as a manifestation of ocular sarcoidosis,[48] as an isolated disorder,[43] or in association with retinal panvasculitis that involves all components of the vascular tree. Ophthalmoscopic and angiographic evidence indicates variable degrees of transmural leakage of plasma and blood cells into the surrounding retinal tissue.

Panvasculitis. The clinical entities responsible for retinal panvasculitis, of which Behcet's disease is a good example,[49] are generally idiopathic.[50] In some parts of the world, such as Japan, Behcet's disease is responsible for disabling a relatively large percentage of the population because of its ocular effects.

Pars planitis. A reasonably discrete (though probably heterogeneous) clinical entity responsible for widespread, low-grade breakdown of the I-BRB is pars planitis, sometimes called vitritis, peripheral uveitis, or chronic cyclitis.[51,52] Pars planitis is characterized by cloudy white deposits in the inferior vitreous, a densely cellular vitreous, disc edema, CME, and widespread retinal vascular leakage (Fig. 13). The blood components entering the vitreous compartment presumably shift slowly downward through the vitreous gel, gravitationally settling in the inferior fundus. Some cases that show circumferential involvement of the entire pars plana have been invoked as evidence against the gravitational theory.[53]

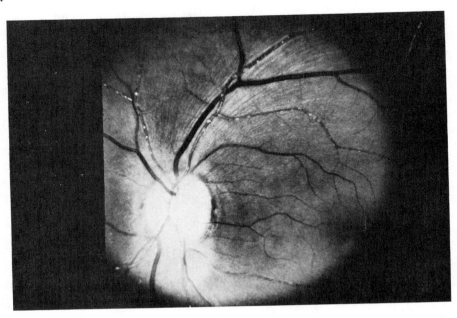

Fig. 11A. Syphilitic periarteritis (red-free view); reprinted from Ref. 45.

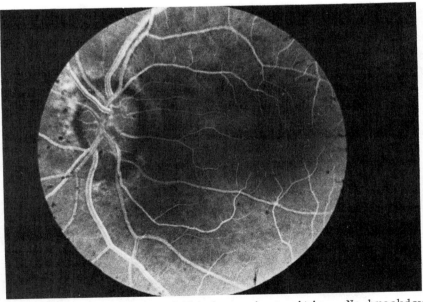

Fig. 11B. Angiography of syphilitic periarteritis. No breakdown of I-BRB and no filling defects are seen in quiescent stage of disease.

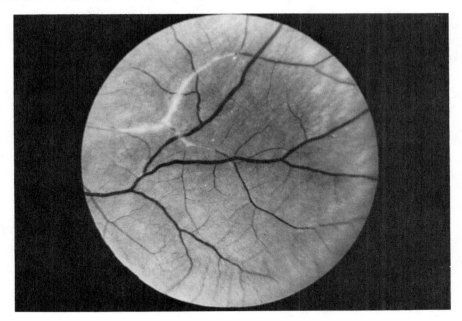

Fig. 12A. Occlusive retinal arteriolitis (red-free view); reprinted from Ref. 47.

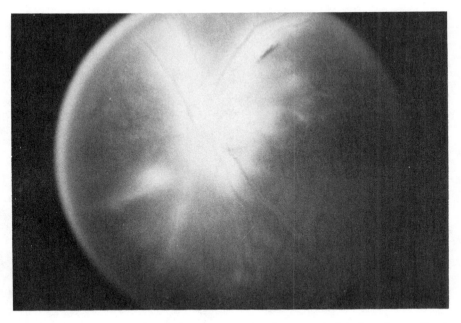

Fig. 12B. Angiogram of occlusive retinal arteriolitis shows leakage from disc and arterioles.

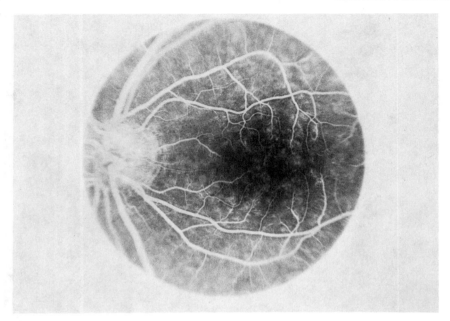

Fig. 13A. Pars planitis and cystoid macular edema, before therapy (late venous phase of angiogram).

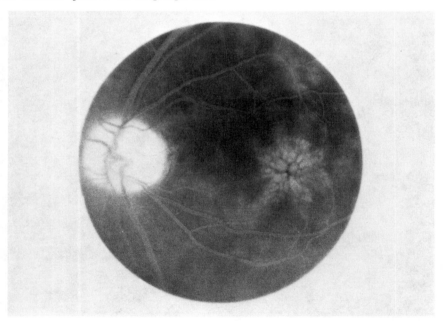

Fig. 13B. Pars planitis and cystoid macular edema, before therapy (very late venous phase of angiogram).

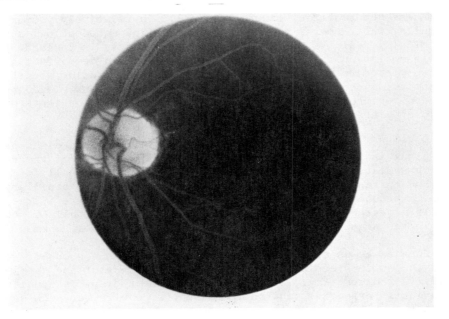

Fig. 13C. One month of corticosteroid therapy is followed by resolution of fluorescein leakage (very late venous phase of angiogram; cf Fig. 13B).

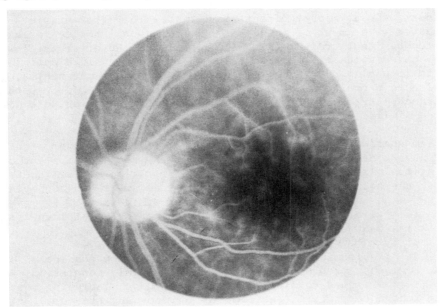

Fig. 13D. One year after Figs. 13A–C, mild recurrence of fluorescein leakage has occurred.

These abnormalities occur chronically in relatively young individuals, who, generally, with some exceptions noted below, appear
systemically healthy. In some cases, particularly in England, there
is an association of retinitis pigmentosa and also demyelinating
disease with pars planitis. Interestingly, perivascular sheathing,
without evidence of pars plana involvement or vitreous cloudbanks,
has been repeatedly observed in the United States in patients with
multiple sclerosis.

Whatever its mechanism and whatever its associated diseases,
pars planitis is characterized by widespread leakiness of the retinal vasculature. Venules histologically show round cell infiltration and cuffing.[53] Arterioles are often spared. The capillary bed
seems invariably to be affected, even when involvement of larger
vessels is either barely visible or not detectable at all by angiographic techniques. Cystoid macular edema is extremely common.

Such cases usually smolder for years. They occasionally re-
spond to corticosteroid therapy, whereupon leaking of the capillaries is reduced (Fig. 13A-C). However, the therapy is usually not
dramatically effective, and pharmacologic side effects, such as
cataract or glaucoma, often supervene.

Cystoid macular edema. Cystoid macular edema from chronically
incompetent perifoveal capillaries not only characterizes pars
planitis, but also complicates an enormous array of other ocular
disorders, whose primary effects may be in either the anterior or
the posterior segment of the eye.[54] CME is even inherited as an
isolated dominant trait[55] (Fig. 14). Whatever the etiology, low-
grade, chronic leakage through the walls of the involved capillaries
results in pooling of plasmoid fluid in the macular parenchyma, giving rise to a characteristic, though generally nonspecific, petaloid
appearance. Breakdown of the outer BRB in the posterior pole may
cause a similar clinical appearance.

The anatomic arrangement of the outer plexiform layer, the
large number of capillaries, and possibly the poor development of
the internal limiting lamina in the macular region may all contribute to the ability of this retinal region to swell and accumulate
a large volume of extravascular fluid. If distention of the cystoid
spaces is severe or chronic enough, lamellar and full-thickness macular holes can result.

From an epidemiologic perspective, CME must be considered one
of the commonest problems affecting the ophthalmic population, because it complicates so many different disorders, including routine,
uncomplicated cataract extraction (the Irvine-Gass syndrome),[56,57]
and because there is no currently accepted, reliable therapeutic regimen. Preliminary evidence, largely from Japan, suggests that a
regimen of antiprostaglandin therapy may minimize the breakdown of

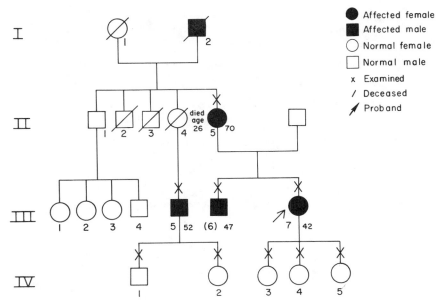

Fig. 14A. Pedigree of family with dominant cystoid macular edema; reprinted from Ref. 55.

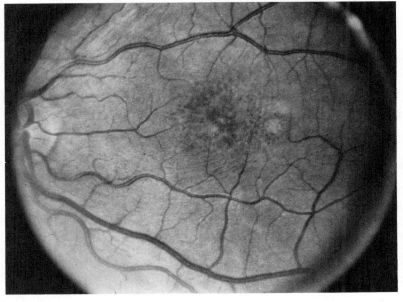

Fig. 14B. Dominant cystoid macular edema (red-free view).

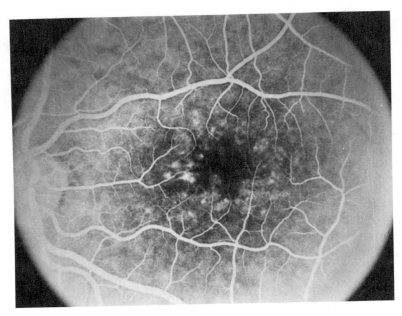

Fig. 14C. Dominant cystoid macular edema   (early venous phase of angiogram).

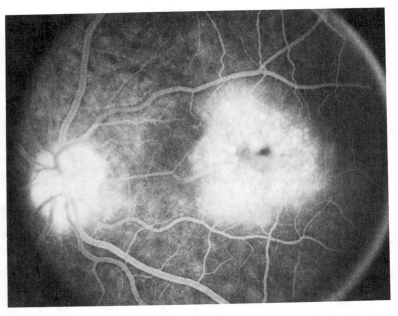

Fig. 14D. Dominant cystoid macular edema (late venous phase of angiogram).

the vascular barrier.[58]

V.   TAPETORETINAL DYSTROPHIES AND RETINOSCHISIS

A fascinating, enigmatic breakdown of the I-BRB has been observed in a variety of tapetoretinal dystrophies. The proposed pathogeneses of these disorders have generally emphasized the photoreceptors and retinal pigment epithelium and have excluded the retinal vasculature as the primarily affected tissue. Yet, evidence is accumulating to suggest that breakdown of the I-BRB may contribute to the characteristic fundus appearance in some of these disorders and may actually cause a reduction of visual acuity in others.

A.   Favre—Goldmann Syndrome

In Favre-Goldmann syndrome diffuse, marked leakage from the retinal vasculature has been documented by fluorescein angiography in several patients[59] (Fig. 15). Two types of breakdown of the I-BRB were noted. One was nonspecific CME, which appeared to contribute to the decreased visual acuity and which might have been responsible for the so-called macular schisis that has previously been reported in Favre-Goldmann syndrome. The other type of vascular incompetence was extensive capillary leakage in areas of extramacular retinoschisis. Other vessels were totally nonperfused. At least two possible pathogenetic sequences can be envisioned in Favre-Goldmann syndrome: (1) the schitic process is primary, and leads to secondary vascular incompetence and/or occlusion, possibly due to kinking or traction on the vessels, or (2) the vascular incompetence (or occlusion) is primary, and fluid accumulating in the extravascular space causes the schitic cavities to form. With either of these courses of events, the relationship between the vascular occlusion and incompetence is unknown, and, as yet, the relationship between either of these courses of events to the photoreceptor and pigment epithelial disease is completely obscure.

Retinal vascular leakage has also been demonstrated in another schitic disease, X-linked (juvenile) retinoschisis, by Green and Jampol.[60] In this disorder, there is no electrophysiologic or other evidence implicating a primary disorder of the photoreceptors and the retinal pigment epithelium. Because scattered intraretinal fluorescein leakage and staining of vessel walls were observed in their patient with X-linked retinoschisis, even in clinically nonschitic portions of the retina, Green and Jampol suggested that the vascular incompetence might precede (and possibly cause) the retinoschisis. Alternatively, it was also considered possible, though unlikely, that the schitic process was primary and led to the vascular incompetence.

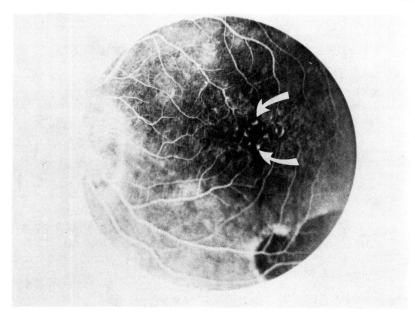

Fig. 15A. Favre-Goldmann syndrome. Early venous phase of angiogram shows leakage from retinal capillaries (arrows).

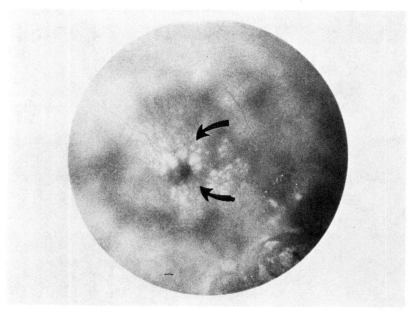

Fig. 15B. Favre-Goldmann syndrome. Late venous phase of angiogram shows cystoid macular edema (arrows) and intense, widespread leakage throughout posterior pole (courtesy of Gerald Fishman, M.D.).

B.   Retinitis Pigmentosa

Fishman et al have found that 14.5% of 110 consecutive, pro-
spectively studied patients with retinitis pigmentosa of different
genetic types had angiographic evidence of CME[61] (Fig. 16).   Bilateral foveal cysts or partial-thickness holes were noteworthy.   All
patients showed variable degrees of macular preretinal membranes and
radial traction lines.   These membranes may have contributed to the
vascular abnormalities, or vice versa.   Macular ischemia may also
have contributed to the pathogenesis of the leakage or the membrane
formation.   In any event, the macular breakdown of the I—BRB appears
responsible, at least in part, for loss of central vision in a disease process customarily attributable to photoreceptor and pigment
epithelial abnormalities.

It is of interest that ffytche[48] has also noted vascular incompetence in retinitis pigmentosa patients, some of whom apparently
had such extensive leakage that the clinical picture of pars planitis
developed (see above).

C.   The Carrier State

Gieser et al[62] have recently shown that female carriers of X-
linked recessive retinitis pigmentosa had normal fluorescein angiograms but abnormally high concentrations of vitreous fluorescein,
as determined by fluorophotometry.   Since retinal vascular abnormalities could not be found, it was concluded that the fluorophoto-
metric abnormality was probably due to a subclinical dysfunction of
the retinal pigment epithelium.   Some leaking from the retinal vascular tree, not detectable by angiography, may also have occurred.

VI.   TRAUMA

Physical trauma of varied types is capable of inducing rapidly
occurring incompetence of the retinal vascular endothelium.   For-
tunately, the I—BRB is usually capable of repairing its barrier function, unless the damage is especially intense.   How it does so is
largely unknown.

A.   Radiation

Radiation retinopathy occurs after excessive exposure of the
retina to external sources of radiation, including x-rays.   Vaso-
occlusion with subsequent formation of leaking microaneurysms and
telangiectatic small vessels may contribute to reduction of central
vision.[63]

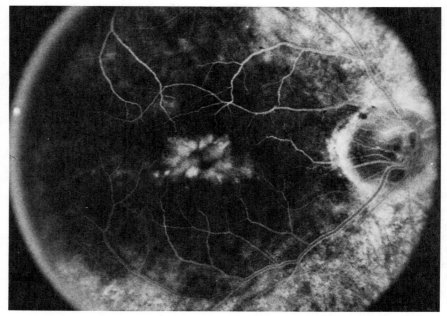

Fig. 16. Retinitis pigmentosa with cystoid macular edema (courtesy of Gerald Fishman, M.D.).

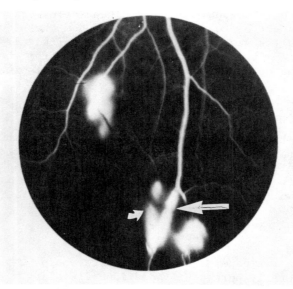

Fig. 17. Argon laser coagulation of arterioles supplying peripheral neovascularization. Note leakage from both the traumatized arterioles (long arrows) and the retinal pigment epithelium (short arrow).

B. Photocoagulation

Mild, diffuse photocoagulation burns can produce leakage, especially from capillaries, even when little or no damage is detectable ophthalmoscopically.[64] If aimed directly at larger retinal
blood vessels, argon laser and xenon arc photocoagulation can cause
gross disruption of the vascular wall[65] (Fig. 17). Fragmentation,
cystoid degeneration, and necrosis of the wall are seen histologically, along with pyknosis of endothelial cell nuclei.[66,67]

With time, initial leakiness or even obstructed flow returns
to normal, unless the initial insult was so intense that permanent
obliteration of the lumen occurs. Restoration of the I-BRB, with
absence of leakiness, is mirrored in the outer BRB by apparently
similar repair mechanisms after photocoagulation of the retinal pigment epithelium.[68]

When photocoagulation is used therapeutically to obliterate
vascular anomalies, such as retinal angiomatosis of the von Hippel-
Lindau type (see below), the immediate transudation that occurs as
the result of photic trauma is often so severe that massive serous
detachment of the retina may develop over several hours. Although
dramatic, this event usually corrects itself or responds to corticosteroid therapy.

C. Cryocoagulation and Diathermy

As a result of thermal damage, both cryocoagulation and diathermy result in leakage of fluid, as well as cells, from retinal
blood vessels. This breakdown of the I-BRB, like that following
photocoagulation, is generally temporary and reversible. Because
the surgical probes delivering thermal energy to the wall of the eye
are held closer to the choroid than to the retina, leakage is most
intense from the choroidal vasculature.[69]

VII. DEVELOPMENTAL VASCULAR ANOMALIES

Marked disruption of the I-BRB characterizes several vascular
anomalies, including Coats' disease and the von Hippel-Lindau syndrome.

A. Coats' Disease

The hallmark of this striking clinical entity is a massive outpouring of lipid-containing plasma products from abnormal telangiectatic and aneurysmal retinal vessels into the retina and subretinal
space (Fig. 18). The disruption of the I-BRB is often so severe
and so prolonged, especially in children, that the accumulated
yellowish-white plasma products may cause a white pupillary reflex

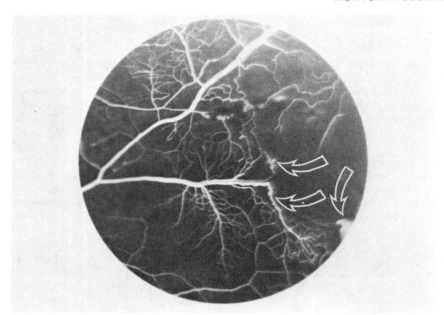

Fig. 18. Coats' disease, demonstrating leaking aneurysms and telangiectases (arrows) and zones of capillary drop-out.

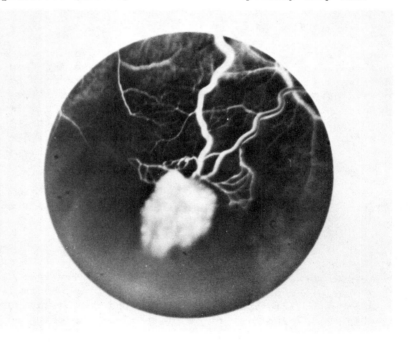

Fig. 19. Von Hippel-Lindau angioma of the retina.

and simulate retinoblastoma. The presence of the anomalous retinal
vessels facilitates the differential diagnosis. This idiopathic
vascular anomaly may be localized to one retinal area, but tends to
be slowly progressive. Occasionally, spontaneous regression occurs.[70]

When the plasma and lipid outpouring is minimal and the vascular
malformation dominates the ophthalmoscopic appearance, the term Leber's miliary aneurysms is often used.[71] It is doubtful that Coats'
disease and Leber's miliary aneurysms are fundamentally distinct
nosologic conditions, but the possibility remains that heterogeneity
exists in this clinical spectrum. Even when the massive collection
of lipid and plasma products does not occur in an individual patient,
fluorescein angiography reveals widespread breakdown of the I-BRB.
The telangiectases and aneurysms affecting arterioles, capillaries,
and venules show leakage that may be mild to severe.

The macula frequently accumulates yellow lipoidal material
that has escaped from even remote portions of the retinal circulation. The reasons for the preferential involvement of the macula
are unknown (see above). Nonetheless, the ophthalmoscopic detection of intramacular lipid is so characteristic, particularly in an
otherwise healthy child, that the entire fundus periphery should be
carefully inspected for the presence of a vascular anomaly such as
Coats' disease or von Hippel-Lindau disease (see below). Therapeutic obliteration of the peripheral vascular anomaly often results
in disappearance of the macular lipid, with improvement in vision.
Sometimes, however, a subretinal disciform nodule persists after the
lipid is resorbed, with concomitant reduction in visual acuity.

Histologically, there are intraretinal and subretinal cholesterol clefts and collections of lipid-filled macrophages. PAS-
positive material is found in thickened vascular walls, due, probably, to the presence of basement membrane—like material and blood
components.[72]

Electron microscopy of a human case of Coats' disease by Tripathi and Ashton has shown the involved vascular walls to be largely devoid of endothelium and pericytes.[72] Where endothelium was present, it showed vacuolated cytoplasm, but intact intercellular junctions. The abnormal vessel walls were invariably infiltrated with
fibrinous and plasmoid material, often including cellular debris.
In some areas the fibrous walls were markedly thinned and even absent,
so that the lumen was bordered only by basement membrane of surrounding glia. It appeared logical to Tripathi and Ashton that a
vascular wall consisting of an acellular porous membrane would become telangiectatic or aneurysmal and would continuously leak copious
quantities of plasma and occasional blood cells into the surrounding
retina. They attributed the primary process to a defect in endothelial permeability, causing so-called plasmatic vasculosis, but
were unable to identify the initial functional or structural

abnormality.

Tripathi and Ashton concluded that telangiectasia and aneurysmal
dilations represented end stages of Coats' disease and not initiating
events, which, they decided, had started in the endothelium.[72] It
remains possible that the reverse sequence might more accurately
characterize the pathogenesis; that is, a developmental aberration
involving the nonendothelial components of the vascular wall might
lead to telangiectases and aneurysms. The stretched endothelium,
which was initially functional, would eventually decompensate and
leak, given sufficient time or severity. The occurrence of Leber's
miliary aneurysms, with prominent vascular abnormalities but minimal
incompetence of the I-BRB, suggests possibly that breakdown of the
endothelial barrier follows, rather than precedes, anatomic degeneration of the vascular wall. Because an animal model for systematic
study of this disorder is not available, knowledge of the precise sequence of events awaits further clinicopathologic correlation.

B. Von Hippel-Lindau Disease

Von Hippel-Lindau disease is a dominantly inherited phakomato-
sis characterized in the retina by hamartomatous development of angiomatous tumors. Although they show no angiographically detectable
vascular incompetence when very small,[73] the tumors tend to enlarge,
and, in the process, characteristically demonstrate leakage of large
amounts of intraluminal fluorescein into the perivascular spaces
(Fig. 19).

Absence of a normal I-BRB in von Hippel-Lindau retinal angiomas
is characterized clinically not only by fluorescein leakage,[74] but
also by exudative or hemorrhagic retinal detachments that occur either
spontaneously or following therapeutic efforts at obliteration by
photocoagulation, cryocoagulation, or scleral diathermy.

Histologic and ultrastructural analysis of von Hippel-Lindau
angiomas was reported by Nicholson et al.[75] They noted that the
angiomatous nodules were composed of tortuous, large capillaries
measuring 8 to 14μ in diameter, lined by normal, flattened endothelium. Electron microscopy showed well-differentiated capillary
ultrastructure with a normal, continuous endothelial lining and intercellular junctions. The capillary basement membrane and invest-
ing pericytes were also normal morphologically. The appearance was
consistent with that of a capillary hemangioma.

The mechanism of fluorescein leakage is not fully understood,
but may be attributed speculatively to functionally abnormal hamartomatous endothelium and also to coexistent new retinal vessels.[9]
As the angiomas enlarge, shunting of arterial blood through the
tumor mass sometimes occurs, and the exposure of the capillary en-

dothelium to a relatively increased hydrostatic pressure may also contribute to loss of competence of the I-BRB to fluorescein.

In nonangiomatous portions of the retina (including the macula) capillary microaneurysms have been observed, and may be at least partially responsible for the formation of CME and lipoidal intra-macular deposits.[9] In most cases, however, angiography has not shown vascular anomalies in the macula, but further angiographic and histologic studies are needed.

VIII.   PRERETINAL NEOVASCULARIZATION

Two major forms of preretinal neovascularization occur: (1) that arising spontaneously, possibly as a consequence of retinal ischemia and hypoxia (Fig. 20 A and B);[76-79] and (2) that arising iatrogenically as a consequence of photocoagulation designed to obliterate pre-existing spontaneous neovascularization.[80] Both types contribute to vitreous syneresis and traction, because of constant, intense leaking of plasma contents into the vitreous gel.

A.   Preretinal Neovascularization

Whatever the underlying ocular or systemic disease, the angio-graphic (or angioscopic) hallmark of preretinal neovascularization is profuse intravitreal leakage. This virtually invariable finding is highly useful in a variety of clinical settings. Diagnostically, the presence of a preretinal, intravitreal cloud of bright green fluorescence is invaluable in ophthalmoscopically confirming the location of each possible patch of true neovascularization, even when the ocular media are cloudy enough to conceal the individual vessels themselves.

Even in the presence of clear media, certain vascular lesions, such as intraretinal microvascular abnormalities (IRMA), shunt ves-sels, and optociliary anastomoses, can be mistaken ophthalmoscopical-ly (but, importantly, not angiographically) for true neovascular tis-sue. The potential of these non-neovascular lesions for deleterious-ly affecting visual function is so far less than that of true new vessels that they ordinarily need not be therapeutically obliterated. In certain cases, such as optociliary anastomoses at the border of the optic disc, focal photocoagulation is not only unnecessary, but is actually contraindicated. The absence of fluorescein leakage in these vascular lesions is thus important therapeutically as well as diagnostically.

Following attempts at ablating neovascular tissue by either focal or indirect photocoagulation, the production of pigmented chorioretinal scars renders the interpretation of the fundus pic-ture somewhat difficult, and neovascular tissue may be difficult to

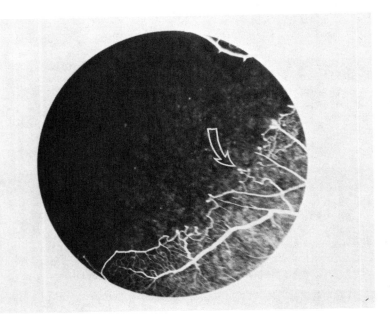

Fig. 20A. Equatorial retina in sickle cell retinopathy. Note total ischemia in periphery. Arrow indicates arteriolar-venular anastomosis and site of future neovascularization (cf Fig. 20B).

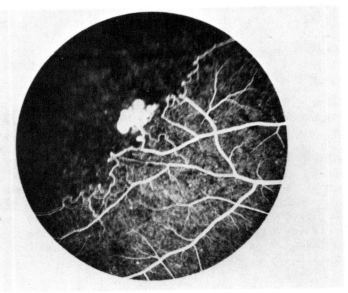

Fig. 20B. Same fundus location shown in Fig. 20A, 3 years later. Note development of leaking fan-shaped neovascularization at border of perfused and non-perfused retinal areas.

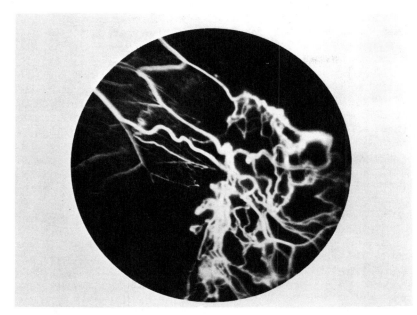

Fig. 21A. Early venous phase of angiogram shows large, fan-shaped neovascular patch in sickle cell retinopathy.

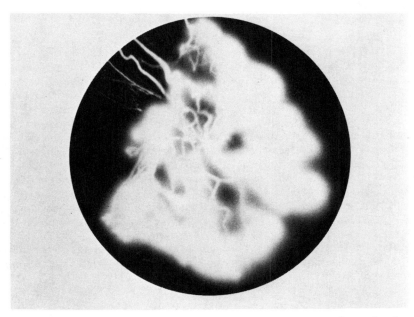

Fig. 21B. Later venous phase of angiogram shows profuse leakage (cf Fig. 21A).

In this circumstance, the use of fluorescein angioscopy or graphy is invaluable for detecting incompletely involuted or cam iflaged neovascular patches.[81]

Although preretinal neovascularization virtually always shows profuse leakage of intraluminal fluorescein into the vitreous (Fig. 21 A and B), some neovascular channels, if allowed to mature, apparently develop some barrier functions. As a result, vessels supplying fan-shaped neovascular patches occasionally lose much of their vascular incompetence over a period of months to years, and profuse leakiness is found only at the peripheral tips of the proliferating neovascular patches.[82] The ultrastructural basis for this functional maturation is unknown, but may include improved intercellular junctions, loss of endothelial attenuations (fenestrations), or development of more normal processes of active transport along the entire endothelial cell membrane.

Ultrastructural studies of human preretinal neovascularization have been extremely limited.[83-85] Neovascular capillaries in diabetics consisted of thinned endothelial cells, pericytes, and basement membrane. The endothelial cells had cytoplasmic fenestrations in one case, as well as abundant pinocytotic vesicles, both of which could represent the anatomic site of breakdown of the I-BRB and fluorescein leakiness. Intercellular junctional complexes were present. In some new capillaries, erythrocytes were found extraluminally, but were bound by the basement membrane.[85]

In a related ultrastructural study of rubeosis iridis, we also observed that new vessels were characterized by the presence of cytoplasmic fenestrations, basement membrane, intercellular junctions, and surrounding pericytes.[86]

In pars planitis Kenyon et al[53] have shown that intravitreal fibrovascular tissue is composed of well-differentiated capillaries with continuous non-fenestrated endothelial cells and junctional complexes. The cells were surrounded by basement membrane and pericytes. Kenyon[87] also studied a fibrovascular preretinal membrane obtained by vitrectomy in a case of presumed BRVO (although the diagnosis was not well documented). The vessels appeared, once again, to be well-differentiated, with a continuous endothelium having occluding junctions, basement membrane, and pericytes. Whether or not these specimens can be considered characteristic of true preretinal neovascularization (such as that occurring in diabetic retinopathy, sickle cell retinopathy, and so on) is questionable; additional specimens for ultrastructural analysis are badly needed.

B. Iatrogenic Choroidovitreal Neovascularization

Following overly intense focal photocoagulation, a florid stalk of choroidally derived blood vessels may erupt through iatrogenic

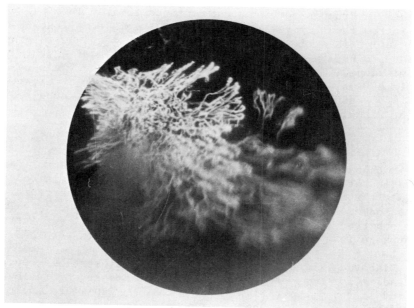

Fig. 22A. Choroidovitreal neovascularization following overly intense photocoagulation and iatrogenic rupture of Bruch's membrane (early venous phase of angiogram).

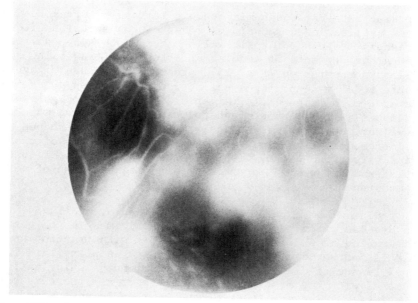

Fig. 22B. Later venous phase of angiogram shows extensive intravitreal leakage of dye (cf Fig. 22A).

defects in Bruch's membrane and continue to grow into the preretinal and intravitreal spaces (Fig. 22).[88,89] This complication of photocoagulation is serious, because the vessels continue to grow, leak plasma profusely, and liberate large quantities of erythrocytes into the vitreous. The frequent resistance of these vessels to all therapeutic attempts at obliteration may be related to a relatively high head of pressure and flow rate with which they are supplied from parent vessels in the choroid.

IX. DIABETES MELLITUS

Both background diabetic retinopathy (BDR) and proliferative diabetic retinopathy (PDR) contribute to markedly impaired vision, largely through mechanisms associated with faulty barrier function. Edema and exudates are often responsible for the poor macular function observed in patients with BDR (Fig. 23),[90,91] and intravitreal hemorrhage is a common blinding event in patients with PDR.[92]

Diabetic retinopathy in its varied manifestations represents a paradigm for many of the types of I-BRB breakdown previously considered in this report(Figs. 24 and 25).[93] Capillary microaneurysms, for example, with stretched, degenerated endothelial cells, characteristically show leakage early in the fluorescein angiogram and perianeurysmal staining late in the angiographic sequence. Lipid and PAS-positive material percolate through the aneurysmal wall and form hard exudates. Localized hemorrhages also tend to occur from microaneurysms, either through microscopic leakage or frank ruptures.[94] Dilated capillaries noted around zones of nonperfusion often show fluorescein staining of their walls. Mural staining can also be marked along segments of venules or arterioles traversing zones of capillary nonperfusion (Fig. 25), presumably because of hypoxia or exposure to as yet undefined vasoactive metabolites generated by or associated with ischemia.[95] Arterioles passing through poorly perfused zones may also show truncated capillary stumps, which show faint fluorescein leakage at their tips.[95] Hairpin-shaped loops of capillaries and veins similarly show local breakdown of their endothelial barrier function, possibly from hypoxic loss of tone (with dilation and stretching) or from external contraction of pericapillary membranes.[96]

If plasma components leak into the macula, pooling of fluorescein dye can often be seen (Fig. 26), sometimes in the petaloid configuration of CME. Premacular fibrosis with traction on the macula is another cause of leakage of intravascular fluid into the retinal tissue of diabetics.[90] Preretinal neovascularization is associated with the most profound leakage of all these vascular abnormalities. The magnitude of the leakage is compounded by the presence of a structurally and functionally incompetent endothelial membrane, a hypoxic surrounding environment, and marked external traction from adherent vitreous membranes.

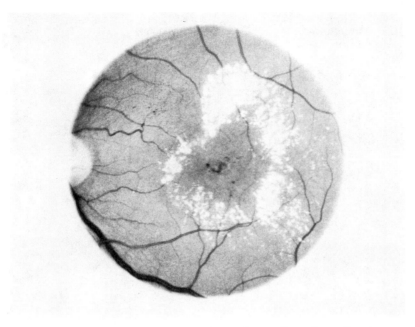

Fig. 23A. Diabetic circinate maculopathy. Parafoveal microaneurysms
cause centrifugal leakage of plasmoid fluid (red-free view).

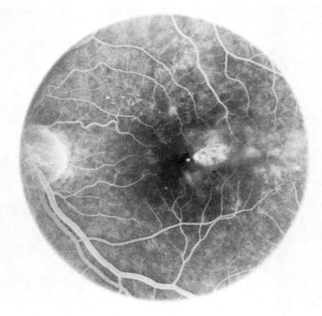

Fig. 23B. Late venous phase of angiogram shows leakage from
parafoveal microaneurysms (cf Fig. 23A). Vision is 20/100.

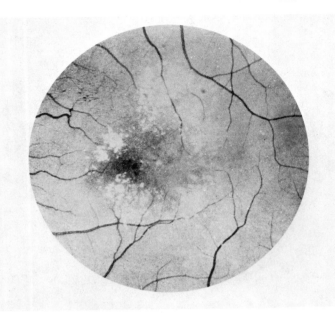

Fig. 23C. Six weeks after argon laser photocoagulation of parafoveal microaneurysms (red-free view).

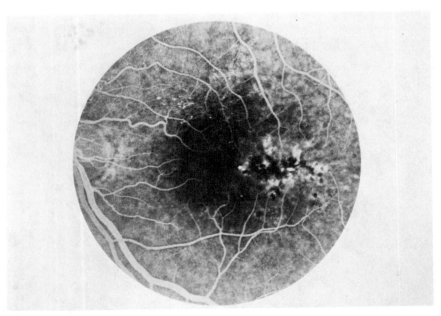

Fig. 23D. Six weeks after photocoagulation, angiogram reveals less fluorescein leakage (cf Fig. 23B). Vision has improved to 20/40

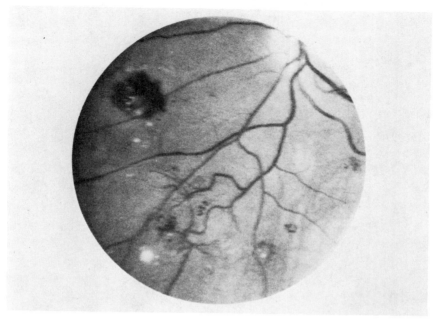

Fig. 24A. Diabetic background and proliferative retinopathy (red-free view; cf Fig. 24B).

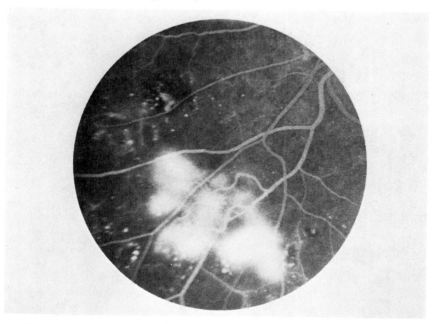

Fig. 24B. Angiographic appearance of leaking punctate microaneurysms, other microvascular anomalies, and new vessels (cf Fig. 24A).

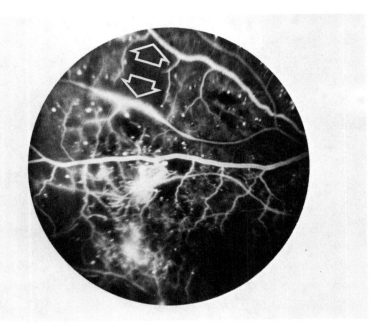

Fig. 25. Diabetic retinopathy with punctate, hyperfluorescent microaneurysms and segmentally staining arteriole and venule crossing ischemic zone (arrows).

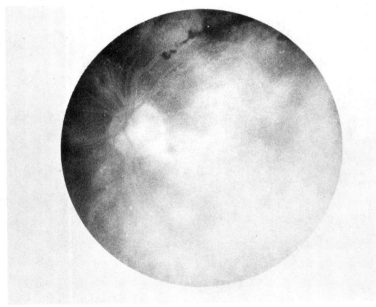

Fig. 26. Diabetic retinopathy with extreme leakage of fluorescein into macula.

CONCLUSION

Dysfunction of the I-BRB is observed in a large variety of ocular diseases. In many of them the mechanism of breakdown of the I-BRB is poorly understood, as is the mechanism of repair. Intercellular junctions remain intact in a surprisingly large number of retinal vascular disorders, and thus cannot be considered invariably responsible for the characteristically increased vascular permeability. Ophthalmoscopic characteristics of individual diseases depend on the location, chronicity, and severity of the barrier breakdown in the retina.[72]

In a few instances, such as branch retinal vein occlusion, embolic diseases, and hypertensive retinopathy, experimental animal models have provided an opportunity for angiographic and ultrastructural analysis. For most disorders of the human retinal vasculature, however (including diabetic preretinal neovascularization), animal models do not exist, and clinicopathologic correlation of individual human cases will remain an important investigative tool.

Fluorescein angiography continues to be an essential methodology for diagnostic and therapeutic assessment of barrier function in retinal vasculopathies.

ACKNOWLEDGMENTS

Supported in part by Core Grant No. EY 1792 and Training Grant No. EY 7038 from the National Eye Institute, Bethesda, Maryland; by an Unrestricted Grant from Research to Prevent Blindness, Inc., New York City; by the Comprehensive Sickle Cell Center of the University of Illinois (Grant No. HL 15168 from the National Heart, Lung, and Blood Institute, Bethesda, Maryland); and by a Macy Foundation Faculty Scholar Award.

REFERENCES

1. Cunha-Vaz, J., _Surv. Ophthalmol._ 23:279-296, 1979
2. Archer, D.B., In Deutman, A.F. (ed.): _New Developments in Ophthalmology, Nijmegen, 1975: Documenta Ophthalmologica Proceedings Series, vol. 7_, The Hague, Dr. W. Junk bv Pub., 1976, pp. 155-167.
3. Wise, G.N., _Am. J. Ophthalmol._ 79:349-365, 1975.
4. Bellhorn, M.B., Friedman, A.H., Wise, G.N., and Henkind, P., _Am. J. Ophthalmol._ 79:366-373, 1975.

5. Sumers, K.D., Jampol, L.M., Goldberg, M.F., and Huamonte, F.U., Arch. Ophthalmol., in press.

6. Tolentino, F.I., Schepens, C.L., and Freeman, H.M.: Vitreo-retinal Disorders: Diagnosis and Management, Philadelphia, W. B. Saunders, 1976, p. 141.

7. Tolentino, F.I., and Schepens, C.L., Arch. Ophthalmol. 74:781-786, 1965.

8. Asdourian, G.K., Goldberg, M.F., Jampol, L., and Rabb, M., Arch. Ophthalmol. 95:624-628, 1977.

9. Goldberg, M.F., and Duke, J.R., Am. J. Ophthalmol. 66:693-705, 1968.

10. Gass, J.D.M., Arch. Ophthalmol. 80:550-568, 1968.

11. Archer, D.B., Ernest, J.T., and Newell, F.W., Trans. Am. Acad. Ophthalmol. Otolaryngol. 78:OP148-OP165, 1974.

12. Joondeph, H.C., and Goldberg, M.F., Am. J. Ophthalmol. 80:253-257, 1975.

13. Orth, D.H., and Patz, A., Surv. Ophthalmol. 22:357-376, 1978.

14. Hamilton, A.M., Kohner, E.M., Rosen, D., Bird, A.C., and Dollery, C.T., Br. J. Ophthalmol. 63:377-387, 1979.

15. Hockley, D.J., Tripathi, R.C., and Ashton, N., Br. J. Ophthalmol. 63:393-411, 1979.

16. Editorial, Br. J. Ophthalmol. 63:375-376, 1979.

17. Clemett, R.S., Br. J. Ophthalmol. 58:548-554, 1974.

18. Goldberg, M.F., and Tso, M.O.M., Ophthalmic Surgery 10(4): 89-123, 1979.

19. Hayreh, S.S., Am. J. Ophthalmol. 72:998-1011, 1971.

20. Hayreh, S.S., van Heuven, W.A.J., and Hayreh, M.S., Arch. Ophthalmol. 96:311-323, 1978.

21. Fujino, T., Curtin, V.T., and Norton, E.W.D., Arch. Ophthalmol. 81:395-406, 1969.

22. Editorial, Br. J. Ophthalmol. 59:1-2, 1975.

23. Keith, N.M., Wagener, H.P., and Barker, N.W., Am. J. Med. Sci. 197:332-343, 1939.

24. Garner, A., Ashton, N., Tripathi, R., Kohner, E.M., Bulpitt, C.J., and Dollery, C.T., Br. J. Ophthalmol. 59:3-44, 1975.

25. Klein, M., Goldberg, M.F., and Cotlier, E., Ann. Ophthalmol. 7:1213-1221, 1975.

26. van Heuven, W.A.J., Hayreh, M.S., and Hayreh, S.S., Trans. Ophthalmol. Soc. U.K. 97:588-617, 1977.

27. Acacio, I., and Goldberg, M.F., Am. J. Ophthalmol. 75:861-866, 1973.

28. Gass, J.D.M., Arch. Ophthalmol. 80:535-549, 1968.

29. Schatz, H., and Drake, M., Ophthalmology 86:468-483, 1979.

30. Shakib, M., and Ashton, N., Br. J. Ophthalmol. 50:325-384, 1966.

31. Ashton, N., and Cunha-Vaz, J.G., Arch. Ophthalmol. 73:211-223, 1965.

32. Peyman, G.A., Bennett, T.O., and Vlchek, J., Ann. Ophthalmol. 7:279-288, 1975.

33. Michels, R.G., and Maumenee, A.E., Am. J. Ophthalmol. 80:379-388, 1975.

34. Ryan, G.B., and Majno, G., Am. J. Pathol. 86:183-276, 1977.
35. Simionescu, N., Simionescu, M., and Palade, G.E., J. Cell Biol. 70(2, pt.2):186a, 1976.
36. Perkins, E.S.: Uveitis and Toxoplasmosis. London, J. & A. Churchill, 1961, p. 85.
37. Aaberg, T.M., Cesarz, T.J., and Rytel, M.W., Am. J. Ophthalmol. 74:407-415, 1972.
38. de Venecia, G., Zu Rhein, G.M., Pratt, M.V., and Kisken, W., Arch. Ophthalmol. 86:44-57, 1971.
39. Wyhinny, G.J., Apple, D.J., Guastella, F.R., and Vygantas, C.M., Am. J. Ophthalmol. 76:773-781, 1973.
40. Minckler, D.S., McLean, E.B., Shaw, C.M., and Hendrickson, A., Arch. Ophthalmol. 94:89-95, 1976.
41. Naumann, G., Gass, J.D.M., and Font, R.L., Am. J. Ophthalmol. 65:533-541, 1968.
42. Brown, R.M., and Mendis, U., Br. J. Ophthalmol. 57:344-346, 1973.
43. Spitznas, M., Meyer-Schwickerath, G., and Stephan, B., A. von Graefes Arch. klin. exp. Ophthalmol. 193:73-85, 1975.
44. Duke-Elder, S. (ed.): System of Ophthalmology, vol. 10, Diseases of the Retina, London, Henry Kimpton, 1967, p. 249.
45. Crouch, E.R., Jr., and Goldberg, M.F., Arch. Ophthalmol. 93:384-387, 1975.
46. Martin, N.F., and Fitzgerald, C.R., Am. J. Ophthalmol. 88:28-31, 1979.
47. Jampol, L.M., Isenberg, S.J., and Goldberg, M.F., Am. J. Ophthalmol. 81:583-589, 1976.
48. ffytche, T.J., Trans. Ophthalmol. Soc. U.K. 97:457-461, 1977.
49. Willerson, D., Jr., Aaberg, T.M., and Reeser, F.H., Am. J. Ophthalmol. 84:209-219, 1977.
50. Wise, G.N., Dollery, C.T., and Henkind, P.: The Retinal Circulation. New York, Harper & Row, 1971, p. 296.
51. Chester, G.H., Blach, R.K., and Cleary, P.E., Trans. Ophthalmol. Soc. U.K. 96:151-157, 1976.
52. Maumenee, A.E., Am. J. Ophthalmol. 69:1-27, 1970.
53. Kenyon, K.R., Pederson, J.E., Green, W.R., and Maumenee, A.E., Trans. Ophthalmol. Soc. U.K. 95:391-397, 1975.
54. Schatz, H., Burton, T.C., Yannuzzi, L.A., and Rabb, M.F.: Interpretation of Fundus Fluorescein Angiography, St. Louis, C.V. Mosby, 1978, pp. 550-631.
55. Fishman, G.A., Goldberg, M.F., and Trautmann, J.C., Ann. Ophthalmol. 11:21-27, 1979.
56. Gass, J.D.M., and Norton, E.W.D., Arch. Ophthalmol. 76:646-661, 1966.
57. The Miami Study Group: Cystoid macular edema in aphakic and pseudophakic eyes. Am. J. Ophthalmol. 88:45-48, 1979.
58. Miyake, K., Sugiyama, S., Norimatsu, I., and Ozawa, T., A. von Graefes Arch. klin. exp. Ophthalmol. 209:83-88, 1978.

59. Fishman, G.A., Jampol, L.M., and Goldberg, M.F., Br. J. Ophthalmol. 60:345-353, 1976.

60. Green, J.L., Jr., and Jampol, L.M.: Br. J. Ophthalmol. 63:368-373, 1979.

61. Fishman, G.A., Maggiano, J.M., and Fishman, M., Arch. Ophthalmol. 95:1993-1996, 1977.

62. Gieser, D.K., Fishman, G.A., and Cunha-Vaz, J., Arch. Ophthalmol., in press.

63. Maumenee, A.E. In L'Esperance, F.A., Jr. (ed.): Current Diagnosis and Management of Chorioretinal Diseases, St. Louis, C.V. Mosby, 1977, pp. 287-294.

64. Kohner, E.M., Dollery, C.T., Henkind, P., Paterson, J.W., and Ramalho, P.S., Am. J. Ophthalmol. 63:1748-1761, 1967.

65. Machemer, R., Am. J. Ophthalmol. 69:27-38, 1970.

66. Apple, D.J., Wyhinny, G.J., Goldberg, M.F., Polley, E.H., and Bizzell, J.W., Arch. Ophthalmol. 94:137-144, 1976.

67. Apple, D.J., Goldberg, M.F., and Wyhinny, G., Am. J. Ophthalmol. 75:595-609, 1973.

68. Noth, J.M., Vygantas, C., and Cunha-Vaz, J.G.F., Invest. Ophthalmol. Vis. Sci. 17:1206-1209, 1978.

69. Amoils, S.P., and Honey, D.P., Arch. Ophthalmol. 82:220-228, 1969.

70. Gass, J.D.M.: Differential Diagnosis of Intraocular Tumors: A Stereoscopic Presentation. St. Louis, C.V. Mosby, 1974, pp. 247-264.

71. Archer, D., and Krill, A.E., Surv. Ophthalmol. 15:384-400, 1971.

72. Tripathi, R., and Ashton, N., Br. J. Ophthalmol. 55:289-301, 1971.

73. Goldberg, M.F., In Peyman, G.A., Apple, D.J., and Sanders, D.R. (eds.): Intraocular Tumors, New York, Appleton/Century/Crofts, 1977, pp. 219-234.

74. Haining, W.M., and Zweifach, P.H., Arch. Ophthalmol. 78:475-479, 1967.

75. Nicholson, D.H., Green, W.R., and Kenyon, K.R., Am. J. Ophthalmol. 82:193-204, 1976.

76. Goldberg, M.F., in Lynn, J.R., Snyder, W.B., and Vaiser, A. (eds.): Diabetic Retinopathy, New York, Grune & Stratton, 1974, pp. 47-63.

77. Archer, D.B., Trans. Ophthalmol. Soc. U.K. 96:471-493, 1976.

78. Archer, D.B., Trans. Ophthalmol. Soc. U.K. 97:449-456, 1977.

79. Henkind, P., Am. J. Ophthalmol. 85:297-301, 1978.

80. Galinos, S.O., Asdourian, G.K., Woolf, M.B., Goldberg, M.F., and Busse, B.J., Arch. Ophthalmol. 93:524-530, 1975.

81. Goldberg, M.F., Trans. Am. Acad. Ophthalmol. Otolaryngol. 75:532-556, 1971.

82. Goldberg, M.F., In Bergsma, D., Bron, A.J., and Cotlier, E. (eds.): The Eye and Inborn Errors of Metabolism: Birth Defects, vol. 12, no. 3, New York, Alan R. Liss, 1976, pp. 475-515.

83. Kimura, T., Jpn. J. Ophthalmol. 18:403-417, 1974.
84. Kimura, T., Chen, C.H, and Patz, A., In The Association for
     Research in Vision and Ophthalmology, Spring Meeting, Sara-
     sota, Fl., 1976, Abstracts, p. 87.
85. Taniguchi, Y., Jpn. J. Ophthalmol. 20:19-31, 1976.
86. Goldberg, M.F., and Tso, M.O.M., Ophthalmology 85:1028-1041,
     1978.
87. Kenyon, K.R., and Michels, R.G., Am. J. Ophthalmol. 83:815-
     823, 1977.
88. Goldbaum, M.H., Goldberg, M.F., Nagpal, K., Asdourian, G.K.,
     and Galinos, S.O., In L'Esperance, F.A., Jr. (ed.): Current
     Diagnosis and Management of Chorioretinal Diseases, St. Louis,
     C.V. Mosby, 1977, pp. 132-145.
89. Goldberg, M.F., Trans. Am. Acad. Ophthalmol. Otolaryngol. 83:
     OP409-OP431, 1977.
90. Gass, J.D.M., Arch. Ophthalmol. 80:583-591, 1968.
91. Patz, A., Schatz, H., Berkow, J.W., Gittelsohn, A.M., and
     Ticho, U., Trans. Am. Acad. Ophthalmol. Otolaryngol. 77:OP34-
92. Myers, F.L., Davis, M.D., and Magli, Y.L., In Goldberg, M.F.,
     and Fine, S.L. (eds.): Symposium of the Treatment of Diabe-
     tic Retinopathy, Airlie House, Warrenton, Va., 1968, Washing-
     ton, D.C., U.S. Public Health Service Publication No. 1890,
     Superintendent of Documents, 1968, pp. 81-85.
93. Michaelson, I.C., In Regnault, F., and Duhault, J. (eds.):
     Colloquium on Cellular and Biochemical Aspects in Diabetic
     Retinopathy, Paris, France, 1978: INSERM Symposium No. 7,
     Amsterdam, North-Holland, 1978, pp. 257-275.
94. Ashton, H., Adv. Ophthalmol. 8:1-84, 1958.
95. Wise, G.N., Dollery, C.T., and Henkind, P.: The Retinal
     Circulation, New York, Harper & Row, 1971, pp. 421-453.
96. Ashton, N., In Amalric, P. (ed.): International Symposium on
     Fluorescein Angiography, Albi, 1969, Basel, S. Karger, 1971,
     pp. 334-345.

SIGNIFICANCE OF ALTERATION OF THE OUTER BLOOD-RETINAL BARRIER

August F. Deutman, M.D.

Institute of Ophthalmology

Nijmegen, Holland

INTRODUCTION

There are two main blood-ocular barriers: the blood-aqueous barrier and the blood-retinal barrier.

The blood-aqueous barrier is formed by an epithelial barrier located in the non-pigmented layer of the ciliary epithelium and in the posterior iridial epithelium and by the endothelium of the iridial vessels. Both these layers have tight junctions of the "leaky" type. The permeability of the blood-aqueous barrier shows a significant degree of pressure-dependent diffusion associated with transport activity, resembling the standing gradient osmotic flow model. The blood-retinal barrier is located at two levels forming an outer barrier in the retinal pigment epithelium and an inner barrier in the endothelial membrane of the retinal vessels. Both these membranes have tight junctions of the "non-leaky" type.[1] The permeability of the blood-retinal barrier resembles cellular permeability in general, diffusion being directly related to the predominant roles of lipid solubility and transport mechanism. Abnormal functioning of the blood retinal barrier is one of the most important factors in the development of retinal diseases. Fluorescein angiography, a qualitative technique, has recently been extended by the use of quantitative vitreous fluorophoto-metry, which can assess the degree of breakdown of the blood-retinal barrier.

In the normal eye, the retinal pigment epithelium is the first cellular layer which opposes the penetration into the retina of any substance originating from the choroid. Light microscopic studies indicated that the penetration of carbon, trypan blue and

fluorescein from the choroid into the retina stops at the level
of the retinal pigment epithelium.[1]

Electron microscopy showed that adjacent pigment epithelial
cells are united by extensive "zonulae occludentes" very similar
to the ones previously described between the endothelial cells of
the retinal vessels.

These junctional complexes present all the morphological and
permeability characteristics of the tight junctions of the "non-
leaky" type. Ion flux and microelectrode experiments performed
on isolated frog pigment epithelium demonstrated that the plasma
membrane at the apex and the base of the epithelial cells has a high
permeability to K^+, an "intra-cellular ion", and a relatively low
permeability to Na^+ and Cl^-, which are "extracellular ions".

In conclusion, the intercellular spaces in the retinal pigment
epithelium are firmly closed, most molecular movements being
forced to take place through the more selective transcellular
route.

It has been demonstrated that Bruch's membrane, located between the choriocapillaris and the pigment epithelium of the retina
does not obstruct the passage of fluorescein nor of tracers like
horseradish peroxidase or ferritin. Bruch's membrane, like most
other vascular basement membranes, acts as a diffusion barrier
only to molecules of large molecular size. The capillaries of the
choroid (the choriocapillaris) have structural characteristics
which are entirely different from those of the retinal vessels.
Their endothelium displays numerous fenestrations which occur
preferentially in the region of the vessel wall that abuts on
Bruch's membrane. Electron microscopic studies using a variety
of tracers have shown that the vessels of the choroid, like those
of the ciliary body stroma, are permeable to macromolecules.

Trypan blue, fluorescein and similar substances permeate
freely this vascular layer of the choroid. In summary, the
choroicapillaris does not appear to have much significance in
barrier function.[1,2]

Decompensation of the outer blood-retinal barrier occurs in
many different disorders.

Acquired conditions well known are conditions such as central
serous choroidopathy where fluorescein leaks from the choriocapillaris through the retinal pigment epithelium in the subretinal
space (Fig. la, b). It has been suggested that a dysregulation
of the autonomous nerve system may play a role in this disease that
occurs most frequently in the 4th decade. Hyperfusion of the
choriocapillaris may result in decompensation of the outer blood

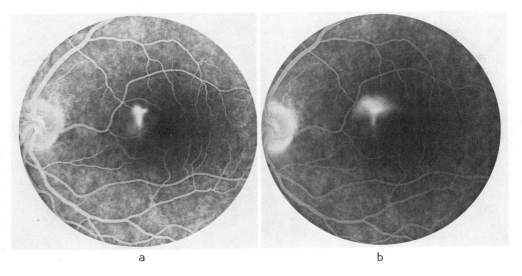

a   b

Fig. 1 ab.   Classical central serous retinopathy showing obvious
              decompensation of the outer blood—retinal barrier.

retinal barrier. It is hard to conceive that damage to the
retinal pigment epithelium alone is the primary cause of this
disorder. Argon laser treatment may be quite successful although
spontaneous recovery generally occurs.

      In serous detachment of the retinal pigment epithelium, the
outer blood retinal barrier appears to be intact and fluid accumulates under a detached but grossly intact retinal pigment epithelium
(Fig. 2a, b). This condition may be idiopathic and benign.
However, in the presence of drusen of the retinal pigment epithelium it is usually the precursor of dreaded disciform response
with subretinal chroidal neovascularization. Photocoagulation
generally will flatten a retinal pigment epithelial detachment,
although spontaneous recovery may occur likewise.

      Subretinal neovascularization leads obviously to a breakdown
of the outer blood—retinal barrier as soon as the new formed
choroidal vessels penetrate the retinal pigment epithelium (Fig.
3ab). In early stages there is sub-pigment epithelial neovascularization with an intact barrier in the beginning. Causes of
subretinal neovascularization are multiple and it appears that
almost any damage to the Bruch membrane - retinal pigment epithelial complex may create the setting for the occurrence of
subretinal neovascularization.

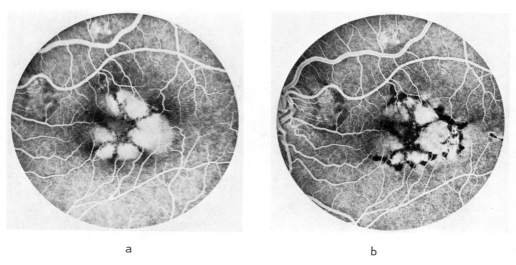

a   b

Fig. 2 ab.   Serous detachment of the retinal pigment epithelium (a)
             and situation after Argon laser treatment with flattening
             of the detachment (b).

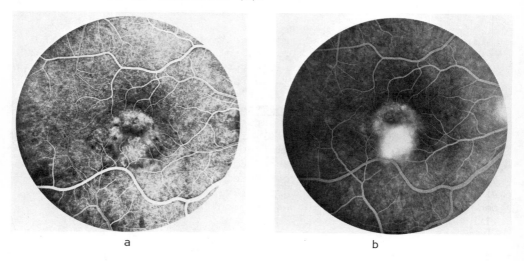

a   b

Fig. 3 ab.   Subretinal neovascularization in vitelliform dystrophy
             with obvious decompensation of the outer blood-retinal
             barrier.

     The following etiological conditions are known in subretinal
neovascularization: presumed histoplasmosis syndrome; angioid
streaks (Fig. 4 ab); myopia; traumatic choroidal rupture (blunt

or directly perforating) (Fig. 5 ab; Fig. 6 abcdef); Argon laser
treatment (high energy, small spot size); choroidal tumors; choroidal
naevi; <u>Toxocara</u> <u>canis</u> infection; toxoplasmosis retinitis; rubella
retinitis;[3] disseminated choroiditis; vitelliform dystrophy (Best)
(Fig. 3 ab); dominant drusen; Sorsby's pseudoinflammatory dystrophy;
polymorphic macular dystrophy; Stargardt's disease; Harada's disease;
idiopathic subretinal neovascularization.

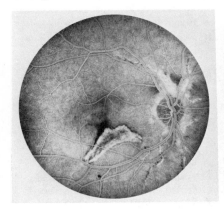
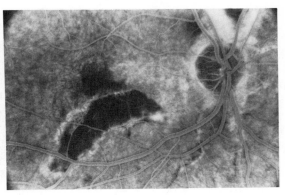

a   b

Fig. 4 ab.   Subretinal neovascularization in angioid streaks before
             and after Argon laser treatment.

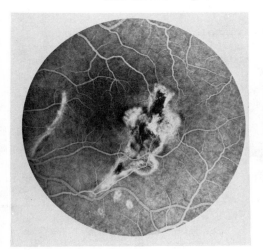
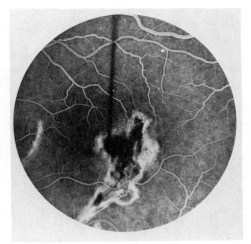

a   b

Fig. 5 ab.   Subretinal neovascularization in traumatic choroidal
             rupture before and after laser treatment of the feeder
             vessels in the scar (temporal to the subretinal neo-
             vascularization). There was complete regression of
             the centrally localized subretinal neovascularization
             and vision improved from 0.2 (20/100) to 1.0 (20/20).

We can conclude from this that any disturbance of the Bruch membrane-retinal pigment epithelial complex may be the beginning of subretinal choroidal neovascularization.

In one of our patients a tiny metal wire, consisting mostly of copper, perforated the globe and hit the retina transvitreally at the posterior pole. Following this, true subretinal neovascularization developed. This appears to be a model for the development of subretinal neovascularization in humans. Argon laser treatment was only temporarily successful in destroying the new formed vessels (Fig. 6 abcdef).

It is well-known, that rather heavy laser coagulation may destroy these neovascular membranes, and this therapy may be quite successful in paracentral subretinal neovascularization (Fig. 4ab).[4] On the other hand, spontaneous disappearance of these vessels has also been seen.

If subretinal neovascularization is too central to treat directly, one may consider the possibility of treating choroidal feeder vessels. In one such case we treated the choroidal feeder vessels of a centrally localized subretinal neovascular membrane in the only eye of a young patient who had subretinal neovascularization secondary to a traumatic choroidal rupture. By coagulation of the paracentral feeding vessels we could obliterate the centrally localized neovascular membrane (Fig. 5 ab).

The pathogenesis of these new vessels is still completely obscure. It appears that neighboring tissues inhibit the outgrowth of cells as long as these tissues are intact. Thus, damage to or interruption of the internal limiting membrane may lead to proliferation of Müller cells or fibroblasts, giving rise to epiretinal fibrosis and macular "pucker".

Holes in the neuroretina give rise to proliferation of retinal pigment epithelial cells, leading ultimately to massive periretinal proliferation (MPP) and decreased integrity of Bruch's membrane seems to lead to outgrowth of the capillaries of the choroid. The exact stimuli to these types of proliferation are completely unknown,

Fig. 6 a-f.   Copper wire (a) accidentally perforating the retina just above the fovea (b) leading to subretinal neovascularization (c). After Argon laser treatment there was a temporary occlusion of these new vessels (d). However, new subretinal neovascularization destroyed central vision (e,f). This appears to be a human model of stimulating subretinal neovascularization in the macular area.

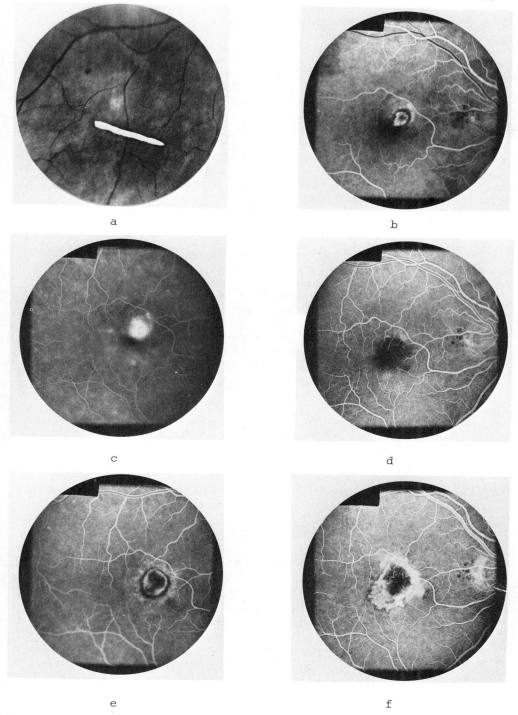

but it appears as if some type of (overreactive (?)) healing
process takes place. Archer[5] (1977) thinks the most likely
possibility is that the outer retinal layers functioning under
stress may provide the needed stimulus to promote choroidal neovascularization. However, it is my feeling that breaks or dehiscences in Bruch's membrane are also necessary.

Inflammation of the neuroretina and retinal pigment epithelium
generally will cause decompensation of the outer blood-retinal
barrier.[6] Leakage and staining of fluorescein is seen in inflammatory retinal conditions such as subacute sclerosing panencephalitis
(SSPE), toxoplasmosis retinitis, Rift Valley Fever retinitis, and
cytomegalic inclusion disease and many others. It seems probable
that there is leakage through the infected and swollen retinal
pigment epithelial cells in these cases although there may be a
breakdown of the tight junctions as well.

Choroidal inflammatory conditions such as Harada's uveomeningeal
syndrome, presumed histoplasmin choroiditis, disseminated choroiditis, will also give rise to obvious decompensation of the outer
blood-retinal barrier. In Harada's disease, this is usually very
prominent with large bullous detachments of the neuroretina.

Obstruction of the flow in the precapillary arterioles of the
choroid as seen in the so-called "acute posterior multifocal placoid
pigment epitheliopathy" leads to definite decompensation of the
outer blood-retinal barrier at the site of the poorly perfused
lobules of the choriocapillaris (Fig. 7 abcdef).[7]

In serpiginous choroiditis a rather similar process may be
observed.[8] Obviously trauma and tumors may lead to decompensation
of the outer blood-retinal barrier as well.

Haemangioma, melanomas, and metastases of the choroid are
well known in this regard. As a rare condition, reticulum cell
sarcoma (mimicking an acute retinitis) may be mentioned.

It is quite striking that inherited retinal dystrophies are
rarely causing an obvious decompensation of the outer blood-retinal
barrier despite extensive atrophy and disappearance of the retinal

Fig. 7 a-f.   Non-perfusion of the precapillary choroidal arterioles
              beautifully seen in the early phases of fluorescein
              angiography (bc) in a patient with acute posterior
              multifocal placoid pigment epitheliopathy (a). In the
              late phases of angiography there is a definite decom-
              pensation of the outer blood-retinal barrier as the
              result of the vascular obstruction.

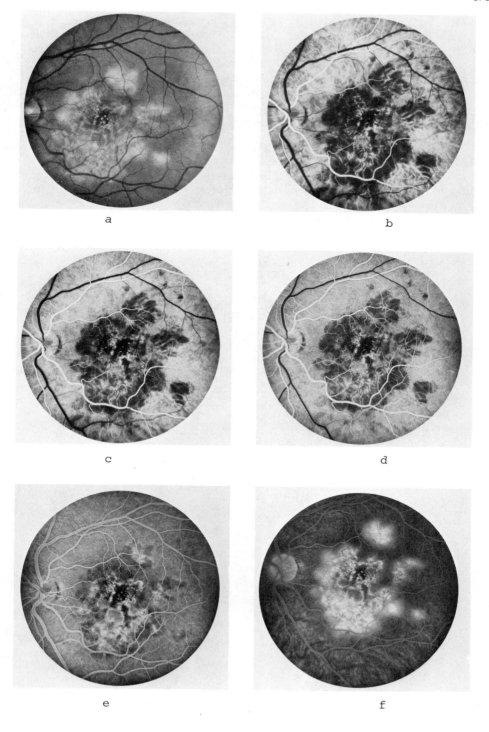

pigment epithelium. In many of these conditions, the choroid becomes atrophic as well and this may be one of the reasons that there is no obvious leakage of fluorescein. Nevertheless, it may be that quantitative vitreous fluorometry will demonstrate discrete leakage of fluorescein in the vitreous in early cases of hereditary retinal dystrophies such as retinitis pigmentosa, although it will be hard to distinguish leakage from the outer and the inner blood-retinal barrier.[2]

In conclusion we can state that alterations of the outer blood-retinal barrier play a very important role in a large variety of ocular diseases. It would be a great step forward if drugs could be developed that may stop decompensation or disruption of the outer blood-retinal barrier. Photocoagulation, laser therapy and steroids have already an important place in this regard, but obviously newer modalities of treatment should be developed.

REFERENCES

1. Cunha-Vaz, J. (1979) Survey Ophthal. 23:279-296.
2. Cunha-Vaz, J., Fonseca, J.R., Abreu, J.F., and Ruas, M.A. (1979) Diabetes 28:16-19.
3. Deutman, A. F. and Grizzard, W.S. (1978) Amer. J. Ophthal. 85: 82-87.
4. Deutman, A.F. and Kovacs, B. (1979) Amer. J. Ophthal. 88:12-17.
5. Archer, D.B. (1977) Trans. Ophthal. Soc. U.K. 97:449-456, part IV
6. Deutman, A.F. (1976) Trans. Amer. Acad. Ophthal. Otolaryngol. 81:472-482.
7. Deutman, A.F. and Lion, F. (1977) Amer. J. Ophthal. 84:652-657.
8. Baarsma, G.S. and Deutman, A.F. (1976) Docum. Ophthal. 40:269-285.

PARTICIPANTS

ABREU, Jose F. de ....Portugal
ANDERS, Juanita ....USA
ALM, Albert ....Sweden
ALGVERE, Peep ....Sweden
ARCHER, Desmond ....Ireland
ATWATER, Illani ....England
BARLAS, Bulent ....Turkey
BEINTEMA, M.R. ....Holland
BEGG, Ian ....Canada
BELHORN, Roy ....USA
BILL. A. ....Sweden
BITO, Laszlo ....USA
BRIGHTMAN, Milton ....USA
BULLOW, Niels ....Denmark
CARDOSO, M. Adelaide ....Portugal
CARVALHO, A. Pato ....Portugal
CARVALHO, Caetana Pato ....Portugal
CLOVER, Gillian ....England
COSCAS, Gabriel ....France
COTLIER, Edward ....USA
CUNHA-VAZ, Jose ....Portugal
DeROUSSEAU, C. Jean ....USA
DEUTMAN, August F. ....Holland
ERGIN, Mehmet ....Turkey
FINKELSTEIN, Daniel ....USA
FLAGE, Thor ....Norway
FLOWER, Robert ....USA
FONSECA, Joaquim A. Reis ....Portugal
FROST-LARSEN, Kim ....Denmark
GAUDRIC, Alain ....France
GIOVANNI, Mann ....England
GOLDBERG, Morton F. ....USA
HENKIND, Paul ....USA
HORNSTRA-LIMBURG, Henriette ....Holland
KERNNEL, Anna ....Sweden
KJAERGAARD, Jens ....Denmark
KLEIN, Ronald ....USA

LAJTHA, Abel ....USA
LASZCZYK, Anna ....Poland
LATIES, Alan ....USA
LIANG, James ....USA
LIMA, J. J. Pedroso de ....Portugal
LUND-ANDERSEN, Henrik ....Denmark
MACEDO, Tice, A. ....Portugal
MALAGOLA, Romualdo ....Italy
MAURICE, David ....USA
MIZUNO, Katsuyoshi ....Japan
MONTEIRO, J. Guilherme ....Portugal
MORALES-S, Julian ....USA
MOSIER, Marjorie ....USA
MOTA, M. Carolina ....Portugal
MURCHLAND, John B. ....Australia
NEWSOME, David ....USA
NIELSEN, Niels Vesti ....Denmark
VAN NOUHUYS, C.S. ....Holland
QUENTEL, Gabriel ....France
QUINTA, M. Emilia F. ....England
RAPOPORT, Stanley ....USA
RASTEIRO, Alfredo ....Portugal
RIASKOFF, Sawa ....Holland
ROJAS, Emilio ....England
RUBIN, Lionel ....USA
SALMINEN, Lotta ....Finland
SOUBRANE, Gisele ....France
TEIXEIRA, Rogerio ....Portugal
TORNQUIST, Per ....Sweden
TSO, Mark ....USA
VAN HAERINGEN, N.J. ....Holland
VYGANTAS, Charles ....USA
WATERBURY, David ....USA